Advanced Topics on Radiosensitizers of Hypoxic Cells

NATO ADVANCED STUDY INSTITUTES SERIES

A series of edited volumes comprising multifaceted studies of contemporary scientific issues by some of the best scientific minds in the world, assembled in cooperation with NATO Scientific Affairs Division.

Series A: Life Sciences

Recent Volumes in this Series

This series is published by an international board of publishers in conjunction with NATO Scientific Affairs Division

A Life Sciences
B Physics

Plenum Publishing Corporation
London and New York

C Mathematical and
   Physical Sciences

D. Reidel Publishing Company
Dordrecht, The Netherlands
and Hingham, Massachusetts, USA

D Behavioral and
   Social Sciences
E Applied Sciences

Martinus Nijhoff Publishers
The Hague, The Netherlands

Advanced Topics on Radiosensitizers of Hypoxic Cells

Edited by

A. Breccia

University of Bologna
Bologna, Italy

C. Rimondi

Malpighi Hospital
Bologna, Italy

and

G. E. Adams

Institute of Cancer Research
Sutton, England

PLENUM PRESS • NEW YORK AND LONDON
Published in cooperation with NATO Scientific Affairs Division

Library of Congress Cataloging in Publication Data

NATO Advanced Study Institute on Radiosensitizers of Hypoxic Cells (1980: Cesenatico, Italy)
    Advanced topics on radiosensitizers of hypoxic cells.

    (NATO advanced study institutes series. Series A, Life sciences; v. 43)
    "Proceedings of the course, Advanced topics on radiosensitizers of hypoxic cells, the second part of the NATO Advanced Study Institute on Radiosensitizers of Hypoxic Cells, held August 27–September 7, 1980, in Cesenatico, Italy." – T.p. verso.
    Includes bibliographical references and index.
    1. Cancer – Radiotherapy – Congresses. 2. Radiation-sensitizing agents – Congresses. 3. Anoxemia – Congresses. I. Breccia, A. II. Rimondi, C. III. Adams, G. E. IV. Title: Radiosensitizers of hypoxic cells. V. Series. [DNLM: 1. Radiation-Sensitizing agents – Pharmacodynamics – Congresses. 2. Anoxia – Congresses. 3. Cells – Drugs effects – Congresses. 4. Neoplasma – Radiotherapy – Congresses. WN 610 N293a 1980]

RC271.R3N28   1980   616.99′40642   82-427
ISBN 0-306-40915-1   AACR2

Proceedings of the course Advanced Topics on Radiosensitizers of Hypoxic Cells, the second part of the NATO Advanced Study Institute on Radiosensitizers of Hypoxic Cells, held August 27 – September 7, 1980, in Cesenatico, Italy

© 1982 Plenum Press, New York
A Division of Plenum Publishing Corporation
233 Spring Street, New York, N.Y. 10013

Printed in the United States of America

FOREWORD

In July 1979, the Faculty of Pharmacy of the University of Bologna received a proposal from Professor Breccia to hold an International Conference on "Nitroimidazoles: Chemistry, Pharmacology and Clinical Application."

Because of the great interest in these drugs in various fields, I was very pleased to accept the proposal and to give the conference the sponsorship of the University of Bologna. It was an added pleasure to accept the chairmanship of the meeting, together with Professors Sensi and Adams.

At the same time, the Minister of Education approved a proposal which also came from the Faculty of Pharmacy, to offer an advanced course on the topic "Radiosensitizers of Hypoxic Cells This course was subsequently approved by a special Committee of the NATO Scientific Programme as an Advanced Study Institute. Since the subject matter of both the conference and the course are closely inter-related, it was logical to plan the conference as part of the overall course.

Bringing together specialists from quite different and apparently unrelated fields of research, but all with an interest in the study and application of one single group of drugs, is a novel idea with intriguing possibilities. The volumes of the proceedings include contributions from experts with such diverse interests as synthetic chemistry, mechanism of drug action, parasitology, anaerobic bacteria and protozoa, pharmacology and toxicology, radiation sensitizers for use in radiotherapy, and the development of drugs for use in cancer in general.

I would like to congratulate the members of the scientific committees on the manner in which they designed the scientific programme. I would also like to thank the committees, the speakers, chairmen, and coordinators for so successfully bringing together such a high standard of scientific and clinical experience from many different countries of the world.

   I would like to say a few words about the region in which the meetings took place. Cesenatico is part of the Romagna, which is one of the most famous of all the Italian Rivieri.   It is, however, not just a holiday area but a scientific one also.   As you may know, one of the most advanced University Centres of Marine Biology is located in this town. Conference initiatives such as this one are fairly frequent; for example, a meeting on polyammines in cancer research will take place in nearby Rimini.

   I am sure that the interest in the topics in these proceedings will not be limited only to the information about research already carried out but will be the basis for a better development of new drugs in cancer therapy.

                              Professor Carlo Rizzoli
                              Rector
                              University of Bologna
                              Italy

P R E F A C E

The Advanced Study Institute sponsored by NATO, on
Radiosensitizers of Hypoxic Cells, was divided into two sections.
The first section of the Institute consisted of an International
Conference on Nitroimidazoles which brought together a broad
range of interests in the chemistry and pharmacology of these
compounds and in their application in various fields in chemical
medicine.

The second section was concerned with a series of papers on
the general subject of Radiosensitizers of Hypoxic Cells. It
included lectures and workshops on the chemical, biological and
clinical developments in this field. For convenience, and also
because of the large number of papers presented, the total proceedings of the Institute are published in two volumes.

A. Breccia

C. Rimondi

G.E. Adams

ACKNOWLEDGEMENTS

The Organizers gratefully acknowledge the following for their generous financial support, including fellowships to some participants:

A.S.I. - N.A.T.O.

Azienda di Soggiorno e Turismo di Cesenatico

Banca del Monte di Bologna

Camera di Commercio di Forli

Istituto De Angeli

Lega Nazionale lotta contro i Tumori sez. di Bologna

Ministero della Pubblica Istruzione

Ospedale "M. Malpighi", Bologna

Provincia di Forli

Regione Emilia-Romagna

Società Carlo Erba Farmitalia

Società Cesenate Corse al Trotto

Società Elettronica, Roma

Società Farmigea

Società Hoffmann-La Roche

CONTENTS

THE CHEMISTRY OF NITROIMIDAZOLE HYPOXIC CELL RADIOSENSITIZERS

C.E. Smithen and C.R. Hardy

Roche Products Limited
Welwyn Garden City
Hertfordshire and
Institute of Cancer Research
Sutton, Surrey, England

1.   INTRODUCTION

It is now well recognised that the imidazole ring system is an important component of many different types of natural products having a wide range of biological activities, including those essential for life itself.   For example, in the form of the amino-acid L-histidine it is present in a variety of peptides, proteins and related macro-molecules and it fulfills an important functional role at the active sites of many different enzymes.   The imidazole-1-β-riboside moiety, present in the purine nucleotides derived from adenine and guanine, forms an essential chiral building block in the macromolecular structure of the nucleic acids whilst other phosphate esters of the corresponding nucleosides, such as ATP, ADP and cyclic-AMP derived from adenosine, have vital functional roles in all living cells. The imidazole ring system is also found in various forms among low molecular weight natural products of animal, plant and microbial origin;   either in simple form, as in the bio-amine histamine, or in much modified form, as in the vitamin biotin.   One of the simplest of biologically active imidazoles is the antibiotic azomycin (I), first isolated in 1953 by the group of Umezawa[1] and identified in 1955 by Nakamura[2] as the hitherto unknown 2-nitroimidazole (Fig. 1).

The simple structure of this natural product and the fact that it exhibited pronounced antiprotozoal activity[3] provided the stimulus for chemists, initially in France and later in Italy and the USA, to devise methods for its synthesis and to attempt to improve upon its therapeutic properties by preparing a variety of synthetic nitro-imidazole compounds.   This approach by the Rhône-Poulenc group in France resulted in the discovery and development of the clinically useful trichomonacide metronidazole (II) and the veterinary histo-monacide dimetridazole (III)[4] (Fig. 1).

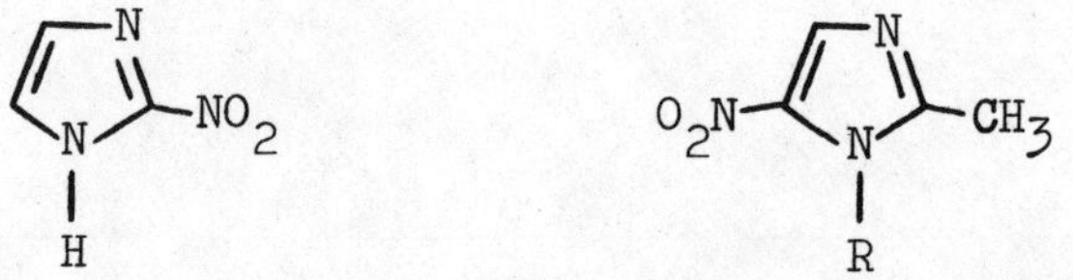

I (azomycin)   II, R = CH$_2$CH$_2$OH (metronidazole)

III, R = CH$_3$ (dimetridazole)

Fig. 1   Prototype nitroimidazoles having antiprotozoal and other
          antimicrobial activities[3] [4]

The success of these two 5-nitroimidazoles attracted the
attention of other research groups which led, from the mid-1960's
onwards, to a rapid expansion of our knowledge of the chemistry and
biology of nitroimidazoles and their use as chemotherapeutic agents.
The present state of this knowledge has been the subject of the
first part of this Conference during which Cavalleri[5] reviewed the
diverse range of chemical methods available for the synthesis of
nitroimidazoles.

The discovery in 1973 by Asquith, Foster and Willson[6] that
metronidazole (II) was able to radiosensitize hypoxic mammalian
cells, but not well-oxygenated cells, to the lethal effects of
ionizing radiation at clinically achievable concentrations opened up
exciting new prospects for the use of nitroimidazoles as adjuncts
in cancer radiotherapy.

It was soon found that 2-nitroimidazoles are generally more
effective than 5-nitroimidazoles as hypoxic cell radiosensitizers[7]
and that the differences in their activity in vitro correlate most
closely with differences in redox properties, in particular their
"electron-affinity" as measured by one-electron (E_7^1) or two-electron
($E_{\frac{1}{2}}^1$) reduction potentials.[8] [9]   For example, several (2-nitro-1-
imidazolyl)alkanols (Fig. 2), notably misonidazole (IV), are
significantly more active on a molar concentration basis than
metronidazole and closely related 5-nitroimidazoles.[8]   The presence
of an additional electron-withdrawing substituent attached directly
to the imidazole ring, as in the case of methyl 1-methyl-2-nitro-
imidazole-5-carboxylate (V)[10] or the corresponding 5-aldehyde (VI)[8]
(Fig. 3), results in further increases in both radiosensitizing
activity and cytotoxicity commensurate with the increased electron-
affinity.

In the course of studying the effect of variations in the
substituent groups within the N-1 side-chain of nitroimidazoles on

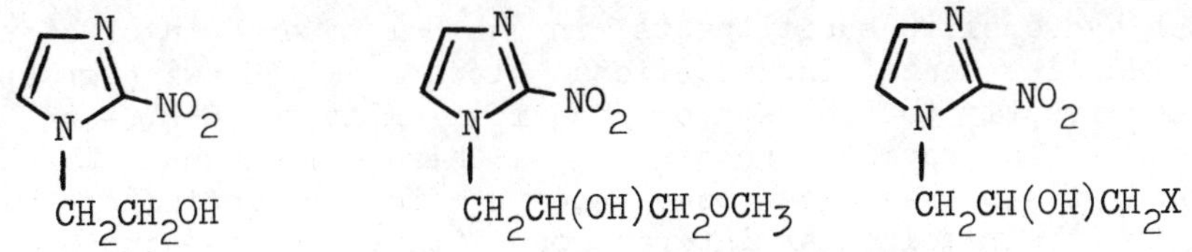

IV (misonidazole)

Fig. 2   (2-Nitroimidazolyl)alkanols having hypoxic cell radio-
         sensitizing activity [where X = hydrogen, halogen, hydroxy
         (desmethylmisonidazole), alkoxy or phenoxy][8]

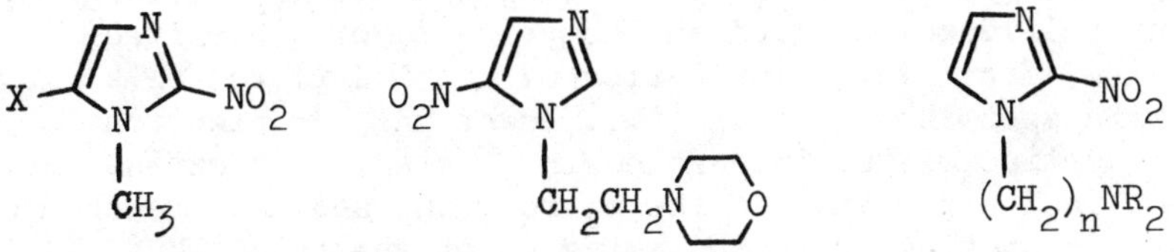

V,   X = CH$_3$OCO   VII (nimorazole)   VIII (n = 2-6)

VI, X = HCO

Fig. 3   Nitroimidazoles having enhanced radiosensitizing activity
         arising from nuclear or side-chain substitution.[8,10]

their radiosensitizing activity it was found that a basic amine
group enhanced activity relative to neutral substituents whereas a
carboxylic acid group resulted in activity much less than predicted
from electron-affinity considerations.   For example, the basic
5-nitroimidazole nimorazole (VII) is more active on a molar
concentration basis than metronidazole[10] whilst several (2-nitro-1-
imidazolyl)alkylamines (VIII) (Fig. 3) show correspondingly higher
activity than misonidazole.[11]   These observations have provided the
basis for the rational design and synthesis of several new series of
nitroimidazoles having the potential for improved therapeutic
properties as hypoxic cell radiosensitizers compared to metronidazole
and misonidazole, both of which are currently undergoing worldwide
clinical evaluation in tumour radiotherapy.

     The present paper reviews the syntheses of those nitroimidazoles
which are of particular interest as hypoxic cell radiosensitizers,
such as analogues of metronidazole and misonidazole containing basic

or other hydrophilic substituents* in the N-1 side-chain or other
nitroimidazoles containing additional electron-withdrawing groups
attached directly to the hetero-aromatic ring at the C-2, 4 or 5
positions.   The chemical reactivity of these compounds is briefly
discussed with emphasis on those aspects which may influence their
stability, their molecular interactions with the endogenous
components of biological systems and their metabolism.   For further
information on these and other aspects of the chemistry of nitroimidazoles the reader is also referred to the recent reviews by
Cavalleri,[5] Breccia,[12] and Monney, Parrick and Wallace.[13]

2.   N-1 SUBSTITUTED NITROIMIDAZOLES

The presence of the strongly electron-withdrawing nitro group
in simple nitroimidazoles, such as azomycin (I) or 4(5)-nitro-
imidazole (IX), facilitates ionization of the N-1 proton (i.e. lower
pKa) and diminishes the basicity (i.e. lower pKb) or electron-
donating properties of the imidazole ring system to an extent that
is dependent on the position of the nitro group and the presence of
other electron-donating or -withdrawing substituents.   Thus (I) is
a stronger acid (pKa 7.15) than (IX) (pKa 9.2) or 2-methyl-4(5)-
nitroimidazole (X) but weaker than 5(4)-chloro-4(5)-nitroimidazole
(pKa 5.85) or 2,4(5)-dinitroimidazole (pKa 2.85).[14]   Consequently
many N-1 unsubstituted nitroimidazoles may be readily converted into
metal salts (e.g. sodium, potassium or silver) or organosilicon
derivatives (e.g. trimethylsilyl) which have proved to be most useful
synthetic intermediates for N-1 substitution reactions, especially
when generated in situ.   In addition, because of the ease of
ionization of the N-1 proton, asymmetrically substituted nitro
imidazoles, such as (IX) and (X), can exist in two tautomeric forms
with the less acidic tautomer predominating.[14]   According to whether
the overall reaction conditions used for N-1 substitution of such
nitroimidazoles are acidic, basic or neutral one may obtain the
products derived from one or both tautomers.[5,13]

---

* An important practical consideration in the evaluation of nitroimidazoles as radiosensitizers is a modest degree of water-
  solubility;   at least ca.100μM.   Many of the side-chain
  substituents reviewed in this paper are included with this factor
  in mind.   Other means of improving the bioavailability of a given
  nitroimidazole, such as by further derivatization of functional
  groups in the side-chain to provide a pro-drug form of the
  sensitizer, are also briefly discussed (see Section 2.3).

4-nitro   5-nitro

IX, R = H

X, R = CH₃

Of greatest interest and utility in the present context are
the N-alkylation reactions of the simplest nitroimidazoles (I), (IX)
and (X) which have been reported using a wide variety of alkylating
reagents and diverse reaction conditions.   The alkyl groups that
have been introduced at the N-1 position of the nitroimidazole range
in complexity from simple unsubstituted lower alkyl or alkenyl (for
example, allyl[15]) to monosubstituted alkyl containing, usually in the
ω-position, functional substituents (for example, hydroxy, alkoxy,
amino, carboxy, halogeno, sulfone or thioether) to di- or polysubstituted alkyl groups containing two or more such substituents.
Among the many N-1 (polysubstituted)alkyl derivatives of nitroimidazoles reported the N-1-glycosides[16-20] are noteworthy as
analogs of the imidazole-1-glycoside moiety mentioned in the
Introduction as widely occurring in Nature.

The reactive groups used in these alkylating reagents include
halide, alkyl- or aryl-sulfonate, acetate (mainly for N-glycosidation),
oxirane, aziridine, 'onium (positive-ion) species derived from ortho-
acetates or ethers and diazoalkane.   Clearly, in the case of di- or
polysubstituted alkylating reagents the choice of reactive group is
generally limited by the chemical reactivity of the other functional
substituents present, in protected form or otherwise, in the same
molecule.

The examples mentioned in the following Sections 2.1, 2.2 and
2.3 have been selected to illustrate the variety of N-1 substituted
nitroimidazoles that are available to the synthetic chemist and are
not intended to be an exhaustive compilation of the literature of
nitroimidazoles.   The extent to which these and other variations
may be combined to devise a synthesis of any desired new nitroimidazole is limited only by the imagination of the reader and the
ingenuity of the chemist.

2.1 N-1 Alkylation of 2-Nitroimidazoles

N-Alkylation of azomycin (I) represents the simplest and most
widely studied reaction of this type.   Due to the symmetry of (I)
and its conjugate base the structure of the product is independent
of the nature of the alkylating reagent or the detailed reaction

mechanism.   The synthetic method of choice is generally determined
by other factors such as the availability of alkylating reagent,
ease of reaction or purification, stability of product, etc.   The
most versatile alkylating reagents have been alkyl halides, using (I)
as a preformed metal salt (Fig. 4),[10][11][14][15][21][22] and substituted
oxiranes where the condensation with (I) is usually carried out in
alcohol containing catalytic quantities of a base (Fig. 5).[21][23][24]
The compounds (XI), (XII) and (XIII) obtained from allyl bromide,[15]
chloroacetic ester[21] and epichlorohydrin[21] respectively are useful
intermediates for further side-chain substitution reactions (see
below, Section 2.3).

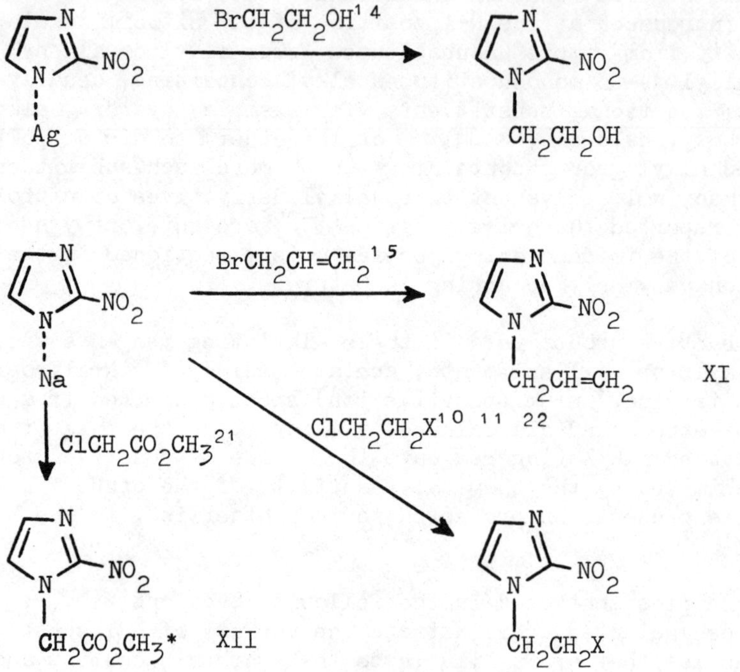

Fig. 4 N-Alkylation of azomycin with alkyl halides [where
        X = halogen,[11] alkoxy,[10] amino[22]]

     Direct N-alkylation of (I) under overall neutral conditions has
been achieved with Meerwein-type 'onium reagents, such as dimethoxy-
carbonium or triethyloxonium tetrafluoroborate,[25] or with diazo-
compounds, such as diazomethane[14] or ethyl diazoacetate,[25] but these
methods offer no major advantage in the 2-nitroimidazole series (Fig. 6

---

*CAUTION: Methyl 2-nitroimidazolyl-1-acetate has <u>explosive</u> properties!

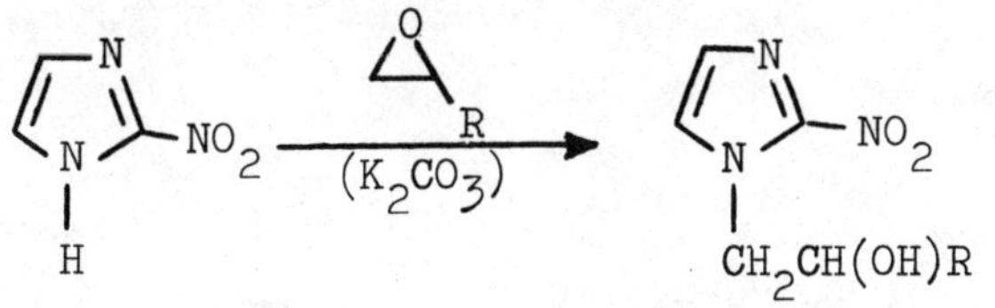

Fig. 5 N-Alkylation of azomycin with substituted oxiranes [where
R = alkyl,[23] halogenomethyl,[21] alkoxycarbonyl,[21] alkoxymethyl,[21] aminomethyl[24]]

A few examples of N-alkylation of 4(5)-alkyl-2-nitroimidazoles[26]
and 4,5-dialkyl-2-nitroimidazoles[15][21] are known; in the former case
the product derived from the 4-alkyl tautomer is significantly
favoured, probably as a result of steric factors (Fig. 6).

N-Glycosidation of (I) is interesting because of the possibility
of producing two stereoisomeric forms of the glycoside-imidazole bond.
Rousseau et al[16] first obtained an azomycin-riboside by acid-catalyzed
fusion of (I) with tetra-O-acetyl-β-D-ribofuranose, followed by
standard deprotection procedures, and tentatively assigned their
product the β-configuration at the glycoside bond (Fig. 7).   Prisbe
et al[19] obtained the same product in higher yield by treating (I)
with 2,3,5-tri-O-benzoyl-D-ribofuranosyl bromide in the presence of
excess mercuric cyanide, followed by deprotection.   Unexpectedly,
the condensation of (I) or its trimethylsilyl derivative with the
corresponding β-D-ribofuranosyl acetate in the presence of excess
stannic chloride/mercuric cyanide gave the α-anomer in good yield
(Fig. 7).   Stereochemical assignments were confirmed by nmr spectroscopy and further chemical studies; for example, the α-anomer
readily underwent a base-catalyzed intramolecular cyclization reaction
with displacement of the nitro group[19] (see below, Section 3.4).

In the glucose series, condensation of (I) with 1,2,3,4,6-penta-
O-acetyl-β-D-glucopyranose in the presence of excess stannic chloride/
mercuric cyanide gave only the corresponding azomycin-1-β-D- gluco-
pyranoside.[19]

2.2 N-1 Alkylation of 4(5)-Nitroimidazoles

Due to the intrinsic asymmetry of 4(5)-nitroimidazoles, such as
(IX) and (X), and their conjugate bases N-alkylation may give either
1-alkyl-4-nitro- or 1-alkyl-5-nitroimidazoles and, in some cases, a
mixture of both products.   The factors which determine the products
of N-alkylation have been discussed in detail by Ridd and
co-workers,[27][28][29] and have been reviewed by others.[5][13][30]   In
summary it may be concluded that N-alkylation under neutral or basic

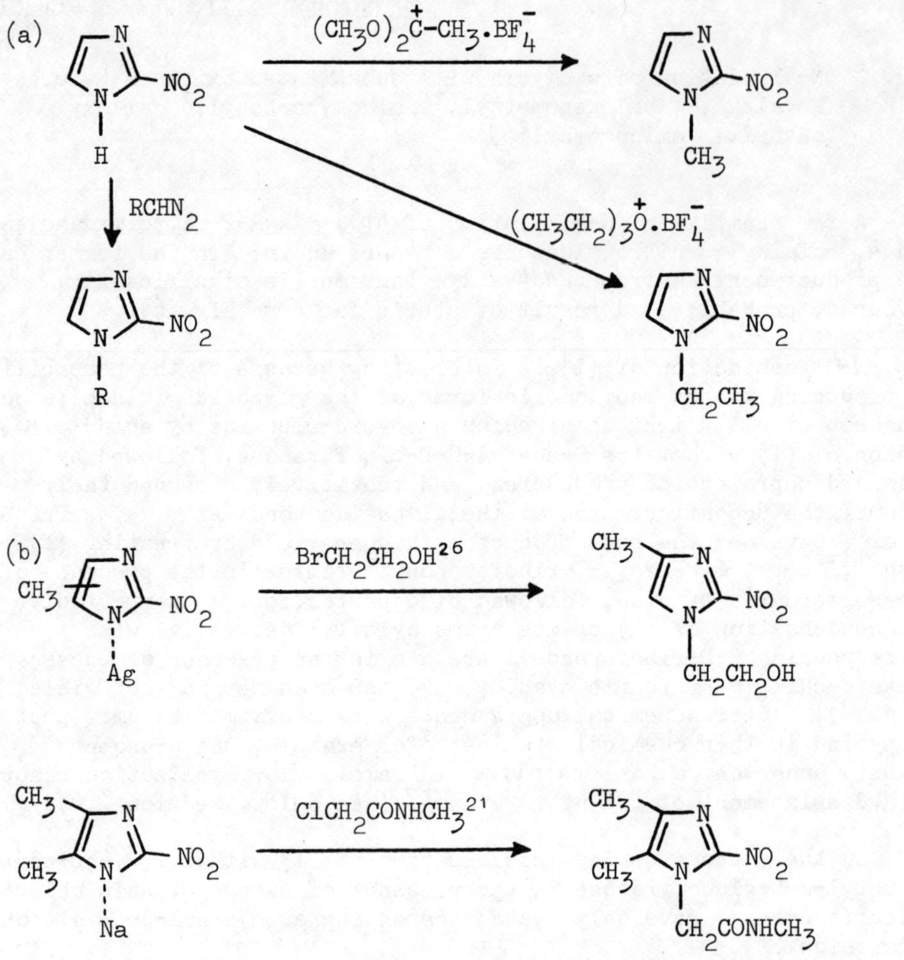

Fig. 6   N-Alkylation (a) of azomycin with Meerwein-type 'onium
reagents[25] and diazoalkanes [where R = hydrogen,[14] ethoxy-
carbonyl[25]] and (b) of 4(5)-alkyl-2-nitroimidazole[26] and
4,5-dialkyl-2-nitroimidazole.[15][21]

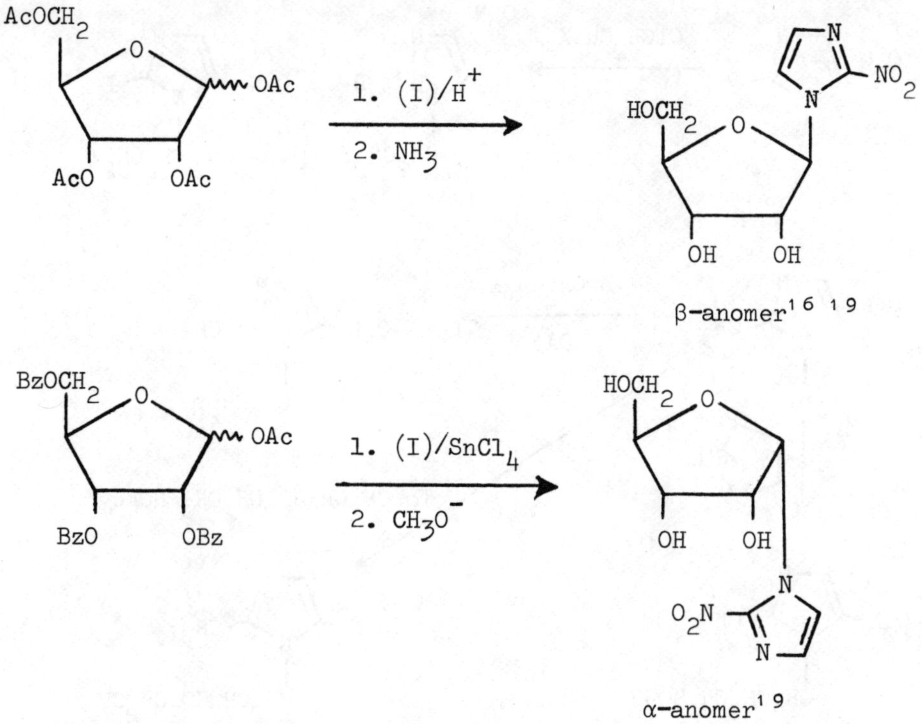

Fig. 7 N-Glycosidation of azomycin.

conditions gives the 4-nitro isomer, as the major or sole product, whereas under strongly acidic conditions the 5-nitro isomer is generally favoured.

A wider range of alkylating reagents have been described[5] for the N-1 alkylation of 4(5)-nitroimidazoles than for 2-nitroimidazoles but amongst the most versatile reagents have been alkyl halides or sulfonates (Fig. 8)[4 30-32] and substituted oxiranes or related hetero-cycles (Fig. 9).[4 30 33-38]   Again, compounds such as the chloro-hydrins (XIV) and (XV), obtained from epichlorohydrin,[34] are useful intermediates for further side-chain substitution reactions (see below, Section 2.3).   2,4(5)-Dinitroimidazole reacted with oxirane to give 2,4-dinitroimidazole-1-ethanol[39] but treatment with various alkyl halides generally led to displacement of the 2-nitro group (see below, Section 3.4).

Direct N-alkylation of 4(5)-nitroimidazoles by means of the electrophilic Meerwein-type 'onium reagents, such as dimethoxy-carbonium tetrafluoroborate,[40] is potentially useful due to the preferred formation of the 5-nitro isomer under overall neutral

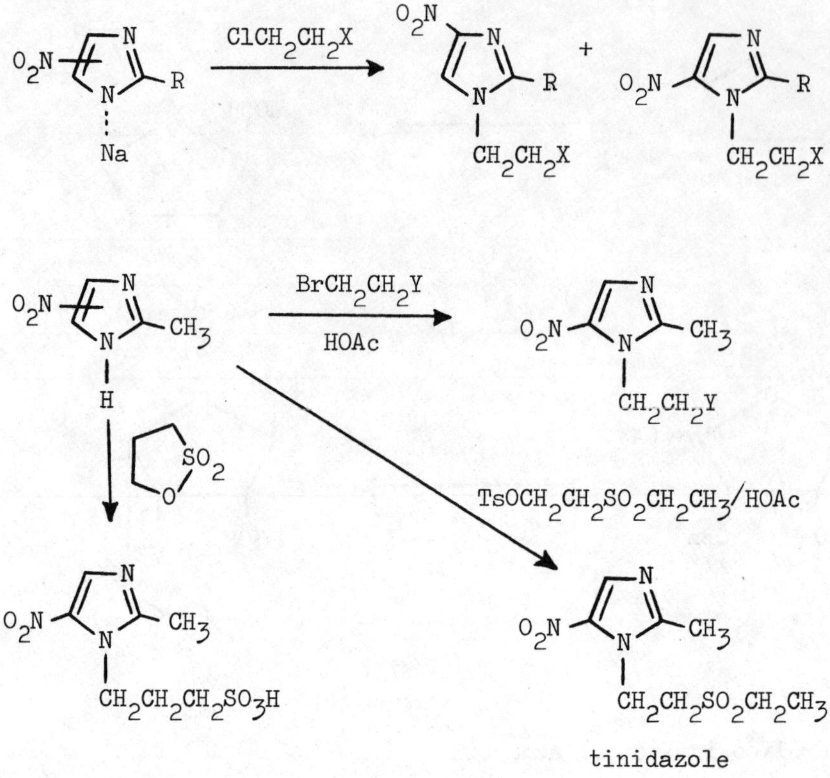

Fig. 8 N-Alkylation of 4(5)-nitroimidazoles with alkyl halides [where R = hydrogen, methyl and X = amino,[31] and Y = alkoxy[32] or thioether[30]] and alkyl sulfonates.[30]

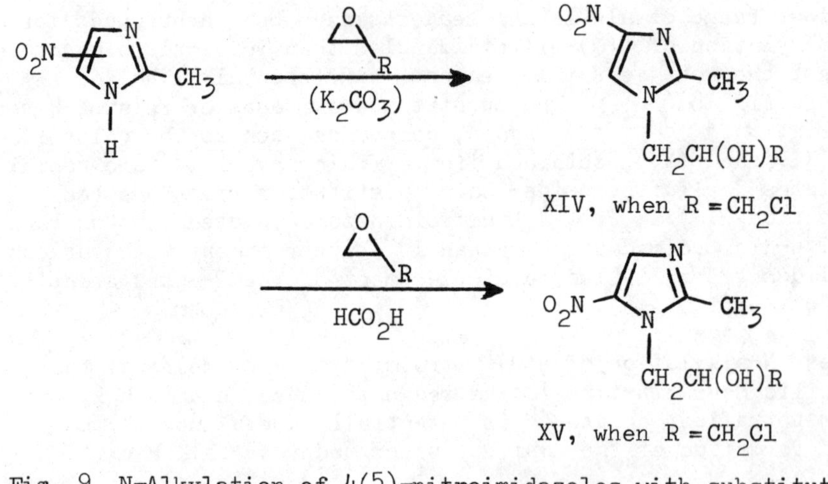

Fig. 9 N-Alkylation of 4(5)-nitroimidazoles with substituted oxiranes [where R = hydrogen[4][33] chloromethyl,[34][37] alkoxymethyl,[36] aryloxymethyl[35]]

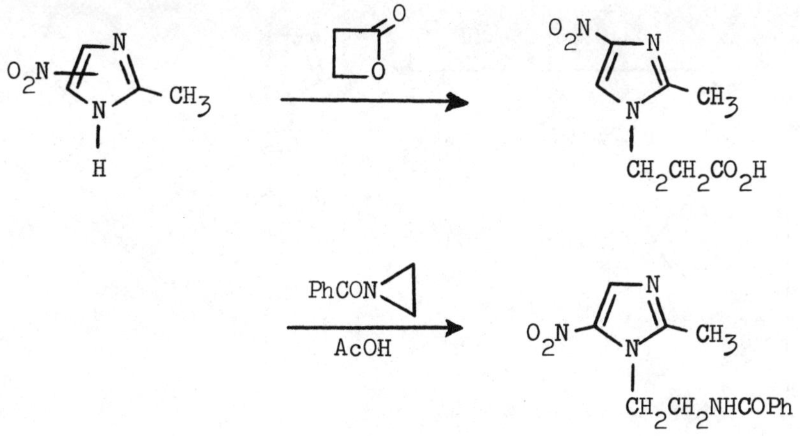

Fig. 9 (continued)   N-Alkylation of 4(5)-nitroimidazoles with propiolactone[30] and N-benzoylaziridine.[38]

reaction conditions (Fig. 10).   Grabowsky et al[40] used this observation to develop the cyclic 'onium analog, 2-methyl-1,3-dioxolenium tetrafluoroborate (XVI), as a novel "acetoxyethylating" reagent of potentially wide utility.   It contributed to an elegant isomer-free synthesis of the 2-aryl-1-hydroxyethyl-5-nitroimidazole flunidazole (XVII) but not as a regioselective alkylating reagent.[40] Reaction of 2,4(5)-dinitroimidazole with diazomethane has been reported to be regioselective and to have given 1-methyl-2,4-dinitro-imidazole as the sole product.[14]   However, a recent investigation of this reaction and that of other 4(5)-nitroimidazoles with diazo-methane has shown that both 4-nitro and 5-nitro isomers are produced[64] (Fig. 10).

N-Glycosidation of 4(5)-nitroimidazoles is especially interesting for two reasons; first, the possible formation of 4 and/or 5-nitro isomers and second, the formation of α- and β-anomers as already noted for 2-nitroimidazoles.   Imbach and co-workers[17,20] have obtained 1-D-ribofuranosyl-4-nitroimidazoles in high yields and with good regiospecificity by the acid-catalyzed fusion of (IX) or (X) with tetra-O-acetyl-β-D-ribofuranose, followed by standard deprotection procedures, with the ratio of α:β anomers equal to 1:9. On the other hand, condensation of (IX) or (X) with penta-O-acetyl-β-D-glucopyranose in the same way gave only low yields of the corresponding 1-β-D-glucopyranosyl-4-nitroimidazoles.[20]   In contrast, condensation of (IX) or (X), as their silver salts, with the corresponding tri-O-acetyl-1-D-ribofuranosyl chloride or tetra-O-acetyl-1-β-D-glucopyranosyl bromide gave mixtures of the 4-nitro and

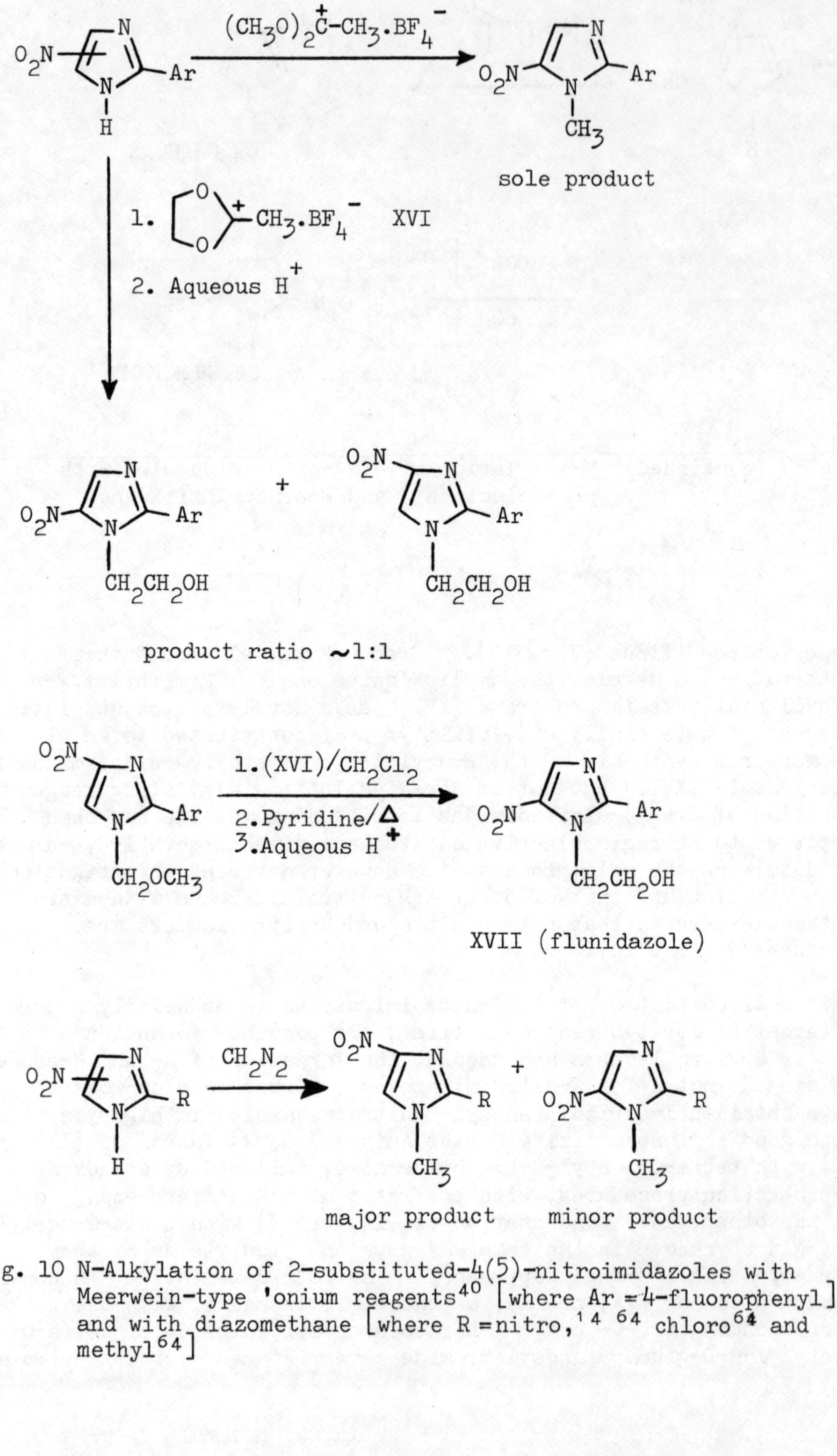

Fig. 10 N-Alkylation of 2-substituted-4(5)-nitroimidazoles with
Meerwein-type 'onium reagents[40] [where Ar = 4-fluorophenyl]
and with diazomethane [where R = nitro,[14] [64] chloro[64] and
methyl[64]]

5-nitro isomers where the product ratio was dependent on the substituent in the 2-position of the parent nitroimidazole[20] (Fig. 11). Methyl 4(5)-nitroimidazole-5(4)-carboxylate similarly gave mixtures of 4-nitro and 5-nitroimidazole nucleosides.[18]

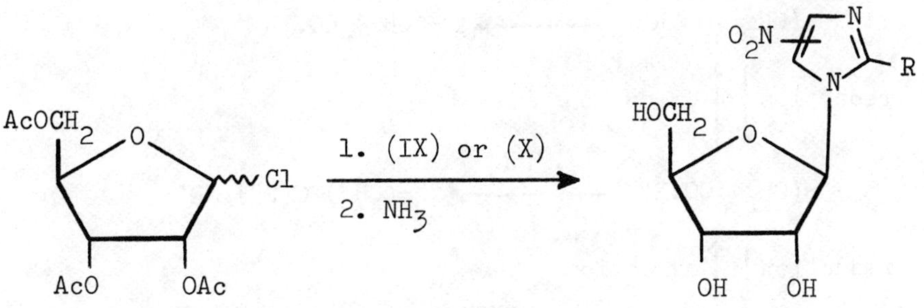
AcOCH2
O
Cl
AcO
OAc
1. (IX) or (X)
2. NH3
O2N
N
N
R
HOCH2
O
OH
OH

Fig. 11 N-Glycosidation of 4(5)-nitroimidazoles.[20]

2.3 Side-Chain Substitution Reactions of N-1-Alkyl Nitroimidazoles

Some of the 1-substituted nitroimidazoles mentioned above, though possibly active as chemotherapeutic agents, have relatively little interest *per se* as potential hypoxic cell radiosensitizers due to their low water-solubility but nonetheless provide versatile intermediates for the synthesis of more hydrophilic 1-substituted nitroimidazoles by means of side-chain substitution reactions. For example, 1-(ω-haloalkyl) or (ω-alkenyl)-nitroimidazoles may be interconverted or otherwise transformed into 1-(ω-epoxyalkyl)nitroimidazoles and their condensation reactions with alcohols, amines or thiols can give rise, in principle, to an almost unlimited range of compounds:

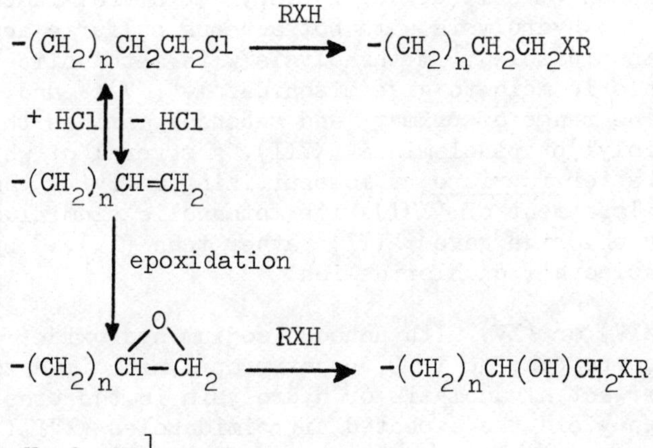
-(CH2)nCH2CH2Cl
RXH
-(CH2)nCH2CH2XR
+ HCl
- HCl
-(CH2)nCH=CH2
epoxidation
O
-(CH2)nCH—CH2
RXH
-(CH2)nCH(OH)CH2XR

where X = O, NR^1 or S

Similarly, 1-substituted nitroimidazoles containing a carboxylic acid, ketone or carbinol function in the side-chain may be interconverted, via oxidation or reduction reactions, or condensed with amines, etc:

$$-(CH_2)_n CO_2 R' \xrightarrow{RXH} -(CH_2)_n CO.XR$$

reduction $\downarrow\uparrow$ oxidation

$$-(CH_2)_n CO.R'' \xrightarrow{R'NH_2} -(CH_2)_n C(R'')=NR'$$

reduction $\downarrow\uparrow$ oxidation

$$-(CH_2)_n CH(OH)R'' \xrightarrow{RXH} -(CH_2)_n CH(XR)R''$$

Adams et al[11] have described the condensation of several 1-(ω-haloalkyl)-2-nitroimidazoles with different secondary amines and Winkelmann et al[41] have described the base-catalyzed condensation of 1-(2-chloroethyl)-2-methyl-5-nitroimidazole with several aryl-thiols to give the corresponding 1-(ω-substituted-alkyl)-nitroimidazoles. Hoffer and Grunberg[34] obtained 1-(2,3-dichloropropyl)-2-methyl-5-nitroimidazole by chlorination of either the corresponding 1-allyl compound with concentrated hydrochloric acid and hydrogen peroxide or the chlorohydrin (XV) with phosphorus pentachloride and phosphorus oxychloride (Fig. 12).

The chlorohydrins (XIII), (XIV) and (XV) have proved to be a versatile series of intermediates. Treatment of (XIII) with aqueous sodium hydroxide gave 1-(2,3-epoxypropyl)-2-nitroimidazole (XVI)[21] which underwent hydrolysis with hot aqueous sulfuric acid to yield desmethylmisonidazole,[21] methanolysis with methanolic boron trifluoride or perchloric acid to give misonidazole (IV)[25] and aminolysis with a wide range of primary and secondary amines to yield (2-nitroimidazolyl)propanolamines (XVII),[24] several of which show significantly better in vitro radiosensitizing activity than (IV)[42] (Fig. 13). Treatment of (XVI) with methanolic aluminium chloride or hydrogen chloride gave (XIII) rather than (IV),[25] by reaction with the nucleophilic chloride ion.

Treatment of (XIV) or (XV) with aqueous sodium hydroxide similarly gave the corresponding 1-(2,3-epoxypropyl)nitroimidazoles (Fig. 12) which underwent alkanolysis or hydrolysis in the presence of perchloric acid to yield the expected nitroimidazoles (XVIII)[36]

XV

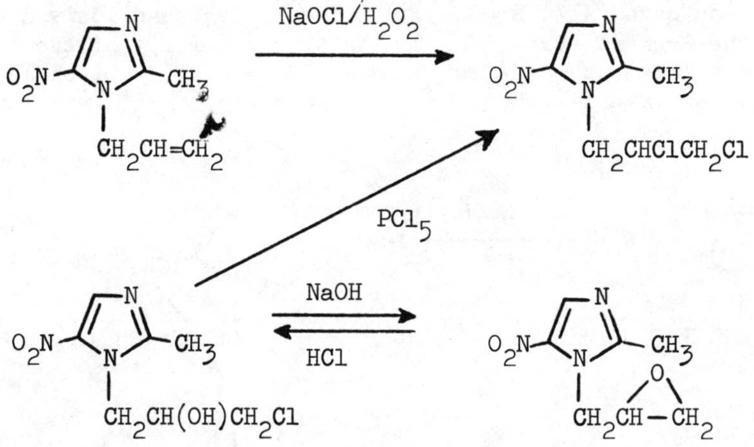

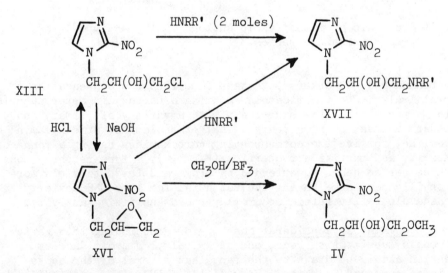

Fig. 12 Some side-chain substitution reactions in the N-1-alkyl 5-nitroimidazole series.[34]

XVI IV

Fig. 13 Some side-chain substitution reactions in the N-1-alkyl 2-nitroimidazole series.[21 24 25]

or (XIX)[37] respectively (Fig. 14).   In the 5-nitro series treatment
with hydrochloric acid gave (XV)[34] (Fig. 12) and treatment with
methoxide ion gave (XIX, R = CH$_3$).[37]   The latter reaction was not
found in the 2-nitro series due to the susceptibility of the nitro
group to displacement (see Section 3.4).[25]   Some (5-nitroimidazolyl)-
propanolamines have also been reported recently.[43]

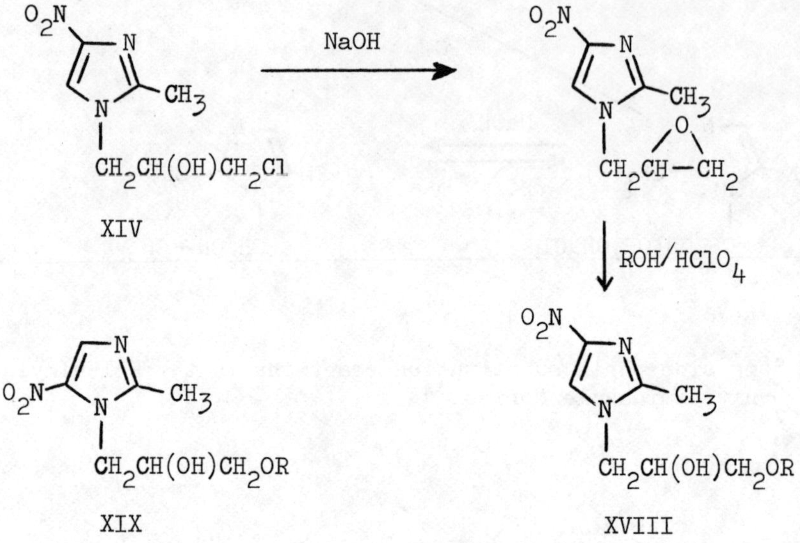

Fig. 14 Synthesis of misonidazole analogs in the 4-nitro[36] and
        5-nitroimidazole series.[37]

Beaman and co-workers[21][44] have described the condensation of
several 1-alkyl-2-nitroimidazoles bearing a carboxylic ester function
in the ω-position of the side-chain with a variety of primary and
secondary amines, such as benzylamine, ethanolamine, dimethylamine or
morpholine, to give the corresponding carboxamides having a range of
solubility and partition properties (Fig. 15).   More recently, one
of these series has been extended by Brown and Lee[45] to yield more
hydrophilic analogs having the potential for less CNS toxicity than
misonidazole whilst retaining similar radiosensitizing activity.

Stereochemical considerations: before continuing this review of
side-chain substitution reactions of N-1-alkyl nitroimidazoles
attention should be drawn to the fact that several of the above
mentioned compounds such as (IV), (XIII), (XIV), (XV) and (XVII), have
a chiral carbon in the side-chain.   Other nitroimidazoles are known
which possess a similar chiral centre in side-chains attached to C-2
or 4(5) of the nitroimidazole ring, such as moxnidazole (XX),[46]

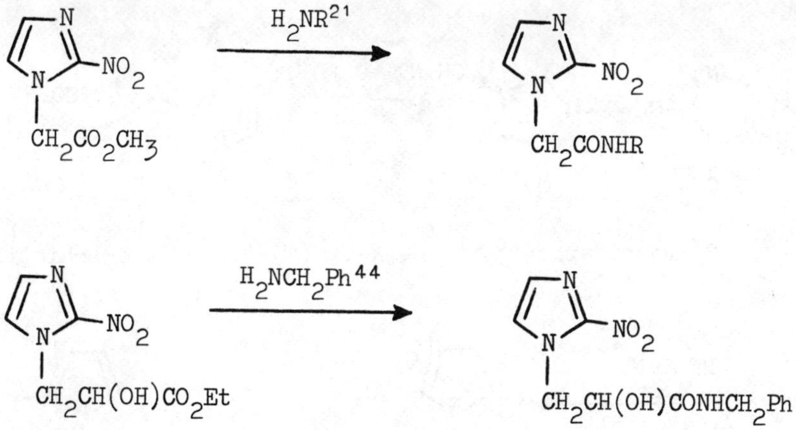

Fig. 15 Aminolysis reactions of some (2-nitroimidazolyl)alkanoic esters.[21] [44]

4(5)-nitrohistidine[47] [48] and 2-nitrohistidine[48] (Fig. 16). The stereochemical consequence of this asymmetry feature is that each compound will generally be obtained as a 50:50 mixture of two different stereoisomers or enantiomers having different (non-superimposable) three-dimensional structures; one being the mirror-image of the other. When separated the two components of the racemic mixture will have equal but opposed chiroptical properties. Separation of the components of the above mentioned pairs of enantiomeric nitroimidazoles can generally be achieved by standard chemical means, such as derivatization or salt formation with an enantiomerically pure chiral carboxylic acid,[49] [50] or by stereospecific synthesis of each enantiomer from an enantiomerically pure chiral compound of known stereochemistry, such as L-histidine.[48] [51] In none of the cases so far studied[49] [50] has there been any significant difference in the biological activity of the resolved enantiomers. Among the series of (2-nitroimidazolyl)propanolamines (XVII) described by Smithen et al[42] there are some examples of compounds having two chiral centres in the N-1 side-chain. The stereochemical consequence of this double asymmetry feature is that each compound will generally be obtained as a mixture of two different pairs of enantiomers (i.e. four different stereoisomers or diastereomers). In some cases it is possible to separate one pair of enantiomers from the other solely by physical means, such as recrystallization, and often such isomers also differ from each other in chemical and biological properties.

In the case of the 1,4-bis-propanolamine (XXI), derived from piperazine,[42] two isomeric forms were isolated by recrystallization and assumed to be the racemic and meso forms by analogy with tartaric

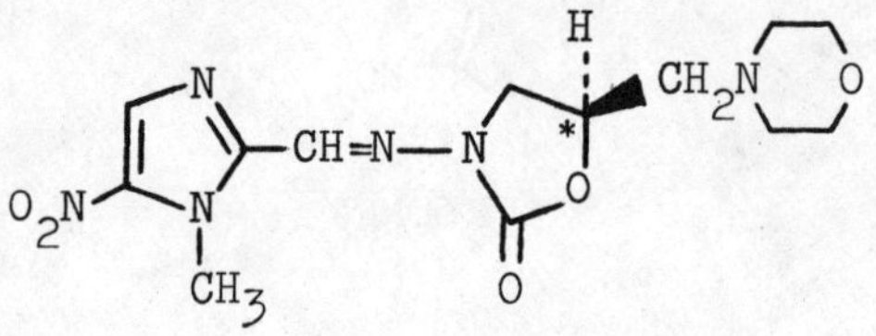

XX, (+)-(R)-moxnidazole[46][49] 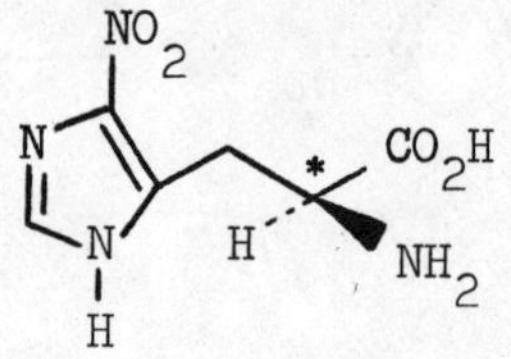   (+)-4(5)-nitro-L-histidine[48]

XVI $\xrightarrow{\Delta/\text{alcohol}}$

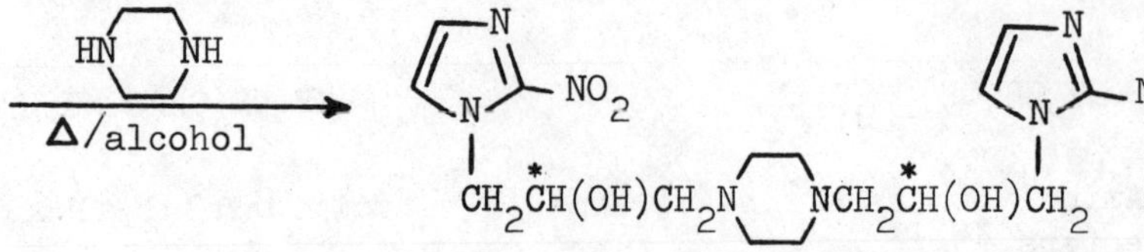

XXI[42]

(R,R)

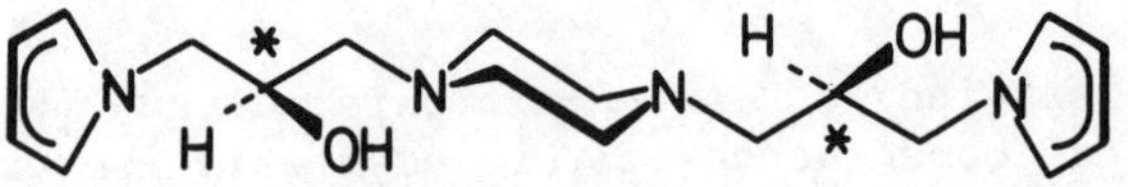

(S,S)

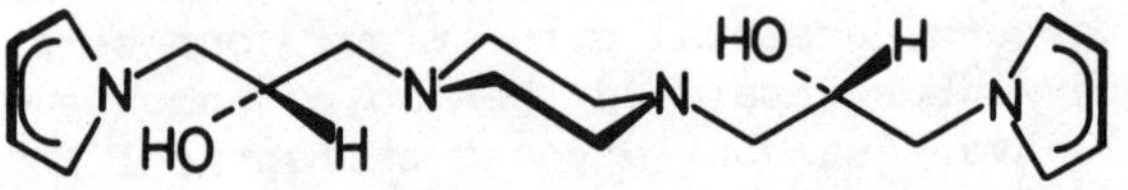

(R,R) + (S,S) = racemic form: mirror-images not superimposable

(R,S)

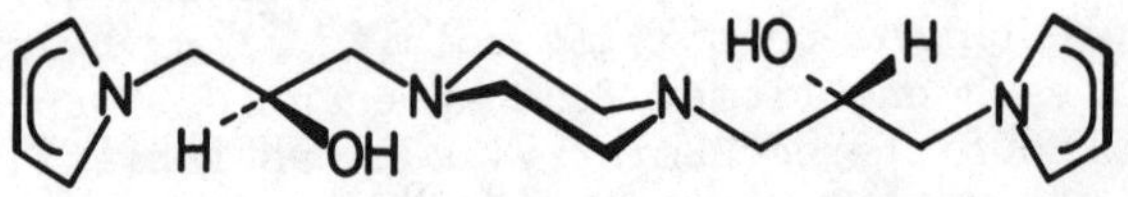

(S,R)

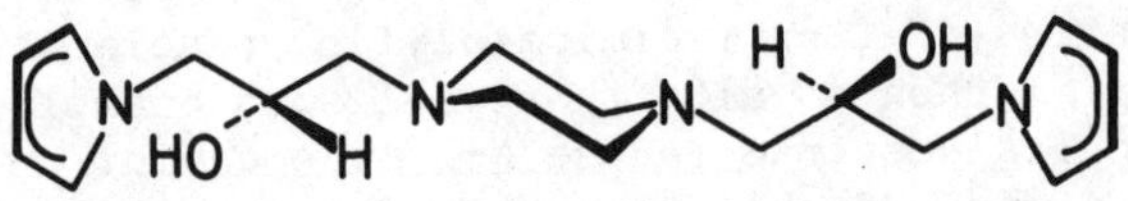

(R,S) + (S,R) = meso form: mirror-images superimposable

$$HO_2C-\overset{*}{C}H(OH)-\overset{*}{C}H(OH)-CO_2H \qquad \text{tartaric acid}$$

Fig. 16 Representative nitroimidazoles having one or two chiral
centres (marked *); in the latter case the stereochemistry
of the four possible diastereoisomers is illustrated by
analogy to the racemic and meso forms of tartaric acid.

acid, a well-known example of a centrosymmetrical molecule containing two equivalent chiral centres substituted with hydroxy groups (Fig. 16 illustrates, in simplified form, the <u>four</u> possible three-dimensional structures and shows that, for symmetry reasons, two stereoisomers of (XXI) are indistinguishable, i.e. <u>meso</u>). It was noteworthy that these isomers of (XXI) showed small but significant differences in their radiosensitizing and cytotoxicity properties which were unrelated to the differences in their physico-chemical properties.[42] This suggested that configurational factors, involving the stereo-chemistry of the side-chain substituents of nitroimidazoles, could make significant and hitherto undetected contributions to their biological properties.

<u>Side-chain oxidation reactions</u>: another class of reactions of N-1-alkyl nitroimidazoles which have potential for the introduction of hydrophilic substituents involve oxidation of existing side-chain substituents, such as hydroxy, amino or thioether.   Beaman et al[21] have described the oxidation of misonidazole (IV) with chromic acid to give the corresponding ketone (Fig. 17) which is capable of further conversion into a range of carbonyl derivatives, such as oximes and semicarbazones.[21]   These derivatives, in turn, are capable of many diverse chemical transformations.[5]

Oxidation of metronidazole (II) with potassium dichromate-acetic acid gave a complex containing unchanged (II) and the unstable 2-methyl-5-nitroimidazolylcarboxaldehyde from which carbonyl derivatives, such as oximes and thiosemicarbazones, were obtained by standard procedures.[52]   Ferric chloride oxidation of such thiosemicarbazones yielded the corresponding amino-1,3,4-thiadiazoles which possess useful chemotherapeutic properties.[52] Oxidation of (II) with chromic acid[53] or a variety of other oxidizing agents[52] gave only 2-methyl-5-nitroimidazolyl-acetic acid, also identified as a metabolite of (II) (Fig. 17).

Oxidation of nimorazole (VII) with hydrogen peroxide-acetic acid gave the corresponding N-oxide,[54] also identified as a metabolite of (VII), which is much more hydrophilic than (VII) but significantly less active <u>in vitro</u> as a radiosensitizer (P Wardman - personal communication).   Side-chain oxidation of 1-(ethylthio-ethyl)-2-methyl-5-nitroimidazole, a more lipophilic nitroimidazole, with aqueous sodium hypochlorite gave the corresponding sulfone tinidazole,[30] which has comparable E_7^1 and radiosensitizing activity <u>in vitro</u> to (VII) though rather more hydrophilic.[10]   Oxidation of several 1-(arylthioethyl)-2-methyl-5-nitroimidazoles with hydrogen peroxide-acetic acid also yielded the sulfone derivatives[41] whereas treatment of 1-(methylthioethyl)-2-nitroimidazole with hydrogen peroxide alone gave mainly the corresponding sulfoxide[45] (Fig. 17).

<u>Pro-drug derivatives</u>: the final class of side-chain substitution reactions of N-1-alkyl nitroimidazoles to be considered in this

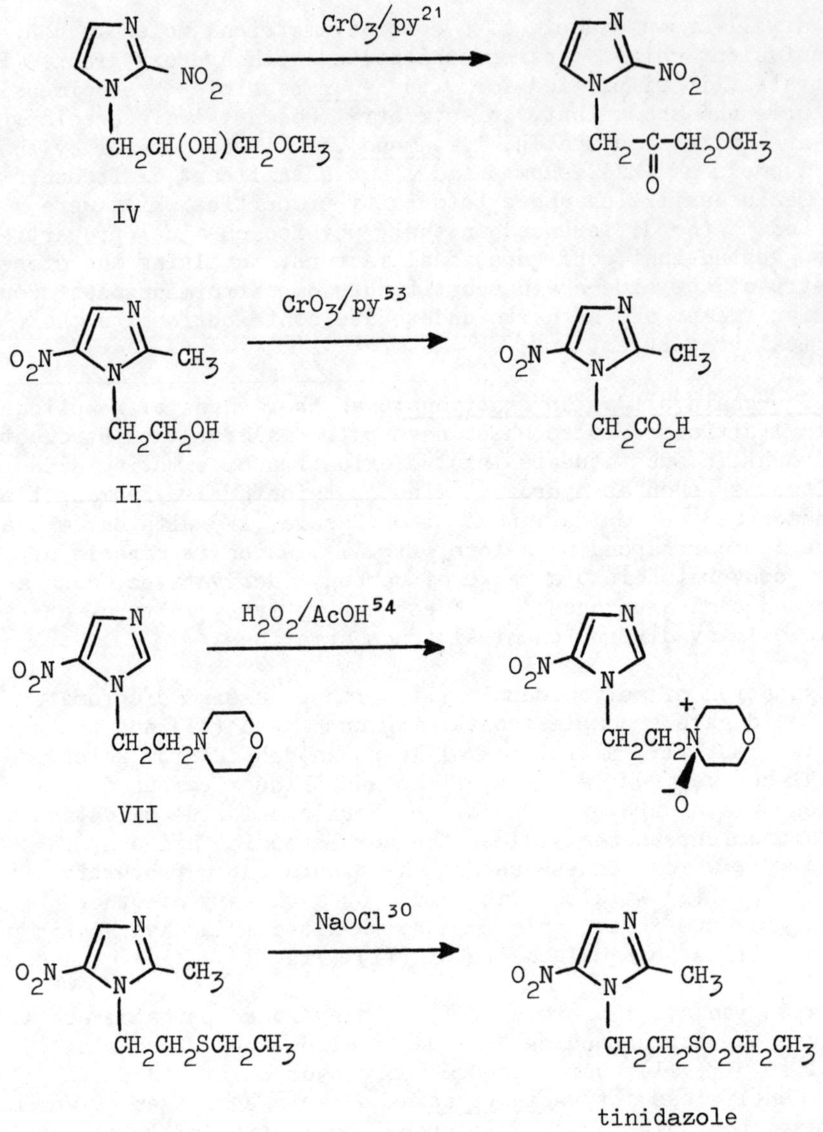

Fig. 17 Some side-chain oxidation reactions of 2-nitro[21] and 5-nitroimidazoles.[30] [53] [54]

Section concerns the derivatization of side-chain hydroxy or amino groups, such as with organic or inorganic acids, in order to modify the bioavailability of the active nitroimidazole. These prodrug forms of nitroimidazoles were generally developed to improve the pharmacokinetic behaviour and therapeutic benefit of clinically important chemotherapeutic agents, such as metronidazole (II),[38] [43] [55] and it remains to be established whether these derivatives and their close analogs (Fig. 18) have the appropriate pharmacokinetic properties to suit their use as radiosensitizers.

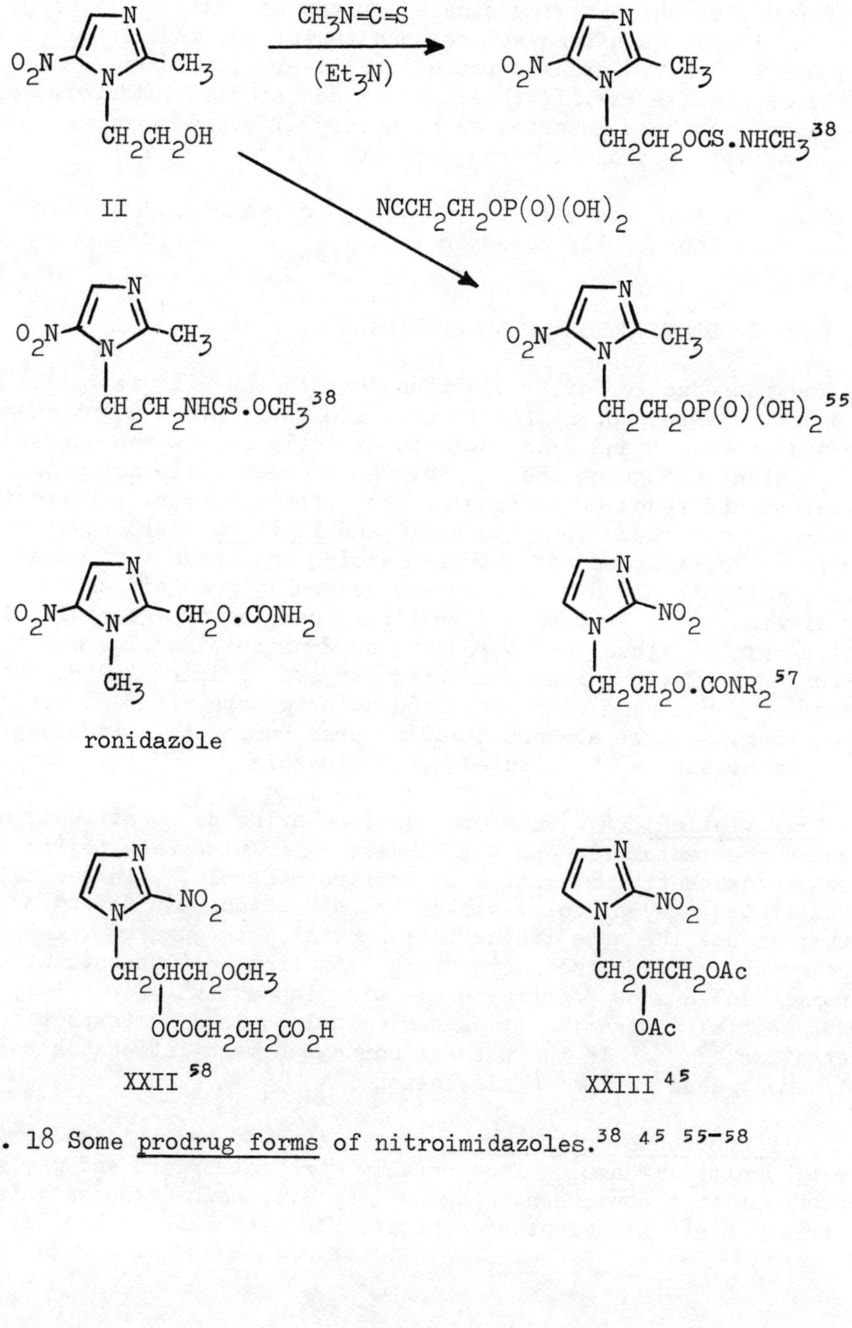

Fig. 18 Some <u>prodrug forms</u> of nitroimidazoles.[38] [45] [55-58]

For example, the base-catalyzed condensation of (II) with methylisothiocyanate gave the corresponding thiocarbamoyl derivative[38] (Fig. 18) and Beaman et al[56][57] have described other acyl and carbamoyl derivatives of (2-nitroimidazolyl)alkanols, such as misonidazole (IV). In most cases there is a substantial change (increase) in lipophilicity which may be expected not to influence radiosensitizing activity significantly.[10] However, Wardman et al[58] have found that the O-hemisuccinate derivative (XXII) (Fig.18) of misonidazole was much less active as a radiosensitizer _in vitro_ than (IV), suggesting diminished bioavailability in this case. The di-O-acetate derivative (XXIII) (Fig. 18) of desmethylmisonidazole, on the other hand, has been reported to be a very effective prodrug form of this relatively hydrophilic radiosensitizer.[45]

Clearly, this approach to the design of improved radiosensitizers remains to be more fully investigated.

3.   RING C-SUBSTITUTION OF NITROIMIDAZOLES

The introduction of C-substituents into the nitroimidazole is an important aspect of nitroimidazole chemistry since substituents attached to C-2, 4 and 5 are able to directly affect the electron distribution throughout the ring system thereby influencing both the ionization and redox properties of the nitroimidazole. Comparison of one-electron reduction potentials and _in vitro_ radiosensitizing data for a large number of nitroimidazoles has shown that more electron-affinic nitroimidazoles are generally more efficient sensitizers.[8][10] 4-Nitro and 5-nitroimidazoles are generally less electron-affinic than the corresponding 2-nitroimidazoles and there is, consequently, particular interest in synthesizing 4(5)-nitro-imidazoles containing electron-withdrawing groups attached directly to the ring. There are essentially three basic steps in the synthesis of such a substituted nitroimidazole:

(a) N-Alkylation: 4(5)-nitroimidazoles having no substituent on nitrogen are tautomeric and N-1 alkylation is necessary to fix the structure as that of a 4-nitro or 5-nitroimidazole. In the case of 2-substituted-4(5)-nitroimidazoles N-1 alkylation can determine whether or not the substituent is essentially conjugated with the nitro group. Furthermore, _in vitro_ data from N-1 unsubstituted nitroimidazoles show poor radiosensitization activity, possibly due to substantial ionization at physiological pH leading to poor cellular penetration.[39][58] In the present context N-methylation has been the most widely used form of N-alkylation.

(b) Introduction of nitro group: nitration of the imidazole ring to give 4(5)-nitroimidazoles is generally straightforward and may be carried out at a convenient stage of the synthesis dependent upon the nature and stability of other substituents present.

(c) Introduction of C-substituent: preparation of C-substituted
nitroimidazoles may involve either replacement of a suitable group
(usually hydrogen or halogen) or modification of a substituent
already present.   Some of the more important examples of such
reactions are now discussed.

3.1 Reactions Involving Replacement of Hydrogen at C-2, 4 or 5

The replacement of hydrogen at C-2,4 or 5 in an imidazole or
nitroimidazole ring occurs in a number of reactions; the most widely
used reaction being halogenation, usually bromination.   Halogenated
4- and 5-nitroimidazoles are generally prepared by nitration of
suitable halogenoimidazoles because halogenation of the nitroimidazole
ring is limited in part due to deactivation of the ring by the
electron-withdrawing nitro group and in part due to instability of
nitroimidazoles under conditions used for halogenation.   Direct
chlorination or iodination of nitroimidazoles is unknown but
bromination has been reported in a few cases.   Thus, bromination of
4(5)-nitroimidazole (IX)[59] and 1,2-dimethyl-4-nitroimidazole[60] gave
the 2,5(4)-dibromo and 5-bromo derivatives respectively but similar
reactions performed on isomeric disubstituted 5-nitroimidazoles gave
only intractable products.   This latter reaction contrasts sharply
with the facile bromination of imidazole to give 2,4,5-tribromo-
imidazole.[61]

Alternative syntheses are available for chloronitro- and iodonitroimidazoles.   For example, the well-known Wallach synthesis has
been available for many years as a route to certain chloronitroimidazoles.   Fusion of a disubstituted oxamide with phosphorus
pentachloride yields a 1-alkyl-5-chloroimidazole (XXIV)[62] which can
be converted (when R is methyl) into the isomeric 1-methyl-4-chloro-
imidazole (XXV) by a transmethylation reaction involving quaternization
with methyl iodide then "dequaternization" by heating above 200°C[63a]
(Fig. 19).   Both chloroimidazoles are readily nitrated to give the
corresponding chloronitroimidazoles (XXVI) and (XXVII).[63b]   The
preparation of chloronitroimidazoles from certain dinitroimidazoles
is discussed elsewhere[64] (see Section 3.4).

Certain iodonitroimidazoles are conveniently obtained by
nitration of 4,5-di-iodoimidazole[65] and N-methylation of the product
under acidic or basic conditions yields the 4-iodo-5-nitro and
5-iodo-4-nitro isomers respectively as major products (Fig. 20).   On
the other hand, attempted nitration of 4,5-dibromoimidazole failed.[61]

The use of organolithium compounds as intermediates for the
synthesis of 2-nitroimidazoles has been discussed already at this
Conference.[5][66]   2-Lithioimidazoles[67] are also an important source

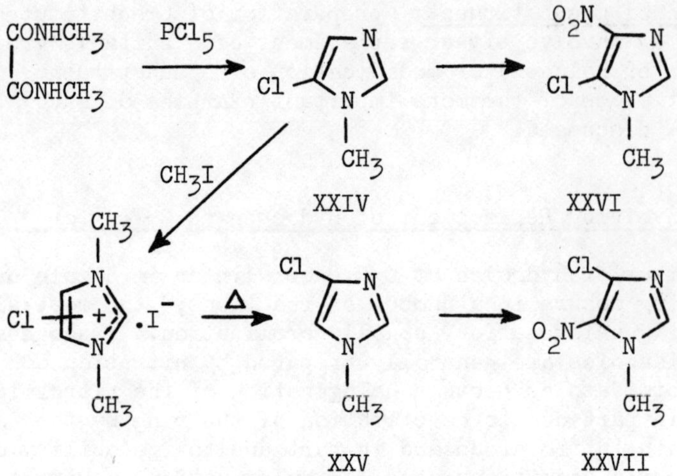

Fig. 19 Syntheses of some isomeric chloronitroimidazoles.[63]

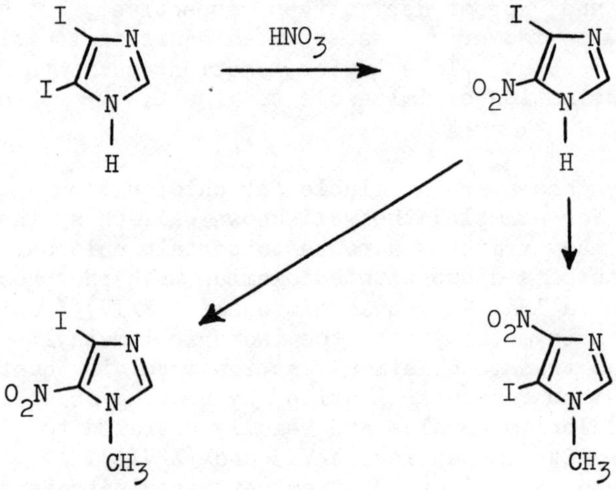

Fig. 20 Syntheses of some isomeric iodonitroimidazoles.[65]

of other 2-substituted imidazoles (Fig. 21).   Nitration of 2-
halogenoimidazoles obtained in this way yields mixtures of 4-nitro
and 5-nitro isomers which are readily separated by chromatography.[68] [6]

Amination of nitroimidazoles using hydroxylamine is another
type of reaction involving replacement of a hydrogen attached to
the imidazole ring.   Good yields of the corresponding amino-nitro-
imidazoles have been obtained in this way from 1,2-dimethyl-4-nitro
and 5-nitroimidazole.[70] [71]   A similar reaction occurs when the same

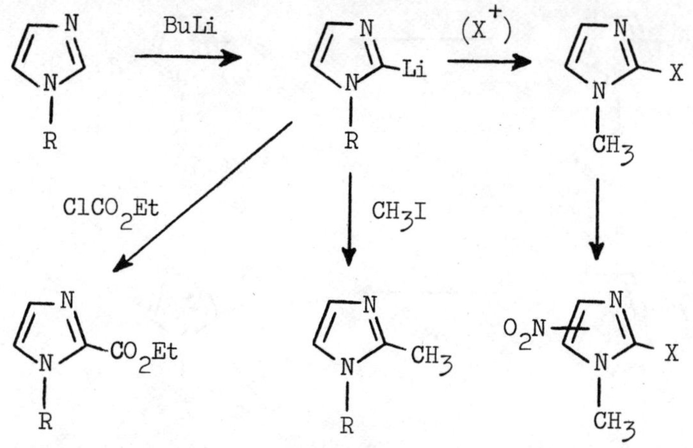

Fig. 21 Syntheses of some 2-substituted-imidazoles via 1-alkyl-2-lithioimidazole[5] [where X = halogen]

nitroimidazoles are heated with potassium cyanide.[70]   In this case, however, simultaneous reduction of the nitro group occurs since cyano-azoxyimidazoles are the only isolated products.[71]

The introduction of the hydroxymethyl group into the C-2 position of certain nitroimidazoles[46] and the range of subsequent chemical transformations have been fully reviewed by Cavalleri.[5]

3.2 Replacement Reactions of Halogenonitroimidazoles

The nucleophilic displacement of a halogen from a halogenonitro-imidazole is an important and versatile reaction in nitroimidazole chemistry and a variety of C-substituents have been introduced in this way (Fig. 22).   The presence of the nitro group appears to be necessary for replacement reactions to occur under mild conditions. Insufficient information is available in the literature, however, to enable conclusions to be drawn regarding the reactivities of halogens at different positions in the nitroimidazole ring and it is only possible to make general observations for individual nucleophiles.

Nitrogen-centred nucleophiles: the reaction of amines with halogenonitroimidazoles reveal differences in reactivity between certain 4- and 5-nitroimidazoles.   Furthermore, it has been observed in some cases that a nitro group in the 5-position is susceptible to replacement by the attacking nucleophile.   Thus, 4-chloro-1-methyl-5-nitroimidazole (XXVII) reacts with morpholine at room-temperature to yield the mono-substituted product (XXVIII)

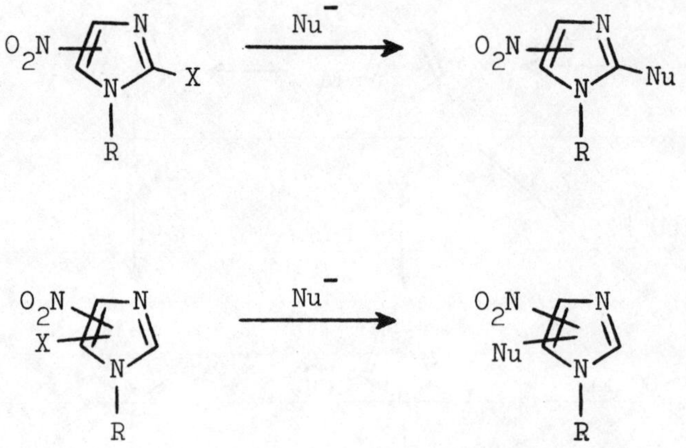

Fig. 22 General reaction scheme for replacement reactions of
halogenonitroimidazoles with nucleophiles [where Nu =
NR'R", OR', SR', CN etc. and X =halogen].

whereas at higher temperatures the disubstituted-imidazole (XXIX) is
the major product.[72]   In contrast, the corresponding 5-chloro-1-
methyl-4-nitroimidazole (XXVI) requires several hours reaction with
morpholine in refluxing alcohol to give the mono-morpholino
derivative (XXX)[72] (Fig. 23).   Bromonitroimidazoles react with
piperidine or ethanolamine to give similar products.[70]

     A few examples are known of the replacement of halogen from
2-halogenonitroimidazoles, mainly the 5-nitro isomers, by amines.[68] [73]
These reactions proceed readily with no evidence of any additional
replacement of the nitro group (Fig. 23).

     Oxygen-centred nucleophiles: the reactions of halogenonitro-
imidazoles with alkoxide and phenoxide ions to yield the
corresponding ethers (Fig. 23) suggest that halogen at either C-4
or 5 position is susceptible to replacement[41] [72] although some
failures have also been reported.[70]   Attempts to produce 5-hydroxy-
1-methyl-4-nitroimidazoles in a similar manner with sodium hydroxide
led only to the isolation of the corresponding sodium salt and
attempts to obtain the free hydroxyimidazole gave only resins.[72]

     Sulfur-centred nucleophiles: nitroimidazolylthiols and
thioethers are prepared by reaction of halogenonitroimidazoles, such
as (XXVI) and (XXVII), with hydrogen sulfide or thiols (Fig. 24). These
reactions proceed very readily at low temperature in the presence of
a suitable base in both the 4- and 5-nitro series and there are no
reports of replacement of the nitro group.[41] [74]   A more convenient
route to 2-sulfur-substituted nitroimidazoles involves the S-alkylatior

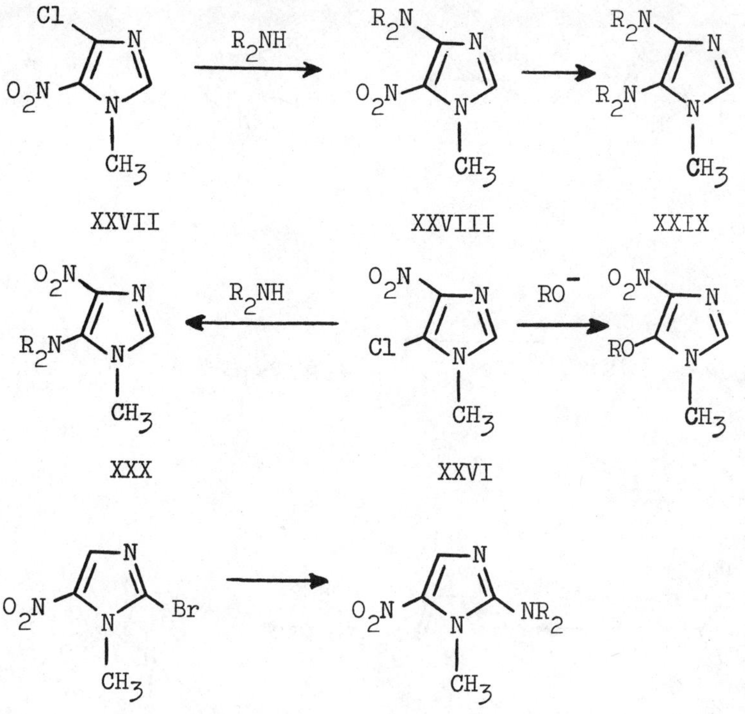

Fig. 23 Some replacement reactions of halogenonitroimidazoles with nitrogen-centred [e.g. R_2N =morpholino or piperidino] and oxygen-centred nucleophiles [e.g. RO =methoxy or phenoxy][72]

of commercially available methimazole (XXXI) to yield the corresponding thioether which, upon nitration, gave a mixture of the 4-nitro and 5-nitro isomers (Fig. 24), readily separable by chromatography.[75][76]

Certain halogenonitroimidazoles are converted into the corresponding 2-sulfonic acids (XXXII) (Fig. 24) by treatment with sodium sulfite, provided that the halogen and nitro groups are in conjugation.[77] In the absence of the nitro group dehalogenation occurs and this reaction was used to good effect to prepare 4-bromo-imidazole from 2,4,5-tribromoimidazole.[61] Some nitroimidazole-4- and 5-sulfonic acids do not behave as normal aryl sulfonic acids and attempts to obtain the corresponding sulfonyl chlorides, using standard methods, have been unsuccessful. This failure may be due, in part, to instability of the sulfonyl chloride per se; in one case, a moderate yield of the chloronitroimidazole (XXVII) was obtained from the corresponding sulfonic acid, presumably due to elimination of sulfur dioxide from the intermediate sulfonyl chloride.[59]

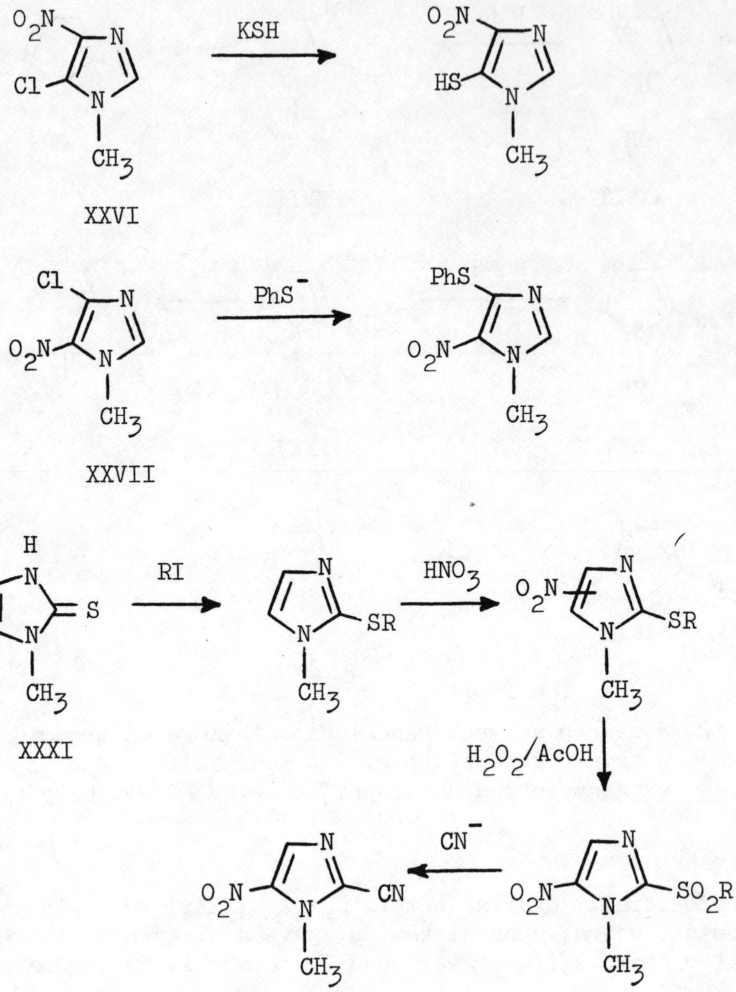

Fig. 24 Some syntheses and reactions of sulfur-substituted nitroimidazoles.[74] [75] [77]

Carbon-centred nucleophiles: the preparation of 2-cyanonitro-
imidazoles is generally limited by the availability of 2-halogeno-
nitroimidazole and alternative methods of synthesis are required
(see Section 3.3). However, the reaction of 2-methanesulfonyl-1-
methyl-5-nitroimidazole with potassium cyanide is reported to give
the corresponding 2-cyanonitroimidazole[78] (Fig. 24).

5-Halogeno-4-nitroimidazoles are apparently susceptible to
attack by cyanide ions giving good yields of 5-cyano-4-nitro-
imidazoles[62 70] whereas the isomeric 4-halogeno-5-nitroimidazoles,
under similar conditions, do not react. However, under more vigorous
conditions cyanation and rearrangement occurs to yield 5-cyano-4-
nitroimidazoles rather than the expected 5-nitro isomer.[79 80] This
rearrangement may be analogous to the transmethylation reaction
discussed above (Section 3.1; Fig. 19) and it has been suggested
that a quaternization/dequaternization mechanism may be involved.

3.3 Modification of C-Substituents in Nitroimidazoles

5-Cyano-4-nitroimidazoles have been converted into the
corresponding carboxylic acid derivatives by hydrolysis of the
cyano group yielding, for example, the carboxamide (XXXIII) or the
free carboxylic acid (Fig. 25). Alternatively, if the cyano group
is first reacted with an alcohol, in the presence of acid, the
resulting carboximidate (XXXIV) can be hydrolyzed to an ester (XXXV)[81]
or aminolyzed to substituted carboxamides (Fig. 25). 2-Cyano-5-
nitroimidazoles may be converted into a range of heterocyclic
derivatives as reviewed by Cavalleri.[5]

Nitroimidazoles substituted with a thioether group are
particularly useful intermediates since oxidation readily provides
the more strongly electron-withdrawing sulfone group.[75 82] (4-Nitro-
5-imidazolyl)thiols are also versatile intermediates and can be
converted into sulfonyl chlorides by treatment at $0°C$ with hypo-
chlorous acid. The resulting sulfonyl chlorides, which slowly
decompose to liberate sulfur dioxide at room-temperature, may be
used to prepare the corresponding sulfonamide (XXXVI) or sulfonate
esters using standard methods[69 74] (Fig. 25).

Methyl groups attached to C-2, 4 and 5 positions of nitroimidazoles are reactive, especially when in conjugation with the
nitro group. For example, 2-methyl-5-nitro- and 5-methyl-2-nitro-
imidazoles undergo base-catalyzed condensations with aromatic
carboxaldehydes, such as benzaldehyde, to give styryl derivatives
where the carbon-carbon double bond may be oxidized by various means,
such as ozone[83] or sodium periodate,[84] to provide the corresponding

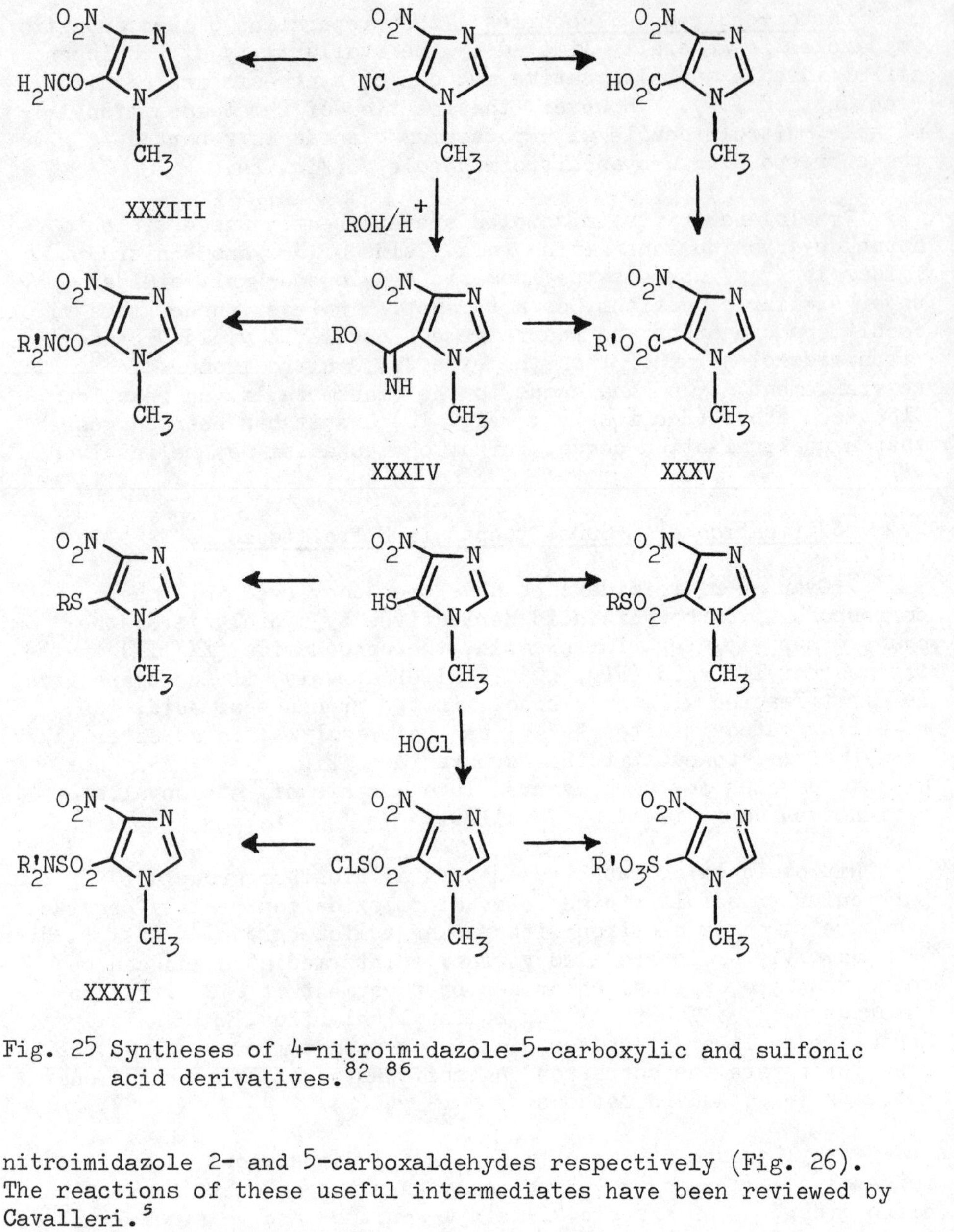

Fig. 25 Syntheses of 4-nitroimidazole-5-carboxylic and sulfonic
       acid derivatives.[82] [86]

nitroimidazole 2- and 5-carboxaldehydes respectively (Fig. 26).
The reactions of these useful intermediates have been reviewed by
Cavalleri.[5]

2-Methyl-4-nitro- and 5-nitroimidazoles have also been reported
to undergo base-catalyzed condensation reactions with diethyl
oxalate[85] or ethyl oxalyl chloride[86] to yield the corresponding ethyl
nitroimidazolylpyruvates (XXXVII).   These esters may be either

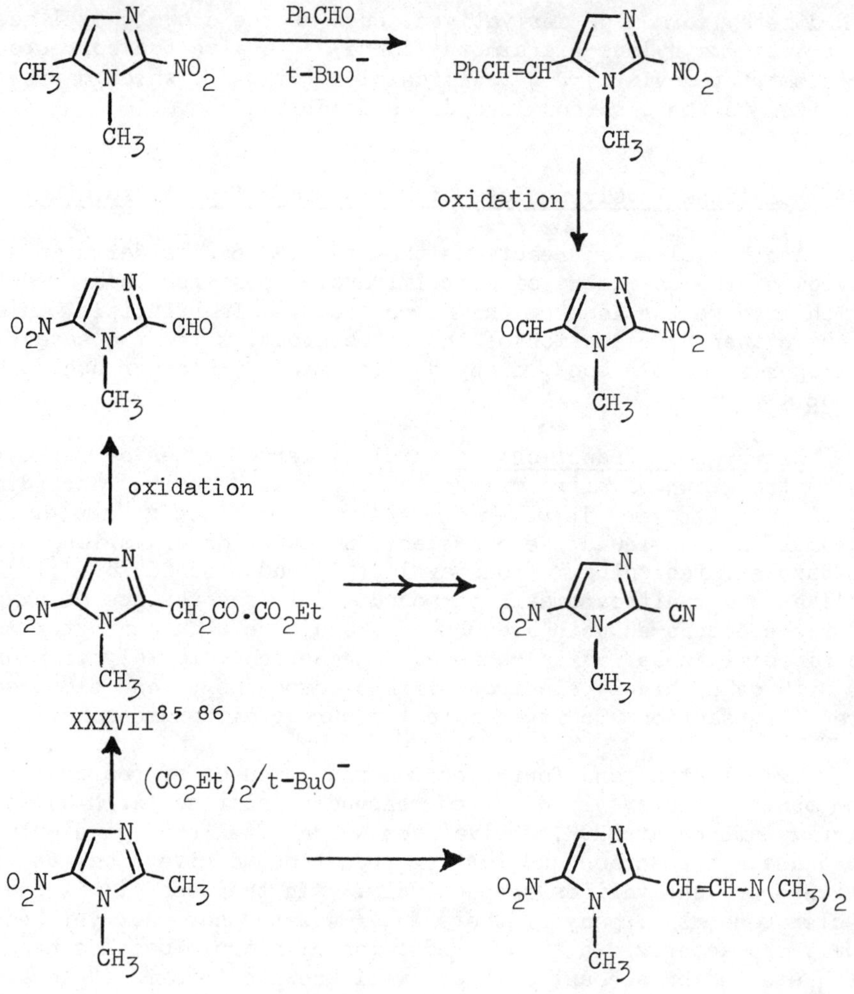

Fig. 26 Some condensation reactions of C-methyl-nitroimidazoles.[83] [85] [86]

similarly oxidized to the 2-carboxaldehyde, for example, using
chlorine and sulfuric acid,[85] or converted into a range of other
2-substituted nitroimidazoles including 2-cyano-1-methyl-5-nitro-
imidazole.[86]   A similar route to the same 2-cyanonitroimidazole
involved base-catalyzed benzoylation of the 2-methyl group followed
by oximination of the resulting ketone and treatment with thionyl
chloride[86] (Fig. 26).

1,2-Dimethyl-5-nitroimidazole also reacts with certain carboxaldehydes and ketones in the presence of acetic anhydride[41] and with

N,N-dimethylformamide derivatives, such as the dicyclohexyl acetal[86] or t-butoxymethylene-bis(dimethylamine),[87] to give the corresponding 2-(substituted-vinyl)-5-nitroimidazoles (Fig. 26) which may be oxidized to the 2-carboxaldehyde as described above.

3.4 Reactions Involving Loss of Nitro Group from Nitroimidazoles

Another class of reactions that should be considered in a review of the chemistry of nitroimidazoles concerns those reactions which involve the loss of the nitro group. In principle, this may occur either by reduction of the nitro group, without cleavage of the nitrogen-imidazole bond, or by displacement by another nucleophilic group.

Nitro-group reduction: several different types of reduction of the nitro group of nitroimidazoles have been described according to th number of electrons involved per molecule of nitroimidazole. Wardman[9] has reviewed the one-electron reduction of various nitro-imidazoles, including metronidazole (II) and misonidazole (IV), as well as other nitroaromatic compounds. In the absence of oxygen stable electron-adducts are observed and have been characterized[9] [88] [8] as nitroimidazole radical-anions. These react rapidly with oxygen or with other highly electron-affinic compounds by one-electron transfer reactions to regenerate the parent nitroimidazole.[9]

Two-electron and four-electron reduction of nitroaromatic compounds formally yield the corresponding nitroso (Ar-N=O) and hydroxylamine (Ar-NHOH) derivatives which often undergo a mutual condensation reaction and further reduction to give azoxy and azo (Ar-N=N-Ar) derivatives respectively. In the case of nitrohetero-cycles generally, many of these intermediates have not yet been fully characterized although reduction of nitroimidazoles has been much studied on account of their well-known cytotoxicity towards anaerobic bacteria, protozoa and hypoxic mammalian cells. In the case of the 2-nitroimidazole misonidazole (IV), this type of reduction has been studied very extensively using chemical,[90] [91] electrochemical,[92] radiolytic[93] and enzymatic[94] [95] means of reduction (Fig. 27). Using zinc dust in aqueous ammonium chloride as the reducing agent Varghese et al[90] have described the putative hydroxyl-amine derivative of (IV) as a labile product which interacts with cellular components, such as DNA and protein. Using zinc dust with aqueous calcium chloride as the reducing agent Josephy et al[91] have isolated and characterized the azoxy and azo derivatives of (IV) as relatively stable products.

Six-electron reduction of nitroimidazoles will formally yield the corresponding aminoimidazole and this has been found to be the case with misonidazole (Fig. 27), where catalytic hydrogenation of

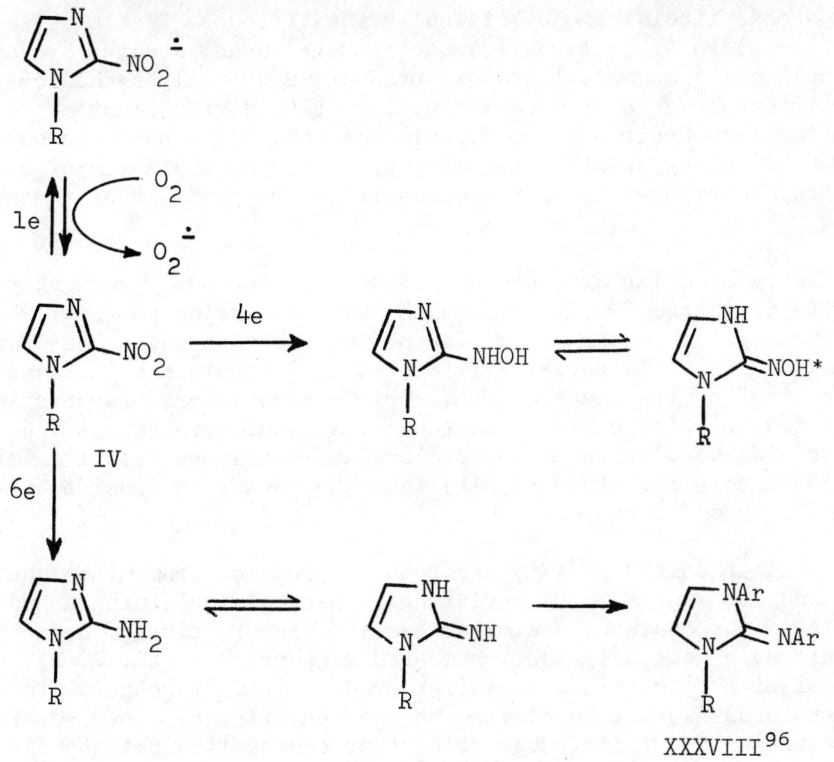

Fig. 27 Nitro-group reduction of misonidazole (IV) [where R = $CH_2CH(OH)CH_2OCH_3$ and Ar = 2,4-dinitrophenyl]

---

* By analogy with acyclic amidoximes and N,N-dialkyl-N'-hydroxy-guanidines the preferred tautomer would possess the exocyclic C=N-OH function.

(IV) gave the 2-aminoimidazole.[96] This fully reduced derivative has been identified as a minor metabolite of misonidazole in some species[96] and its further chemical characterization as the N,N'-bis-(2,4-dinitrophenyl) derivative[96] (XXXVIII) (Fig. 27) suggests that substantial tautomerism to the 2-imino-imidazoline structure (compare 2-imidazolinones; see below, Fig. 28) can occur in these reduced nitroimidazoles. In contrast, the corresponding 5-amino-imidazole derivative of metronidazole (II) appears to be highly unstable.[97][98]

Nitro-group displacement: the first report of this reaction of nitroimidazoles arose from the attempted N-hydroxyethylation of 2,4(5)-dinitroimidazole, by condensation with chloroethanol, which

gave a mononitroimidazole originally identified by Lancini et al[99]
as 5(4)-chloro-4(5)-nitroimidazole.   More recent studies by Hardy[69]
and Suwinski[64] suggest that this product is actually 2-chloro-4(5)-
nitroimidazole arising from the nucleophilic displacement of the
more reactive 2-nitro group by chloride ion.   The products obtained
by Sehgal and Agrawal[100] from attempted N-cyanoethylation of 2,4(5)-
dinitroimidazole with chloropropionitrile are probably of the same
type.

Intramolecular displacement of the nitro group (presumably as
nitrite ion) from 2-nitroimidazoles have been reported (Fig. 28) where
a hydroxy group in the β-position of the N-1 side-chain has provided
the attacking nucleophile.   Prisbe et al[19] obtained a "2,2'-anhydro-
nucleoside" by treatment of 2,3,5-tri-O-benzoyl-D-ribofuranosyl-2-
nitroimidazole (of unknown stereochemical configuration at the
N-glycoside bond) with methoxide ions and concluded from its imidazo-
[2,1-b]oxazole structure (XXXIX) that the parent D-riboside had the
α-anomeric configuration.

Similar compounds (XL) are readily prepared from misonidazole
(IV) and its analogs by refluxing in alcohol containing anhydrous
potassium carbonate or a similar base;[25] interestingly, desmethylmisonidazole gave only the 5-membered ring product (XL, R = H).
Agrawal et al[39] obtained a similar product (XLI) together with 2,4-
dinitroimidazole-1-ethanol from the condensation of 2,4(5)-dinitro-
imidazole with oxirane, suggesting that conjugation between the two
nitro groups is an important factor in the displacement of the
2-nitro substituent.

Photochemical reactions: although it is widely recognized that
most nitroimidazoles are sensitive to actinic light in the solid-
state, undergoing increasingly yellow to brown discoloration and
overt deterioration, there is almost no information available on the
chemical changes that occur at the surface of the solid.   Nitrite
ion has been detected qualitatively in misonidazole (IV) powder
after several months exposure in air to daylight and standard
laboratory lighting but this could arise from slow nitro group
displacement reactions of the type discussed above and not arise from
specifically photochemical processes.[25]

However, some photochemical reactions of nitroimidazoles in
solution have been investigated.   A novel photochemical displacement
reaction of 1-methyl-5-nitroimidazole has been reported where photolysis in aqueous solution containing cyanide ions gave 1-methyl-5-
cyanoimidazole in good yield (Fig. 28) whereas the 2-nitro and 4-nitro
isomers gave little or none of the corresponding displacement
product.[101]   It has been suggested that the 5-nitroimidazole reacts
via its (π,π^*) excited state which is less readily available in the
isomeric nitroimidazoles.   The electronic structure of a range of

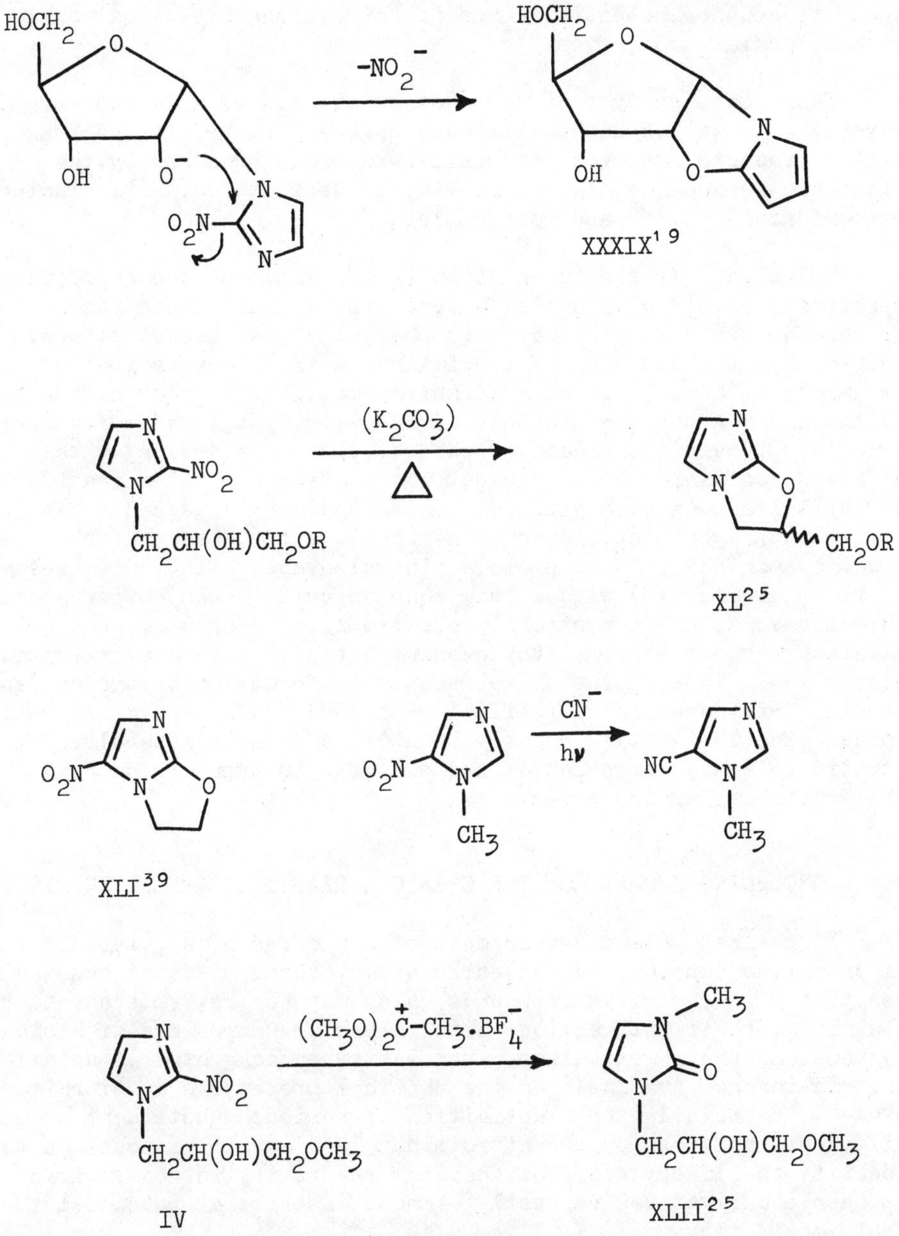

Fig. 28 Miscellaneous reactions of nitroimidazoles involving
displacement of nitro group.

nitroimidazoles has been investigated using photoionization spectroscopy as another potential means of correlating biological activity with molecular properties.[102]

It is noteworthy that the photosensitized oxygenation (singlet oxygen, $^1O_2$) of 1,2-dimethylimidazole gave a range of ring-fragmented products[103] which are similar to those produced by the anaerobic metabolism of several 5-nitro derivatives,[104] including metronidazole (II)[98] and ronidazole.[105]

Relatively little information is available on the chemical reactivity of nitroimidazoles under strongly acidic conditions (pH $<$2) or towards strongly electrophilic reagents.   As discussed above (see Section 2), the basicity of the imidazole ring (unsubstituted imidazole, pKb 6.95) is considerably diminished by the introduction of the nitro group (1-methylnitroimidazoles, pKb's range from 2 to -1; 1-methyl-2,4-dinitroimidazole, pKb -7.5).[14]   By analogy with other nitrogen-containing heterocycles, protonation or quaternization of the N-3 of N-1 substituted nitroimidazoles would be expected to increase the reactivity of the ring-carbon substituents towards displacement reactions or possibly to promote ring-cleavage.   In fact, treatment of misonidazole (IV) with strong aqueous acids, such as perchloric or sulfuric acid, or with strongly electrophilic reagents, such as dimethoxycarbonium or triethyloxonium tetrafluoroborate, resulted generally in loss of the nitro group with formation of the corresponding 2-imidazolinones (XLII)[25] (Fig. 28).   The 4-hydroxy-5-nitroimidazoline derivative recently identified[106] as a metabolite of ipronidazole may represent an example of this type of reactivity in the 5-nitroimidazole series.

4.   CONCLUDING SUMMARY OF THE CHEMICAL REACTIVITY OF NITROIMIDAZOLES

In the design and development of new drugs of any type it is important to consider, at an early stage, those sites of chemical reactivity in the given compounds which may be most relevant to their stability, their interactions with molecular components of biological systems and their metabolism.   Against the background of detailed information now available on the chemical properties of nitroimidazoles,   especially the reactivities of various substituent groups in different positions on the nitroimidazole ring, it is possible to identify the likely sites of chemical reactivity in those nitroimidazole derivatives currently of most interest as potential tumour radiosensitizers.

We conclude the present review of the synthesis and chemistry of nitroimidazoles as hypoxic cell radiosensitizers by summarizing, in diagrammatic form, the sites of chemical reactivity in metronidazole (Fig. 29) and misonidazole (Fig. 30) which may be relevant to their stability, biological interactions and metabolism.

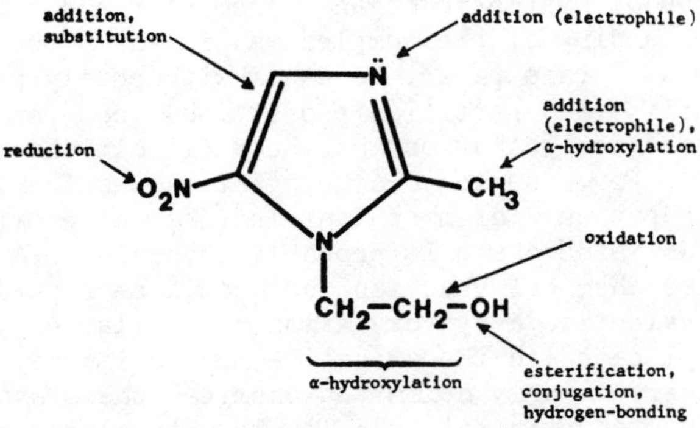

Fig. 29 Sites of chemical reactivity in metronidazole.

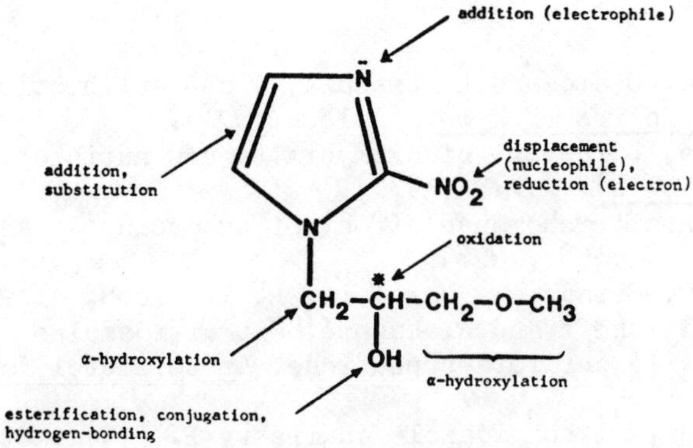

Fig. 30 Sites of chemical reactivity in misonidazole.

The results of drug metabolism studies of these two compounds and several other closely related nitroimidazoles have been reviewed at this Conference by Schwartz[104] and Marten.[107]   It will be readily apparent, from a comparison of these data obtained from the different fields of synthetic organic chemistry and drug metabolism, that our understanding of the complex way in which the chemical factors reviewed in this paper, together with purely physical factors (such as solubility and partition properties), combine to determine the overall biological behaviour of these nitroimidazoles remains far from complete.   For example, O-demethylation was found[96] to be a major metabolic pathway for misonidazole (IV) and enzymatic hydroxylation of the N-1 side-chain is probably involved.   At present there is no definitive chemical reaction that could be regarded as a valid synthetic equivalent to α-hydroxylation or similar enzymatic reactions that may be implicated in the oxidative metabolism of nitroimidazoles. Consequently there is only a limited chemical basis available at present on which to anticipate the likely metabolism of other nitroimidazoles.

Nonetheless, it is hoped that any increase in the knowledge of the chemistry of nitroimidazoles[108] will provide for a better understanding of the use of these drugs in therapy and assist the development of new radiosensitizers having improved therapeutic properties.

REFERENCES

1.   K. Maeda, T. Osato and H. Umezawa, A new antibiotic, azomycin, J. Antibiotics (Tokyo), 6A:182 (1953).
2.   S. Nakamura, Structure of azomycin, a new antibiotic, Pharm. Bull. (Tokyo), 3:379 (1955).
3.   H. Horie, Antitrichomonas effect of azomycin, J. Antibiotics (Tokyo), 9A:168 (1956).
4.   C. Cosar, C. Crisan, R. Horclois, R. M. Jacob, J. Robert, S. Tchelitcheff and R. Vaupré, Nitroimidazoles: preparation et activité chimiothérapeutique, Arzneimittel Forsch., 16:23 (1966).
5.   B. Cavalleri, Nitroimidazole chemistry I.   Synthetic methods, in Proc. Conf. on Nitroimidazoles, Cesenatico, Italy, (1980).
6.   J. C. Asquith, J. L. Foster and R. L. Willson, Radiosensitization of hypoxic cells by metronidazole (Flagyl), Brit. J. Radiol., 46:648 (1973).
7.   J. C. Asquith, M. E. Watts, K. B. Patel, C. E. Smithen and G. E. Adams, Electron-affinic sensitization V.   Radiosensitization of hypoxic bacteria and mammalian cells in vitro by some nitroimidazoles and nitropyrazoles, Radiat. Res., 60:108 (1974).

8.   G. E. Adams, I. R. Flockhart, C. E. Smithen, I. J. Stratford,
     P. Wardman and M. E. Watts, Electron-affinic sensitization
     VII.   A correlation between structures, one-electron
     reduction potentials and efficiences of nitroimidazoles as
     hypoxic cell radiosensitizers, Radiat. Res., 67:9 (1976).
9.   P. Wardman, The use of nitroaromatic compounds as hypoxic cell
     radiosensitizers, Curr. Topics Radiat. Res. Quart., 11:347
     (1977).
10. G. E. Adams, E. D. Clarke, I. R. Flockhart, R. S. Jacobs,
     D. S. Sehmi, I. J. Stratford, P. Wardman, M. E. Watts,
     J. Parrick, R. G. Wallace and C. E. Smithen, Structure-
     activity relationships in the development of hypoxic cell
     radiosensitizers I.   Sensitization efficiency, Int. J.
     Radiat. Biol., 35:133 (1979).
11. G. E. Adams, I. Ahmed, E. D. Clarke, P. O'Neill, J. Parrick,
     I. J. Stratford, R. G. Wallace, P. Wardman and M. E. Watts,
     Structure-activity relationships in the development of
     hypoxic cell radiosensitizers III.   Effects of basic
     substituents in nitroimidazole side-chains, Int. J. Radiat.
     Biol., 38:613 (1980).
12. A. Breccia, Nitroimidazole chemistry II.   Chemical properties
     and reaction mechanisms, in Proc. Conf. on Nitroimidazoles,
     Cesenatico, Italy (1980).
13. H. Monney, J. Parrick and R. G. Wallace, Nitroimidazole radio-
     sensitizers: approaches to their chemical synthesis,
     Pharmacol. Therapeutics, in press (1981).
14. G. G. Gallo, C. R. Pasqualucci, P. Radaelli and G. C. Lancini,
     The ionization constants of some imidazoles, J. Org. Chem.,
     29:862 (1964).
15. A. G. Beaman, W. Tautz, T. Gabriel, O. Keller, V. Toome and
     R. Duschinsky, Studies in the nitroimidazole series I.
     Synthesis of azomycin A and related compounds, Antimicrobial
     Agents and Chemotherapy 1965, 469 (1966).
16. R. J. Rousseau, R. K. Robins and L. B. Townsend, The synthesis
     of 2-nitro-1-β-D-ribofuranosylimidazole (azomycin riboside),
     J. Heterocyclic Chem., 4:311 (1967).
17. J. L. Barascut, C. Tamby and J. L. Imbach, Synthetic nucleosides
     V.   Ribofuranosides of some nitroazoles, J. Carbohydr.,
     Nucleosides, Nucleotides, 1:77 (1974).
18. H. Guglielmi, Imidazole nucleosides II.   Nucleosides of 4(5)-
     nitroimidazole-5(4)-carboxamide, Justus Liebigs Ann. Chem.,
     1286 (1973).
19. E. J. Prisbe, J. P. H. Verheyden and J. G. Moffatt, 5-Aza-7-
     deazapurine nucleosides 2.   Synthesis of some 8-(D-ribo-
     furanosyl)imidazo[1,2-a]-1,3,5-triazine derivatives, J. Org.
     Chem., 43:4784 (1978).
20. C. Chavis, F. Grodenic and J. L. Imbach, Nucléosides de synthèse
     XVII.   Obtention de glycosyl-1-nitro-5-imidazoles et
     pyrazoles, Eur. J. Med. Chem., 14:123 (1979).

21. A. G. Beaman, W. Tautz and R. Duschinsky, Studies in the nitro-
     imidazole series III.   2-Nitroimidazoles substituted in the
     1-position, Antimicrobial Agents and Chemotherapy 1967, 520
     (1968).
22. A. G. Beaman and W. Tautz (F Hoffmann-La Roche & Co., Inc.),
     U. S. Patent 3,793,317 (1974).
23. A. G. Beaman (F Hoffmann-La Roche & Co., AG), U. K. Patent
     1,066,409 (1967).
24. C. E. Smithen (Roche Products Ltd.), U. K. Patent 2,003,154
     (1979).
25. C. E. Smithen, unpublished data, Synthesis, chemistry and
     metabolism of misonidazole and closely related 2-nitro-
     imidazoles (Poster), presented at 6th Internat. Symposium
     on Medicinal Chemistry, Brighton, U. K. (1978).
26. G. C. Lancini, E. Lazzari, V. Ariole and P. Bellani, Synthesis
     and relationship between structure and activity of 2-nitro-
     imidazole derivatives, J. Med. Chem., 12:775 (1969).
27. A. Grimison and J. H. Ridd, The mechanisms of methylation of
     4(5)-nitroglyoxaline with methyl sulphate, Chem. Industry,
     983 (1956).
28. A. Grimison, J. H. Ridd and B. V. Smith, The mechanisms of
     N-substitution in glyoxaline derivatives I.   Introduction
     and study of prototropic equilibria involving 4(5)-nitro-
     glyoxaline, J. Chem. Soc., 1352 (1960).   II.   The methy-
     lation of 4(5)-nitroglyoxaline by methyl sulphate, J. Chem.
     Soc., 1357 (1960).
29. J. H. Ridd and B. V. Smith, The mechanisms of N-substitution in
     glyoxaline derivatives III.   Factors determining the
     orientation of N-methylation in substituted glyoxalines and
     benzimidazoles, J. Chem. Soc., 1363 (1960).
30. M. W. Miller, H. L. Howes, R. V. Kasubick and A. R. English,
     Alkylation of 2-methyl-5-nitroimidazoles: Some potent anti-
     protozoal agents, J. Med. Chem., 13:849 (1970).
31. P. N. Giraldi, V. Mariotti, G. Nannini, G. P. Tosolini, E. Dradi,
     W. Logemann, I. de Carneri and G. Monti, Studies on anti-
     protozoans II.   Synthesis and biological activity of some
     N-alkylamino-nitroimidazoles, Arzneimittel-Forsch., 20:52
     (1970).
32. F. Kajfez, V. Sunjic, D. Kolbah, T. Fajdiga and M. Oklobdzija,
     1-Substitution in 2-methyl-4(5)-nitroimidazole I.   Synthesis
     of compounds with potential antitrichomonal activity, J. Med.
     Chem., 11:167 (1968).
33. K. Butler, H. L. Howes, J. E. Lynch and D. K. Pirie, Nitro-
     imidazole derivatives: relationship between structure and
     antitrichomonal activity, J. Med. Chem., 10:891 (1967).
34. M. Hoffer and E. Grunberg, Synthesis and antiprotozoal activity
     of 1-(3-chloro-2-hydroxypropyl)-substituted nitroimidazoles,
     J. Med. Chem., 17:1019 (1974).

35. V. Sunjic, D. Kolbah, F. Kajfez and N. Blazevic, 1-Imidazolyl
    derivatives of 2-hydroxy-3-phenoxypropane, J. Med. Chem.,
    11:1264 (1968).
36. J. Suwinski, E. Salwinska, J. Watras and M. Widel, Synthesis and
    some physico-chemical properties of 1-(2-hydroxy-3-alkoxy-
    propyl)-4-nitroimidazoles (Polish), Acta Pol. Pharm., 35:529
    (1978).
37. J. Suwinski, A. Rajca, J. Watras and M. Widel, Nitroimidazoles
    II.   Synthesis and physico-chemical properties of N-sub-
    stituted 4 and 5-nitroimidazoles (Polish), Acta Pol. Pharm.,
    37:59 (1980).
38. J. Heeres, J. H. Mostmans, B. Maes and L. J. J. Backx,
    Synthesis and antiprotozoal activity of nitroimidazoles:
    carbamates and thiocarbamates, Eur. J. Med. Chem., 11:237
    (1976).
39. K. C. Agrawal, K. B. Bears, R. K. Sehgal, J. N. Brown, P. E. Rist
    and W. D. Rupp, Potential radiosensitizing agents: dinitro-
    imidazoles, J. Med. Chem., 22:583 (1979).
40. E. J. J. Grabowski, T. M. H. Liu, L. Salce and E. F. Schoenewaldt,
    An efficient and selective method for the synthesis of 2-(4-
    fluorophenyl)-1-(2-hydroxyethyl)-5-nitroimidazole
    (Flunidazole), J. Med. Chem., 17:547 (1974).
41. E. Winkelmann, W. Raether, U. Gebert and A. Sinharay, Chemo-
    therapeutically active nitro compounds IV.   5-Nitroimidazoles
    (Part 1), Arzneimittel-Forsch., 27:2251 (1977).
42. C. E. Smithen, E. D. Clarke, J. A. Dale, R. S. Jacobs,
    P. Wardman, M. E. Watts and M. Woodcock, Novel (nitro-1-
    imidazolyl)alkanolamines as potential radiosensitizers with
    improved therapeutic properties, in "Radiation Sensitizers:
    Their Use in the Clinical Management of Cancer", L. W. Brady,
    ed., p. 22, Masson, New York (1980).
43. E. Gattavecchia and D. Tonelli, Thin-layer chromatography of some
    5-nitroimidazoles of pharmaceutical interest, J. Chromatography,
    193:340 (1980).
44. A. G. Beaman, N. Caldwell, R. Duschinsky, N. J. Montclair and
    W. Tautz (F Hoffmann-La Roche & Co., AG), U. K. Patent
    1,138,529 (1969).
45. J. M. Brown and W. W. Lee, Pharmacokinetic considerations in
    radiosensitizer development, in "Radiation Sensitizers: Their
    Use in the Clinical Management of Cancer", L. W. Brady, ed.,
    p. 2, Masson, New York (1980).
46. C. Rufer, H. J. Kessler and E. Schroeder, Chemotherapeutic nitro-
    heterocycles VI.   Substituted 5-aminomethyl-3-(5-nitro-2-
    imidazolylmethylene)amino-2-oxazolidinones, J. Med. Chem.,
    14:94 (1971).
47. G. E. Trout, Synthesis of some histidine analogs and their effect
    on the growth of a histidine-requiring mutant of Leuconostoc
    mesenteroides, J. Med. Chem., 15:1259 (1972).

48. W. Tautz, S. Teitel and A. Brossi, Nitrohistidines and nitro-
    histamines, J. Med. Chem., 16:705 (1973).

49. H. J. Kessler, C. Rufer and K. Schwarz, Chemotherapeutische
    nitroheterocyclen XXI.   Synthese und antimikrobielle
    Eigenschaften der Enantiomeren von Furaltadon und einem
    analogen Nitroimidazolderivat (Moxnidazol), Eur. J. Med.
    Chem., 11:19 (1976).

50. W. Hofheinz, C. E. Smithen, P. Wardman and M. E. Watts,
    unpublished data (1980).

51. H. C. Beyerman, A. W. Buijen van Weelderen, L. Maat and
    A. Noordam, Imidazole chemistry II.   Synthesis and chir-
    optical properties of (-)-(S)-2-chloro-3-(5-imidazolyl)-
    propanol, Rec. Trav. Chim., Pays-Bas, 91:246 (1972).

52. S. S. Berg and B. W. Sharp, Derivatives of 4- and 5-nitro-2-
    methylimidazolylacetaldehyde, Eur. J. Med. Chem., 10:171
    (1975).

53. R. M. J. Ings, G. L. Law and E. W. Parnell, The metabolism of
    metronidazole (1-2'-hydroxyethyl-2-methyl-5-nitroimidazole),
    Biochem. Pharmacol., 15:515 (1966).

54. P. N. Giraldi, G. P. Tosolini, E. Dradi, G. Nannini, R. Longo,
    G. Meinardi, G. Monti and I. de Carneri, Studies on anti-
    protozoans III.   Isolation, identification and quantitative
    determination in humans of the metabolites of a new
    trichomonacidal agent, Biochem. Pharmacol., 20:339 (1971).

55. M. J. Cho and J. J. Biermacher (Upjohn Co.), U. K. Patent
    2,013,683 (1979).

56. A. G. Beaman (F Hoffmann-La Roche & Co. Inc.), U. S. Patent
    3,468,902 (1969).

57. A. G. Beaman (F Hoffmann-La Roche & Co. Inc.), U. S. Patent
    3,865,823 (1975).

58. P. Wardman, E. D. Clarke, R. S. Jacobs, A. Minchinton,
    M. R. L. Stratford, M. E. Watts, M. Woodcock, M. Moazzan,
    J. Parrick, R. G. Wallace and C. E. Smithen, Development of
    hypoxic cell radiosensitizers: the second and third
    generations, in "Radiation Sensitizers: Their Use in the
    Clinical Management of Cancer", L. W. Brady, ed., p. 83,
    Masson, New York (1980).

59. A. W. Lutz and S. DeLorenzo, Novel halogenated imidazoles:
    chloroimidazoles, J. Heterocyclic Chem., 4:399 (1967).

60. P. M. Kochergin, A. M. Tsyganova and V. S. Shlikhunova,
    Imidazoles XLIII.   Synthesis of 4(5)-nitro-5(4)-bromo-
    imidazoles (Russian), Khim. Farm. Zh., 2:22 (1968).

61. I. E. Balaban and F. L. Pyman, Bromo-derivatives of glyoxaline,
    J. Chem. Soc., 947 (1922).

62. P. M. Kochergin, Imidazole series XV.   Reaction products of
    N,N'-dimethyloxamide with pentahalo-phosphorus compounds
    (Russian), Zh. Obshch. Khim., 34:3402 (1964).

63a. P. M. Kochergin, Imidazole series XVIII.   1-Alkyl or 1,2-di-
    alkyl-4-chloroimidazoles (Russian), Khim. Geterotsikl.
    Soedin., 754 (1965).

63b. Imidazole series XIX. Nitrochloroimidazoles (Russian), <u>Khim. Geterotsikl. Soedin.</u>, 761 (1965).

64. J. Suwinski, E. Salwinska, J. Watras and M. Widel, Chloronitro-imidazoles and 4,5-dinitroimidazoles: potential radio-sensitizers (Poster), Proc. Conf. on Nitroimidazoles, Cesenatico, Italy (1980).

65. M. Hoffer, V. Toome and A. Brossi, Nitroimidazoles II. Synthesis and reactions of iodonitroimidazoles. <u>J. Heterocyclic Chem.</u>, 3:454 (1966).

66. D. P. Davis, K. L. Kirk and L. A. Cohen, A new synthesis of 2-nitroimidazoles (Poster), Proc. Conf. on Nitroimidazoles, Cesenatico, Italy (1980).

67. K. L. Kirk, Facile synthesis of 2-substituted imidazoles, <u>J. Org. Chem.</u>, 43:4381 (1978).

68. G. B. Barlin, The relative electron-releasing power of a singly bound and the electron-attracting power of a doubly bound nitrogen atom when present in the same five-membered ring, <u>J. Chem. Soc. (B)</u>, 641 (1967).

69. C. R. Hardy, unpublished data (1980).

70. V. Sunjic, T. Fajdiga, M. Japelj and P. Rems, Nucleophilic substitutions in some derivatives of 4- and 5-nitroimidazoles, <u>J. Heterocyclic Chem.</u>, 6:53 (1969).

71. V. Sunjic, T. Fajdiga and M. Japelj, Reactions of some 1-(carboxyalkyl)nitroimidazole derivatives in polyphosphoric acid, J. Heterocyclic Chem., 7:211 (1970).

72. P. M. Kochergin, A. M. Tsyganova, V. S. Shlikhunova and M. A. Klykov, Imidazoles LVI. Nucleophilic substitution of 4(5)-nitro-5(4)-chloro or bromoimidazoles (Russian), <u>Khim. Geterotsikl. Soedin.</u>, 7:689 (1971).

73. L. F. Miller and R. E. Bambury, 2-Amino-5-nitroimidazoles, <u>J. Med. Chem.</u>, 14:1217 (1971).

74. F. F. Blicke and C. M. Lee, Derivatives of 7-methyl-6-thia-1,6-dihydro and 7-methyl-6-thia-1,2,3,6-tetrahydropurine-6,6-dioxide, <u>J. Org. Chem.</u>, 26:1861 (1961).

75. R. C. Tweit, E. M. Kreider and R. D. Muir, Synthesis of anti-microbial nitroimidazolyl 2-sulfides, sulfoxides and sulfones, <u>J. Med. Chem.</u>, 16:1161 (1973).

76. R. C. Tweit, R. D. Muir and S. Ziecina, Nitroimidazoles with antibacterial activity against <u>Neisseria gonorrhoeae</u>, <u>J. Med. Chem.</u>, 20:1697 (1977).

77. F. L. Pyman and G. M. Timmis, Bromo-derivatives of 4-methyl-glyoxaline, <u>J. Chem. Soc.</u>, 494 (1923).

78. Merck & Co., Inc., Neth. Appl. 6,409,120 (1965).

79. E. C. Taylor and P. K. Loeffler, Studies in purine chemistry IX. A new pyrimidine synthesis from o-aminonitriles, <u>J. Amer. Chem. Soc.</u>, 82:3147 (1960).

80. J. Baddiley, J. G. Buchanan, F. E. Hardy and J. Stewart, Chemical studies in the biosynthesis of purine nucleotides III. The synthesis of 5-amino-1-(β-D-ribofuranosyl)glyoxa-line-4-carboxyamide and 4-amino-1-(β-D-ribofuranosyl)glyoxa-line-5-carboxyamide, <u>J. Chem. Soc.</u>, 2893 (1959).

81. D. W. Henry (Merck & Co., Inc.), U. S. Patent 3,644,392 (1972).

82. L. L. Bennett and H. T. Baker, Synthesis of potential anti-cancer agents IV.   4-Nitro and 4-amino-5-imidazole sulfones, J. Amer. Chem. Soc., 79:2188 (1957).

83. G. Asato and G. Berkelhammer, Nitroheterocyclic antimicrobial agents: 1-methyl-2-nitro-5-imidazolyl derivatives, J. Med. Chem., 15:1087 (1972).

84. D. W. Henry and D. R. Hoff (Merck & Co., Inc.), Belg. Patent 661,262 (1965).

85. H. Hagen and R. D. Kohler (BASF AG.), Ger. Offen 2,827,351 (1980).

86. J. D. Albright and R. G. Shepherd, Reactions of 1,2-dimethyl-5-nitroimidazole: novel methods of conversion of the 2-methyl group to a nitrile, J. Heterocyclic Chem., 10:899 (1973).

87. C. Rufer, K. Schwarz and E. Winterfeldt, Chemotherapeutic nitro-heterocycles XIX.   Synthesis of 5-nitroimidazoles substituted in the 2-position by heterocycles, Justus Liebigs Ann. Chem., 1465 (1975).

88. P. B. Ayscough, A. J. Elliot and G. A. Salmon, In situ radio-lysis electron spin resonance study of the radical-anions of substituted nitroimidazoles and nitroaromatic compounds, J. Chem. Soc., 74:511 (1978).

89. E. Perez-Reyes, B. Kalyanaraman and R. P. Mason, The reductive metabolism of metronidazole and ronidazole by aerobic liver microsomes, Mol. Pharmacol., 17:239 (1980).

90. A. J. Varghese and G. F. Whitmore, Binding of nitroreduction products of misonidazole to nucleic acids and protein, in "Radiation Sensitizers: Their Use in the Clinical Management of Cancer", L. W. Brady, ed., p. 57, Masson, New York (1980).

91. P. D. Josephy, B. Palcic and L. D. Skarsgard, Synthesis and properties of reduced derivatives of misonidazole, in "Radiation Sensitizers: Their Use in the Clinical Management of Cancer", L. W. Brady, ed., p. 61, Masson, New York (1980).

92. R. C. Knight, D. A. Rowley, I. M. Skolimowski and D. I. Edwards, Mechanism of action of nitroimidazole antimicrobial and antitumour radiosensitizing drugs: effects of reduced misonidazole on DNA, Int. J. Radiat. Biol., 36:367 (1979).

93. D. W. Whillans and G. F. Whitmore, The radiation chemical reduction of misonidazole (Abstract), Radiat. Res., 83:467 (1980).

94. E. D. Clarke, P. Wardman and K. H. Goulding, Anaerobic reduction of nitroimidazoles by reduced flavin mononucleotide and by xanthine oxidase, Biochem. Pharmacol., 29:2684 (1980).

95. P. D. Josephy, B. Palcic and L. D. Skarsgard, Reduction of misonidazole and its derivatives by xanthine oxidase, Biochem. Pharmacol., 30:849 (1981).

96. I. R. Flockhart, P. Large, D. Troup, S. L. Malcolm and T. R. Marten, Pharmacokinetics and metabolic studies of the

hypoxic cell radiosensitizer misonidazole, Xenobiotica, 8:97 (1978).

97. J. E. Stambaugh, L. G. Feo and R. W. Manthei, The isolation and identification of the urinary oxidative metabolites of metronidazole in man, J. Pharmacol. Exp. Ther., 161:373 (1968).

98. P. Goldman, R. L. Koch and E. J. T. Chrystal, Anaerobic metabolism of metronidazole and its consequences, in "Radiation Sensitizers: Their Use in the Clinical Management of Cancer", L. W. Brady, ed., p. 225, Masson, New York (1980).

99. G. C. Lancini, N. Maggi and P. Sensi, Synthesis of some derivatives of 2-nitroimidazole with potential antitrichomonal activity, Farmaco, Ed. Sci., 18:390 (1963).

100. R. K. Sehgal and K. C. Agrawal, Hydroxymethylation and cyano-methylation of nitroimidazoles, J. Heterocyclic Chem., 16:871 (1979).

101. C. Oldenhof and J. Cornelisse, Photoreactions of aromatic compounds XXXVI. Nucleophilic photosubstitution reactions of some derivatives of imidazole and pyrazole, Rec. Trav. Chim., Pays-Bas, 97:35 (1978).

102. F. Kajfez, L. Klasinc and V. Sunjic, Application of photo-electron spectroscopy to biologically active molecules and their constituent parts IV. Methylnitroimidazoles, J. Heterocyclic Chem., 16:529 (1979).

103. T. Matsuura and M. Ikari, Photoinduced reactions XXVII. Photosensitized oxygenation of alkylated imidazoles (Japanese), Kogyu Kagaku Zasshi, 72:179 (1969).

104. D. E. Schwartz and W. Hofheinz, Metabolism of nitroimidazoles, in Proc. Conf. on Nitroimidazoles, Cesenatico, Italy (1980).

105. C. Rosenblum, N. R. Trenner, R. P. Buhs, C. B. Hiremath, F. R. Koniuszy and D. E. Wolf, Metabolism of ronidazole (1-methyl-5-nitroimidazol-2-ylmethylcarbamate), J. Agric. Food Chem., 20:360 (1972).

106. G. Weiss, N. R. Felicito, P. D. Duke and T. Williams, The isolation of a major rat fecal metabolite of ipronidazole, Xenobiotica, in press (1981).

107. T. R. Marten, R. J. Ruane, J. A. White and L. Clarke, Pharmaco-kinetics of nitroimidazoles, in Proc. Conf. on Nitroimidazoles, Cesenatico, Italy (1980).

108. Our own studies of the chemistry of nitroimidazoles have been greatly facilitated by the advice and support of numerous colleagues at Roche, at CRC Gray Laboratory, Mount Vernon and at ICR Sutton.

We would also like to gratefully acknowledge the pioneering research efforts of Dr Arnold Brossi and his colleagues at Hoffmann-La Roche, Nutley, New Jersey, USA during the 1960's. Without their fruitful studies of nitroimidazoles the field of hypoxic cell radiosensitizers may not have reached its present exciting state of development.

We are indebted to Miss Penny Gray for her skill and patience in typing this manuscript.

DISCUSSION (on paper by Smithen and Hardy)

DR SRIDHAR: The perspective with which you have viewed nitro-
imidazole-glycosides is very interesting.   Do you have any other
information on the synthesis or biological activity of compounds
containing both nitroaromatic and glucose-analog moieties?
Dr K C Agrawal at Tulane University has recently reported compounds
of this type [M Sakaguchi, M W Webb and K C Agrawal, Potential
radiosensitizing agents IV.   2-Nitroimidazole nucleosides, Abstract
MEDI-54, 179th Meeting Amer. Chem. Soc., 1980].

At Oklahoma City we are investigating nitrobenzene-type
derivatives of 2-deoxy-D-glucose as agents for hypoxic cell killing
as well as for hypoxic cell radiosensitizion.   A compound having an
electron-affinic nitroaromatic system linked to a glucose antimetabolite will have the ability to act against hypoxic tumour cells
by two different mechanisms and may offer some significant advantage.

DR SMITHEN: On the synthetic aspects there is very little to
add.   About a year ago Harmon described some 2- and 4-nitroimidazole
derivatives of 2'-deoxyribonucleosides, obtained by reacting nitroimidazole metal salts with 5'-halogeno of 5'-tosyloxy-2'-deoxyribo-
nucleosides [R E Harmon, J L Hansen and M Gortiz, Synthesis of some
radiosensitizing agents, Abstract CARB-51, 178th Meeting Amer. Chem.
Soc., 1979]:

E.g.

I have no further information on the chemical or radiosensitizing properties of these compounds and the only other nitroimidazole glycoside that has been studied as a hypoxic cell radiosensitizer, to my knowledge, is the azomycin-riboside of Townsend[16]
which was investigated by Dr J D Chapman at Edmonton, Canada [data
subsequently presented at this Conference].

Kimler and coworkers at Kansas City have reported modest radiosensitizing activity in vitro for 5-nitrouridine but the cytotoxicity
aspect of this and related nucleosides especially towards hypoxic

cells, is apparently unknown [B F Kimler, T McDonald, C C Cheng, E G Podrebarac and C M Mansfield, Development and testing of new hypoxic cell radiosensitizers, _Radiology_, 133:515 (1979)]

In view of the recently reported inhibitory action of 5-nitro-uridine-monophosphate on thymidylate synthetase [Y Wataya, A Matsuda and D V Santi, Interaction of thymidylate synthetase with 5-nitro-2'-deoxyuridylate, _J. Biol. Chem._, 255:5538 (1980)], it seems likely that these and closely related nitroaromatic nucleosides may possess rather general cytotoxicity. Your own current studies should prove informative.

MOLECULAR STRUCTURE AND BIOLOGICAL ACTIVITY OF HYPOXIC CELL

RADIOSENSITIZERS AND HYPOXIC-SPECIFIC CYTOTOXINS

Peter Wardman

Cancer Research Campaign Gray Laboratory
Mount Vernon Hospital
Northwood, Middlesex HA6 2RN, England

INTRODUCTION

It has been suggested (1) that if we were to seek an anticancer drug by randomly testing compounds, some 400 million compounds might need to be examined before a successful drug were found.   This paper outlines briefly some of the methods which should prove useful in optimising the chemical properties of a series of compounds in which some activity has been demonstrated, thus reducing the burden to perhaps one-millionth of that which would otherwise be necessary. We shall also comment on the problem of identifying potential 'new-lead' compounds, where the basis for potential activity is not well understood, as distinct from optimising the properties of an already active series.

The concepts and techniques introduced in this paper have already been used successfully in other branches of medicinal chemistry and we shall therefore concentrate on illustration of the application of these ideas to the problem of the development of com- pounds which are of potential therapeutic value specifically against hypoxic cells, either as an adjunct to radiotherapy or in combination chemotherapy.   The potential application of quantitative structure- activity relationships (QSARs) to this area has already been intro- duced (2,3) and some applications to in vitro studies of radio- sensitization and cytotoxicity have been published (4-8).   Some earlier papers, whilst not treating the data in the way now generally used in QSARs, were of great importance in demonstrating the importance of redox properties in radiosensitization (9-11).

The nature of the problem might well be illustrated in Fig. 1. Here we plot data for 25 observations of a dependent variable Y on

49

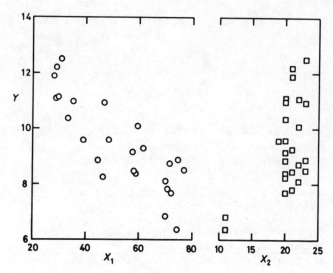

Fig. 1.   The influence of individual variables in multivariate
           analysis. Data from Draper and Smith (12) (see text).

two independent variables X_1 and X_2.   One does not need to resort
to statistics to conclude that   Y is correlated with X_1;   however,
the variable X_2 appears at first sight to have little   influence
on Y.   In fact, using multiple linear regression, some 85 percent
of the variation in Y about the mean $\bar{Y}$ can be accounted for by the
regression equation (1)(12) :

$$Y = 9.1266 - 0.0724 \, X_1 + 0.2029 \, X_2 \tag{1}$$

whilst ignoring X_2 explains only about 71 percent of the variation.
The data illustrated in Fig. 1 are actually the variables $X_1(Y)$, X_8
$(X1)$ and $X_6(X2)$ from the worked example in Draper and Smith's
excellent text: a good illustration of how a variable which has a
significant influence on response could be overlooked if we were
to make judgements purely by eye.

We give this illustration here because it represents a situation commonly encountered in the present application.   Several
biological properties of nitro-aryl compounds are now well known to
be predominantly influenced by their redox properties, as quantified,
e.g. by their reduction potential.   If we are to optimise their
other properties for potential clinical application, then we will
often need to examine the influence of these other variables in
situations where the response is already dominated by the redox
relationship.

We shall first outline those molecular properties which might usefully be measured if we are to identify, and quantify the individual properties which have a significant influence on biological response.   The mathematical techniques useful for analysing multivariate data will then be illustrated from the current Gray Laboratory data files.   It should be assumed from the outset that we shall have to test many compounds expecting that their performance in the biological test system could well be inferior to that of contemporary lead compounds.   Only by exploring the widest possible data space can we expect to progress rationally in this field: we hope this paper will help in the design of experiments and help minimise duplication and wastage, not least in the use of experimental animals.

CHEMICAL PROPERTIES LIKELY TO INFLUENCE BIOLOGICAL RESPONSE

The benefit of hindsight and experience, both of observations of the activity of hypoxic cell radiosensitizers (4-11) and of many QSARs in the biochemical (13), medicinal chemistry (14) and cancer chemotherapy (15) fields help us to identify the following chemical properties which are likely to influence the biological properties of potentially useful radiosensitizers.   It appears that a similar approach would be useful in the application of nitroaryl compounds as chemotherapeutic agents specific against hypoxic cells, since redox properties again dominate the cytotoxic properties of the compounds (5,8).   Since we have already reviewed (16) or outlined (2,3) for a multidisciplinary readership some of the chemical properties of nitroaryl compounds of special interest in the field of hypoxic cell sensitizers, the present survey will cover mainly those aspects necessary to understand the material described later in this paper, or will simply update previously-established (2,4,5) relationships to include all relevant data presently available from the Gray Laboratory group.   The first 3 properties to be considered involve direct measurements of equilibria and therefore offer particular advantage in theoretical treatments.

<u>Reduction Potentials</u>

Reduction potentials, expressed in volts, give us a quantitative measure of the relative electron affinities of molecules.   Since free-radical one-electron transfer reactions may well be important in radiosensitization, it is especially useful that one-electron reduction potentials E may be measured directly using the pulse radiolysis technique (17).   The equilibrium constant K_2 of the one-electron transfer reaction (2) is measured (18-21):

$$S^- + R \rightleftharpoons S + R^- \tag{2}$$

where S is the sensitizer and R is the reference compound of known E.   The difference in potential, ΔE, between unknown and reference

is logarithmically related to K so that ca. 0.06 V difference in E
corresponds to an order of magnitude change in the position of the
equilibrium (2).   For nitroaryl compounds, values of E are generally
between ca. -0.6 and -0.2 V when expressed relative to the hydrogen
electrode, i.e. covering a range of equilibrium constants of reactions such as (2) of ca. 10^7.   Misonidazole has E = -0.389 V and
metronidazole -0.486 V(20,21), the less negative value (i.e.
misonidazole) corresponding to the higher electron affinity.

Molecular modifications of nitroaryl compounds which influence
E have been described elsewhere (2,3,4,20,21,22).   These include
the position of the nitro group in an aromatic ring, the nature of
the ring itself, additional electron-withdrawing or -donating groups,
prototropic and steric properties.   The low activity of some
4-nitropyrazoles compared to 2-nitroimidazoles (23) is now explained
by a recent measurement by E. D. Clarke (unpublished) of E = -0.56 V
at pH 7 for the 4-nitro-1-pyrazolyl analogue of misonidazole, a
compound kindly supplied by Dr J. Parrick.   A recent demonstration
(24) that nitro radical-anions could be generated by flash photolysis
techniques (and hence K_2 measured) was most welcome.

We shall see later that several biological properties have a
dependence on E equivalent to a change in the concentration C needed
to achieve a defined response by about an order of magnitude when E
is changed by 0.1 V.   In principle, replicate pulse radiolysis
measurements of K_2 can achieve a precision of perhaps $\pm$ 2 percent,
corresponding to a precision in ΔE between unknown and reference of
about $\pm$ 0.5 mV.   In practice, there are two major sources of
potential systematic error in the measurement of E by pulse radiolysis, which could give errors in E of perhaps 0.02 V, corresponding
to a change in C by about 50-60 percent.   Hence the usual assumption
that deviations of the dependent variable Y, e.g. - log C, from
fitted QSARs arise from variance in Y only may not be entirely valid.
We may have undertainty in the independent variable which is not
negligible in the present application.

Wardman and Clarke (21) measured a 25 percent increase in K_2
when the ionic strength was increased from 0.008 to 0.2 (S =
misonidazole, R = 9,10-anthraquinone-2-sulphonate).   Whilst a
correction for the influence of ionic strength on electron-transfer
equilibria such as (2), or on the rates of individual reactions,
can only be made if the charge on the individual reactants are
known.   Whilst this will usually be known for the ground state of
the sensitizer, it is unknown for potential biomolecules or radicals
reacting with S or S⁻.   All values of ΔE published by the Gray
Laboratory refer to zero ionic strength.

An equally important source of uncertainty in E is the use of
different reference compounds, R.   For practical reasons (17,20,21)
a single reference compound cannot be used to measure changes in K_2

covering 7 orders of magnitude.   Both quinones (19,20,21) and
viologens (21) have been found useful as reference compounds, and
although they can be interrelated (21), Clarke and Wardman (unpublished) have found that the use of methyl viologen as a reference,
using E = -0.447 V often gives values of E for nitroaryl compounds
ca. 0.015 V lower than that measured using benzyl viologen or
anthraquinone sulphonate.   A systematic error of ca. 0.015 V for
one group of compounds included in a QSAR spanning ca. 0.4 V is
perhaps not too serious.   However, the indiscriminate analysis of
data for one group nominally of very similar E but in fact including
compounds measured against different redox indicators, possibly also
at different ionic strengths, could give rise to difficulties in
quantifying the influence on the biological response of less
important chemical properties.

In an introductory review (16) we were somewhat biased against
the use of polarographic half-wave potentials as substitutes for E
measured from equation (2), for use in QSARs with nitroaryl compounds.   Although a correlation between published polarographic
measurements and E was noted (16), more recent work by Breccia et al.
(25) and unpublished data of Dr C. J. Little demonstrate rather a
good correlation between E and polarographic potentials.   Several
successful QSARs (26-28) using polarographic potentials have been
reported.   Thermodynamic E values from K_2 measurements are preferable for some theoretical uses.

Partition Coefficient (Hydrophobicity)

Reduction potential is a measure of the position of an electron-
transfer equilibrium : partition coefficient a measure of a distribution equilibrium in a biphasic system.   Hansch and Leo (29) list
nearly 15,000 partition coefficients in a most useful compilation;
the introductory material for an earlier list (30) of the Pomona
College data bank gives much useful information concerning the
measurement and use of partition coefficients.   Octanol has emerged
as a preferred model for the organic (lipid) phase;   0.1 mol dm^{-3}
phosphate buffer, pH 7.4 for compounds negligibly ionized or protonated at that pH is usually used as the aqueous phase.

Fig. 2 displays the values for the octanol : water partition
coefficient, P, and the one-electron reduction potential at pH 7,
E, for some of the neutral nitroaryl compounds which have been
investigated in the Gray Laboratory.   The concentration $C_{1.6}$
required to achieve a sensitizer enhancement ratio (SER) of 1.6
with hypoxic Chinese hamster cells, line V79-379A in vitro has been
measured for every compound: most of the data have been published
(4,22,31,32).   The majority of the compounds are 2-nitroimidazoles;
many of these are analogues of misonidazole (E,P = -0.389 V, 0.43)
(20,21,31) but with P varying over 3 orders of magnitude.   A 100-
fold range of P has also been investigated for metronidazole

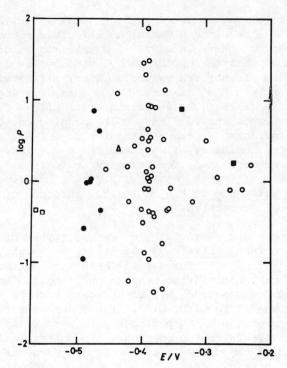

Fig. 2.   Range of values of E and P for some neutral nitroaryl
          compounds studied at the Gray Laboratory.   o = 2-nitro-
          imidazoles;   ● = 5-nitroimidazoles;   ▢ = 4-nitroimidazoles;
          ■ = 5-nitrofurans;   Δ = nitrobenzenes.

analogues (E,P = -0.486, 0.96)(21,31).   Such a diagram suitably
annotated with, e.g., file numbers, is extremely useful in selecting
compounds for further study and as a preliminary exercise in
ensuring E and P are not correlated.   With the experience accrued
by the Gray Laboratory group in the successful use of substituent
constants (see below), many values of E and P for compounds of
potential interest can be calculated prior to synthesis, avoiding
unnecessary duplication.

     For acids HA or bases B we have to define the conditions under
which P is measured, for in aqueous solution the ionic or protonated
conjugate A^- or BH^+ will be present to an extent defined by pH and
pK_a (see below), and the ionic forms will generally be extremely
hydrophilic.   Normally, P refers to undissociated acids or unproton-
ated bases;   a distribution coefficient, D, can be defined:

     D = (1 - α) P   (3)

where α is the degree of ionization or protonation (see below)(33,
34).   D is then pH-dependent.

Ionization and Protonation

  We now turn to prototropic equilibria, involving either acids
HA or bases B :

$$HA \rightleftharpoons H^+ + A^- \tag{4}$$

$$BH^+ \rightleftharpoons H^+ + B \tag{5}$$

with, in both instances, a characteristic pK_a defined as pK_4 or pK_5
as appropriate ($p \equiv -\log_{10}$).   It is easily shown that the fraction
ionized or protonated, α, is given by :

$$\alpha = [A^-]/([A^-] + [HA]) = (1 + 10^{pK-pH})^{-1} \tag{6}$$

$$\alpha = [BH^+]/([BH^+] + [B]) = (1 + 10^{pH-pK})^{-1} \tag{7}$$

Hence at pH 7.4, acids with pK < 6.4 are at least 90 percent dis-
sociated (A^-) and bases with pK > 8.4 are at least 90 percent protonated (BH^+). When a base has pK << 7.4 it is essentially a neutral
compound at pH 7.4; 5-nitroimidazoles such as metronidazole have a
basic centre with pK $\simeq$ 2.5 (the unsubstituted imidazolyl nitrogen)
(35).   In the present paper we neglect this latter type of basic
centre, generally referring only to the pK of basic residues on

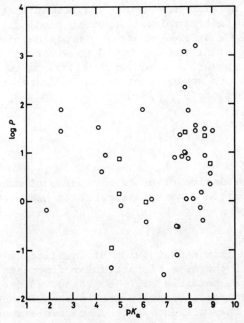

Fig. 3. Range of values of P and pK_a for some 2-nitroimidazoles
         (o) and 5-nitroimidazoles (□) substituted at N-1 with
         alkyl- or alkanol-amine functions.

substituents on the imidazole ring and not to the ring itself.

Fig. 3 illustrates the values of P and pK for some nitroimidazoles carrying a sidechain on N-1 which terminates in a basic
residue, which have all been investigated by the Gray Laboratory
group, i.e. values of $C_{1.6}$ are available in every case.   Most of
the compounds are (2-nitro-1-imidazolyl)-propanolamines (36), i.e.
misonidazole analogues with the terminal $-OCH_3$ replaced by $-NR^1R^2$,
or are the corresponding -ethylamines or -propylamines (6); much
of the data are published (6,36).   We have investigated bases with
pK > 7.4 extending over 3 orders of magnitude in the values of P
(measured as the free bases, at pH > (pK + 2)).   Bases with pK
< 6.4 can be considered essentially neutral at pH 7.4 and are in fact
included in the compounds in Fig. 2.   Not included in Fig. 3, for
this reason, are some hydrazones (37) derived from 1-methyl-2-nitro-
imidazole-5-carboxaldehyde which are very weak bases with pK ca. 2
(6).   There seems little point in studying bases with pK > 9 since
they are already > 97.5 percent protonated at pH 7.4.

Protein-binding of Drugs

Drug-receptor binding is the basis for many models of drug
action in medicine: none-selective drug-protein binding generally
serves simply to reduce the amount of free drug able to diffuse
from the plasma to the tumour and hence to the site of action (33,
38).   Clarke and Wardman have begun a systematic study of the
factors controlling nitroimidazole/protein binding.   Preliminary
results (32) showed that some neutral nitroimidazoles of high
lipophilicity were significantly bound to 4 percent w/v bovine
serum albumin.   Drug/protein equilibrium constants (K_8) have not
yet been measured, but would be expected to be related to P by an
equation of the form of (9): (38,39).

$$D + Pr \rightleftharpoons DPr \tag{8}$$

$$\log K_8 = b_0 + b_1 \log P \tag{9}$$

An interesting correlation of protein binding of some metronidazole
analogues with electron density distribution has been reported (40).

Steric Properties

We now depart from a discussion of equilibrium properties.
Whilst estimates of the size of particular fragments of nitro-aryl
radiosensitizers are possible (29), e.g. the van der Waals radii of
the methoxy and analogous substituents in the sidechain in misonidazole analogues, the influence of such possible steric effects has
not been investigated.   One of the reasons for the lack of emphasis
on steric properties is the frequently high degree of collinearity
between the lipophilicity parameter log P and any steric parameter
(29).   Consider, for example, Fig. 1 of Wardman et al.(2) which

demonstrated the (expected) increase in log P as the size of the
terminating alkoxy group in misonidazole analogues was increased.

Another reason for the difficulty in investigating the influence
of steric parameters on radiosensitization is simply the lack of
suitable parameters. Many of the molecules of interest carry
substituents such as OH, OR, halogen, CF_3, CN which are either not
amenable to measurement of substituent constants (see below) by the
Taft method, or are poorly fit by the Charton radius method (29).
It seems likely, therefore, that an attempt to use conventional
steric substituent constants in the analysis of radiosensitization
data would not be successful. A better approach is to compare the
behaviour of groups of compounds where E, P, etc. are known to cover
a similar range but where, e.g., the NO_2 group is clearly more
accessible to reactants in one group than another. This appeared
successful in demonstrating (5) a difference between 2-nitroimida-
zoles with either a N-methyl substituent or a rather longer N-1
sidechain, often carrying a 2-hydroxy function (as in misonidazole)
which could hydrogen-bond to the NO_2 group.

This latter feature (the importance of a single functional
group in a particular position) can most easily be examined using
the "dummy-variable" technique (12) in multiple regression (see
below), applied unsuccessfully to one case (4) but nevertheless a
powerful tool.

The Use of Substituent Constants : Predictive Relationships for Chemical Properties

Much of the above discussion has assumed that chemical properties such as E, P, pK are measured experimentally. In fact, the
properties of many analogues can be calculated with good reliability
using existing chemical information. The 15,000 partition coefficients in the literature (29) contain only a few (nitrobenzene)
radiosensitizers: but the information can be used to predict the
partition properties of numerous analogues of, e.g., metronidazole
and misonidazole. Possibly the majority of QSARs between biological
response and chemical properties involve the use of substituent
constants (29) such as Hammett sigma or Hansch pi valies.

The basis for the definition of a substituent constant S_X for
a group X is the measurement of an equilibrium constant for a suitable reaction or other equilibtium in a model system. If we define
as K_O the equilibrium constant of a parent molecule, ArH (substituent H in parent fragment Ar), and K_X the constant for an
analogue with H replaced by a substituent X, then :

$$S_X = \log(K_X/K_O) = \log K_X - \log K_O \qquad (10)$$

Thus electronic substituent constants (Hammett sigma, σ)(41) are
defined by :

$$\sigma_X = pK_O - pK_X \tag{11}$$

where pK refers to the pK_a, e.g. for the ionization of substituted benzoic acids. The higher the Hammett σ, the more electron-withdrawing the substituent. The lipophilicity constants (Hansch pi, π) (42) are defined by :

$$\pi_X = \log P_{ArX} - \log P_{ArH} \tag{12}$$

where Ar = phenyl, for example. Thus π_X is a measure of the alteration in lipophilicity caused by the substituent X.

If all the compounds were of a single general type, we could use, e.g. σ or π as an independent variable in place of E or log P, respectively, as independent variables in QSARs. More use-fully in the present application, we can use σ or π to estimate values of E or P for other analogues in a series once "baseline" values for 2 or 3 analogues are measured directly. Of course, the precision or reliability of such estimates is of great importance and we consider this in the examples below.

We presented previously (16,21) some experimental data for the increase in E resulting from the substitution of electron-withdrawing groups in the 5-position of 1-methyl-2-nitroimidazole. Together with more recent unpublished measurements of Clarke and Wardman, these establish the relationship :

$$E/V = (-0.406 \pm 0.005) + (0.146 \pm 0.008) \sigma_p^- \tag{13}$$

where the uncertainties are standard errors and σ^- is that appropriate for an electron-rich transition state (29,41). A similar approach using data (20,43-5) for 6 4-nitrobenzenes yields:

$$E/V = (-0.484 \pm 0.011) + (0.168 \pm 0.014) \sigma_p^- \tag{14}$$

Thus for these two classes of compounds, E can be predicted with a standard error for the value of E of an individual compound of about 0.013 and 0.020 V respectively. The similarity in slope in equations (13) and (14), i.e. between the heteroaryl system and the benzene system, is noteworthy.

Wardman et al. (2) first applied π substituent constants to the problem of predicting P for nitroimidazole radiosensitizers. Fig. 4 illustrates more complete data for the alterations in lipo-philicity (log P) caused by the variation of the substituent R in analogues of misonidazole (n = 1) or the 2-(2-nitro-1-imidazolyl)-ethyl analogues (n = 0). Values of π_R were obtained (29) from the benzenoid system, but apply equally well at the end of a 2- or 3-carbon chain in these examples. Values of log P, for π within the limits shown, can be predicted with standard errors for an

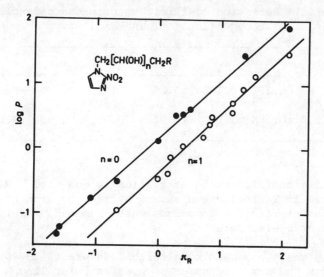

Fig. 4.   Relationship between measured P (octanol:water) and
          the Hansch π substituent constant.

individual observation of about 0.09 for these two classes of
compounds.   In both series, the literature values (29) of π for
N-piperidino and N-morpholino substituents underestimated log P by
about 0.5, and may be in error.

The form of the relationships in Fig. 4 is :

$$\log P = b_0 + b_1 \pi_R \tag{15}$$

and in Table 1 we list estimated values of b_0 and b_1 for the eight
nitroimidazoles shown in Fig. 5, obtained from similar relationships (43).   Compounds in group (c) are of the form R = CH_2R'
(except for R = H) and compounds in group (f) are the hydrazones
(6,37) previously referred to, i.e. R = NR'R".   Group (h) includes
the compounds directly ring-substituted with powerful electron-
withdrawing groups included in equation (13).   In this instance
there is clear evidence of an electronic effect on P, indicated by
the marked decrease in b_1 from 0.8-0.9 for the other examples to
ca. 0.5, and by a doubling of the standard error of the estimate.
Attempts to include this electronic effect in an equation (42) :

$$\log P = b_0 + b_1 \pi_R + b_2 \sigma_R \tag{16}$$

Table 1.   Partition coefficients of nitroimidazoles
(see equation (15) and Fig. 5).

Formula	(a)	(b)	(c)	(d)	(e)	(f)	(g)	(h)
b_0	-0.367	0.164	0.191	0.06	0.59	0.779	-0.4	0.336
b_1		0.914	0.884	0.860	(0.91)	(0.88)	0.792	(0.91)	0.487

did not yield a coefficient b_2 statistically non-zero. Values of b_1 in parentheses in Table 1 are assumed, by analogy with the other series, since insufficient compounds were examined.   Full details will be presented elsewhere.

Recently there has been considerable interest (29,46) in predicting log P from the sum of fragmental constants for lipophilicity, rather like assembling a jigsaw from scratch rather than adding the last piece.   Using Hansch and Leo's (29) FRAGMENT method, values and nomenclature, values of log P for 9 of the misonidazole analogues illustrated in Fig. 4 (cf. Fig. 1 of Wardman et al. (2)), we derive:

$$\log P = (0.09 \pm 0.05) + (1.08 \pm 0.08) \; (f_R + F_{P2}) \qquad (17)$$

where f_R is the fragmental constant similar to π, and F_{P2} is a proximity correction for the effect on lipophilicity of the presence of two hydrogen-bonding polar groups separated by 2 carbon atoms. In virtually all the derivatives this interaction between the 2-hydroxy group and the substituent R must be taken into account, causing especial problems with highly polar groups.   Whilst apart from the latter groups, equation (17) provides a reasonable fit to the data, the simpler equation (15) is superior.

Of the 134 values of P of nitroaryl radiosensitizers currently in the Gray Laboratory data files, 23 have been estimated by comparison with close analogues using equations such as (15) and/or the π values or fragment constants (29).   Obviously, having now clearly demonstrated the usefulness of these predictive relationships in the types of molecules of interest, we shall make increasing use of them. Some of the values of E, P and pK for compounds featured in Figs 2 and 3 were therefore estimated using the substituent constant concept, but only where it was considered that the risk of serious error was very low.

Interrelation Between Chemical Properties

An electronic effect on pK is implicit in the Hammett σ definition (11), which can be applied equally well to the effect of

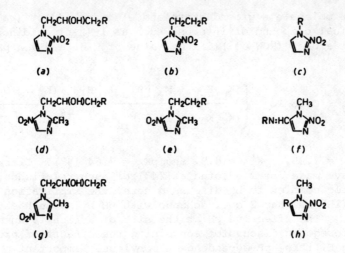

Fig. 5.   Structure of the nitroimidazoles with partition
properties estimated by equation (15), see Table 1.

electron-withdrawing groups (such as a 2-nitro-l-imidazolyl group)
on the ionization constants pK_5 of bases B.   The base strengths of
the amine groups in the (2-nitro-l-imidazolyl)-alkylamines or
-alkanolamines which have been studied as radiosensitizers (6,36)
are considerably lower than those of the free bases.   If the
2-nitro-l-imidazolyl group is separated from the basic group NR^1R^2
by a C_2 chain, shifts in pK compared to that for HNR^1R^2 of between
3.5 and 1.0 are observed, depending on the nature of the base;   a C_3
chain decreases the shift to between 2.4 and 0.9 in those studied
(6,36)..   These trends are quite systematic and enable the pK of
other analogues to be estimated if the pK of the free base HNR^1R^2 is
known.   Such estimates have now been made for 21 nitro-l-imidazolyl
amines studied at the Gray Laboratory;   most of the experimental
measurements have been published (4,6,36).

There is also a dependence of E on the ground state pK of the
basic group in, e.g., (2-nitro-l-imidazolyl) amines.   If E is
measured at pH 7 (E_7), then E_7 is generally close to -0.35 V if
pK $\simeq$ 8 but decreases steadily to ca. -0.39 V if pK $\simeq$ 5.   Again,
the clear trend permits interpolation and estimation of some values
if the pK is known, although this procedure is not too reliable for
the following reason.   E is a function of both pH and the several

pKs of the molecule's ground state and electron-adduct (radical).
For a typical compound of interest such as 1-(2-piperidinoethyl)-
2-nitroimidazole, (RGW-603)(6) the value of E at a given pH is given
by (47) :

$$E \simeq E_7 + 0.06 \log \left\{ \frac{(K_{r1}K_{r2} + K_{r1}[H^+] + [H^+]^2)(K_o + 10^{-7})}{(K_{r1}K_{r2} + 10^{-7}K_{r1} + 10^{-14})(K_o + [H^+])} \right\} \quad (18)$$

where pK_{r1} = 4.95, pK_{r2} = 8.9, and pK_o = 7.64 (43). Clarke and
Wardman have made detailed studies (43) of such relationships and
although too complex to be discussed here, the implication of
equation (18) is that E could change with pH by as much as 0.06
V/pH unit.   The effective pH at the site of action is unknown, but
from the foregoing discussion concerning the effects of errors in
estimaging E, this pH-dependence is obviously important.

The effects upon E of ionization of acidic functions substituted
on nitroimidazole rings or sidechains can be quite dramatic. A
good example was presented by Wardman et al. (22) : replacement of
the imidazolyl-methyl group in 8-nitrocaffeine by a proton (giving
8-nitro theophylline, ground state pK for ionization of acidic
imidazolyl proton = 2.3) decreased E_7 by ca. 0.3 V, with a consequent
dramatic effect on biological properties. A pH-dependent E for
azomycin was reported earlier (21).

MEASUREMENT OF THE DEPENDENT VARIABLE: THE BIOLOGICAL RESPONSE

We note here two important points. Firstly, there are sound
theoretical reasons why it is preferable to define a standard
response and then measure the concentration C required to achieve
this response, if the data from QSARs for radiosensitizers are to be
useful in modelling possible reactions (13-15,29,34,48).   Studies
(10,49) which measure the extent of response at a fixed concentration of sensitizer are obviously valuable in establishing relationships but the results are more difficult to use in theoretical
models for radiosensitization (16,48,50).

Secondly, the nature of the response/concentration curve is
important in estimating the deviations from predictions which might
arise from experimental uncertainty.   Data from an earlier analysis
(34 compounds)(4) show that for radiosensitization in the in vitro
test system most commonly used, compounds with E similar to misonidazole or metronidazole generally require ca. 3 times higher concentrations to increase the SER from 1.4 to 1.6.   Thus an uncertainty in ± 0.1 in a measurement of SER around this level might
result in an uncertainty in log C of around ± 0.25, values which
might be borne in mind when considering the data summarized
below.

Model: $Y = B_0 + B_1 X_1 + B_2 X_2 + ... B_m X_m + \varepsilon$ $Y = X\beta + \varepsilon$

Solution: $\hat{Y} = b_0 + b_1 X_1 + b_2 X_2 + ... b_m X_m$ $Y = Xb$

$$\begin{bmatrix} n & \Sigma X_1 & \Sigma X_2 & .... & \Sigma X_m \\ \Sigma X_1 & \Sigma X_1^2 & \Sigma X_1 X_2 & ... & \Sigma X_1 X_m \\ \Sigma X_2 & \Sigma X_2 X_1 & \Sigma X_2^2 & ... & \Sigma X_2 X_m \\ \vdots & & & & \\ \Sigma X_m & \Sigma X_m X_1 & \Sigma X_m X_2 & ... & \Sigma X_m^2 \end{bmatrix} = X'X$$

$$\begin{bmatrix} \Sigma Y \\ \Sigma X_1 Y \\ \Sigma X_2 Y \\ \vdots \\ \Sigma X_m Y \end{bmatrix} = X'Y$$

$$\begin{bmatrix} b_0 \\ b_1 \\ b_2 \\ \vdots \\ b_m \end{bmatrix} = b \qquad \begin{bmatrix} 1 & X_1 & X_2 & ... & X_m \end{bmatrix} = X'_k$$

$\Sigma Y^2 = Y'Y$

$$\begin{aligned} b &= (X'X)^{-1}X'Y \\ V(b) &= (X'X)^{-1}\sigma^2 \\ s^2 &= (Y'Y - b'X'Y)/(n-m-1) \\ \hat{Y}_k &= X'_k b \\ V(\hat{Y}_k) &= X'_k(X'X)^{-1}X_k \sigma^2 \end{aligned}$$

Fig. 6.   Matrix formulation of the multiple linear regression problem.

CORRELATING BIOLOGICAL RESPONSE WITH CHEMICAL PROPERTIES

The Technique of Multiple Linear Regression

The available data suitable for analysis by QSAR will probably include the concentration C required to achieve a fixed biological response, together with measurements or reliable estimates of chemical properties such as E, P, pK.   Hansch analysis (13-15) usually involves examining the correlations between these properties using multiple linear regression (12,34,51-54).   Since this technique may be useful in analysing multivariate responses in any branch of experimental science, we outline the principles of the method, aiming especially to stress the simplicity of the basic require- ments for a program suitable for computer calculation.

Stating the problem and expressing the solution in matrix terms is especially valuable since even the smallest computers now often have matrix ROM's which greatly facilitate matrix algebra.   In Fig. 6 we outline both the model and solution in linear and matrix form (12).   We have a model of n data sets with a dependent variable Y, together with m independent variables X, each with para- meters β, and an amount ε by which Y deviates from the regression line.   The solution uses the least-square procedure to provide

estimates b of β. Writing the transpose of a matrix M as M' and
the inverse as M$^-$, the matrix B giving values of the coefficients
b is obtained by multiplying the inverse of the matrix X'X (the
sums and cross-products of the X-variables) by the matrix X'Y (the
sums and cross-products of Y and X). With a simple BASIC program,
these two matrices can be generated by looping statements occupying
only two lines, and the matrix inversion and multiplication completed in a third line using the matrix algebra ROM.   Hence most
of the information necessary for quite sophisticated regression
analyses can be obtained in only 3 or 4 lines of program.   The
estimated standard errors (the square root of the variance V) on
the coefficients b or on predicted values of Y, $\hat{Y}$ for given values
of X are then readily obtained by substituting s for   . Other
useful statistics such as the square of the multiple correlation
coefficient, R^2 can be obtained equally simply (12).

It is hoped the above outline will encourage others to use this
powerful technique.   A common problem is roundoff errors (12), which
can be minimized by 'centering' the data, i.e. by regressing not
Y upon X but $(Y-\bar{Y})$ upon $(X-\bar{X})$.   Slight modifications to the calcula-
tions are then involved (12,54).   The use of the correlation
coefficient R in simple linear regression as a measure of "goodness
of fit" has been criticised (55) and a common method of assessing
the usefulness of adding a variable X to the equation is the use of
a sequential F test.   Also useful is a 2-sided t-test, examining
the estimated standard error on the coefficient b to test whether
the latter is significantly non-zero.   Such methods are discussed
extensively in the texts listed earlier.

An Illustration of Multiple Regression Analysis

The following example is not particularly suitable since one
variable dominates the response, but it serves to illustrate the
principles.   We use the Gray Laboratory data file, accumulated
over a 5-year period, and largely published (4-6, 22,32,36).   In
part it is an extension of earlier analyses (2,4-6) but then intro-
duces some concepts previously unexplored in this application.

If we consider the radiosensitization efficiencies, $C_{1.6}$,
measured in the Chinese hamster in vitro system, of 59 neutral
nitroaryl compounds (including those with basic substituents with
pK < 6.4) we obtain the following equations on adding the variables
log P and $(\log P)^2$ successively to E :

$$-\log C_{1.6} \;=\; b_0 \;+\; b_1\, E \tag{19}$$

$$-\log C_{1.6} \;=\; b_0 \;+\; b_1\, E \;+\; b_2 (\log P) \tag{20}$$

$$-\log C_{1.6} \;=\; b_0 \;+\; b_1\, E \;+\; b_2 (\log P) \;+\; b_3 (\log P)^2 \tag{21}$$

(The latter equation corresponds to the form :

$$-\log C = b_0 + b_1\sigma + b_2\pi + b_3\pi^2 \tag{22}$$

often successful in earlier QSARs (13-15).   Values of b_0= 6.94 $\pm$ 0.28
and b_1 = 9.56 $\pm$ 0.71 V^{-1} if C is in mol dm^{-3} were obtained from
equation (19), and rather similar values for (20) and (21).   For
equation (21) we found b_2= 0.20 $\pm$ 0.06 and b_3= -0.14 $\pm$ 0.06, i.e. a
quadratic dependence on log P with coefficients non-zero at the 0.05
probability level.   The values of R^2 increase from 0.759 for (19)
to 0.799 for (21) and s decreases from 0.348 to 0.323.

In an earlier analysis (4) (n = 38, partition coefficient P
> 0.05) we could not demonstrate a statistically-significant effect
of P on radiosensitization.   (This is not the same as demonstrating
no effect of P.)   Now, however, it appears that a dependence is
apparent at the 0.05 probability level although still explaining
only a few percent of the variance in log $C_{1.6}$.   The quadratic
dependence predicts an optimum log P = $-b_2/2b_3 \simeq 0.7 \pm 0.4$. However,
such conclusions are probably abuses of the method, as we now see
from a more detailed examination.

Three of the 59 compounds have log P < -1 and 2 of these 3 have
a much lower radiosensitization efficiency than would be predicted
by equation (19).   A similar marked lowering of efficiency with
very low P has been observed in a bacterial strain (56).   Together
with incomplete data for one or two other compounds these results
leave us with no doubt in our minds that values of P in the region
of 0.05 or less often result in a marked decrease in radiosensitization efficiency.   However, if we exclude these 3 compounds, i.e.
n = 56, log P > -1 and repeat the regression we now find

$$-\log C_{1.6} = (6.96 \pm 0.22) + (9.54 \pm 0.56)\ E \tag{23}$$

with R^2 increased to 0.844 and s decreased to 0.272.   Further, no
statistically-significant effect of P can now be demonstrated
even though P covers about 3 orders of magnitude.   Hence, there is
no evidence for an optimal P, i.e. a turndown in the efficiency at
high P.   It is hoped that this example will discourage the mis-
leading use of algebraic forms when the data are best described in
simpler or alternative ways.

There are two immediate explanations why -log C might appear to
be invariant with log P over quite a wide range and then suddenly
decrease as log P is decreased below a critical value in the range
-1 to -2.   Firstly, the data could conceivably fall on the rising
edge of a parabolic response, but the effective C at high log P is
reduced because of removal of free drug from the medium (which contains serum protein) by drug-protein binding, expected to increase
linearly with log P (32,38,39,43).   Alternatively, a very simple

model for drug partitioning yields an algebraic form possibly more
applicable to the present data.   Consider the drug to be partitioned
between an aqueous phase, volume V_{aq} and an organic phase, volume
V_{org}, with actual partition coefficient P' (i.e., not the octanol:
water coefficient, P).   If the potency is proportional to the
fraction of total drug in the organic phase, then :

$$potency \; \alpha \; (1 + \left[V_{aq}/V_{org}P'\right])^{-1} \tag{24}$$

and using the Collander equation (30) :

$$\log P' \; = \; a \log P + b \tag{25}$$

we derive, after including the redox term E, an equation of the
form :

$$-\log C = b_0 + b_1 E + b_2 (\log P) + b_3 \log (cP^a + 1) \tag{26}$$

with $b_2 = a$, $b_3 = -1$ and $c = 10^b V_{org}/V_{aq}$.   Such an approach was
used by Kubinyi (57) and with minor modifications by Martin et al.
(34).   It also resembles the form of the equation proposed by
Hyde (58).   Preliminary analysis of the data for 59 neutral compounds, using equation (26), gives a slightly superior fit compared
to the alternative (21) but the values of log P are poorly distribu-
ted in the data space for such an analysis.   A more serious
objection is that the fall-off in efficiency occurs at such low log P
values that improbably high values of c, i.e. V_{org}/V_{aq} are required.
However, Kubinyi's time-dependent (non-equilibrium) model (57) may
offer an alternative explanation.

The Examination of Residuals

In Fig. 7 we plot the data for 56 neutral compounds with log P
> -1.   The solid line is the least-squares' fit, equation (23).
If we denote $-\log C_{1.6} = Y$ and the value predicted from (23) as $\hat{Y}_n$,
then the residual is $(Y-\hat{Y}_n)$.   The open circles in Fig. 8 are
these residuals, plotted for convenience against $\hat{Y}_n$.   We earlier
explained that the nature of the response/concentration curve could
easily give residuals of ca. $\pm$ 0.2 unless a number of replicate
measurements were made;   a few compounds were also measured under
conditions which cannot now be repeated (32).   The mean residual is
of course zero (12).

However, the residual plot is especially useful to illustrate
the effects of ionization or protonation, i.e. the behaviour of
acids and bases, not included in Fig. 7.   The closed circles in
Fig. 8 are the values of $(Y-\hat{Y}_n)$ calculated from equation (23), for
bases with pK > 7.4.   We see that 25 of the 27 bases have residuals
> 0.   The squares are the corresponding data for acids, pK < 7.4;
6 of the 7 acids have residuals < 0.   The enhanced sensitization

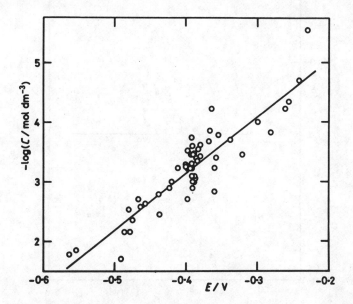

Fig. 7.   Radiosensitization of Chinese hamster cells in vitro
          by neutral nitroaryl compounds.

efficiency of bases (6,36,59) and the decreased efficiency of acids
(23) (after allowing for the effect of E) have been previously
referred to.   Let us now consider a possible explanation.

    In earlier summaries (3,22) we mentioned the physico-chemical
backgrounds to the rationale for the emphasis on the development of
basic molecules by the Gray Laboratory group (6,36).   Apart from
the unusual activity expected (59), it was considered a useful method
of decreasing the tissue exposure to compound (and hence, possibly,
neurotoxicity, cf. Disch et al.(60) and Brown and Workman(61)) by
enhancing renal clearance.   Consider now a more general model, of
which Fig. 10 (33) of the earlier discussion (3) is a specific
example.   If we have two aqueous phases 1 and 2 separated by a lipid
membrane, through which neutral molecules B or HA can pass, but not
charged conjugates BH^+ or A^-, then a pH differential between phases
1 and 2 will induce a concentration gradient C_2/C_1 defined by :

$$C_2/C_1 \;=\; \frac{10^{-pH_2} \;+\; 10^{-pK}}{10^{-pH_1} \;+\; 10^{-pK}} \tag{27}$$

for a base, with $C = [B] + [BH^+]$.   For an acid, $C = [HA] + [A^-]$,
we derive the same function multiplied by the factor $10^{(pH_2 - pH_1)}$.

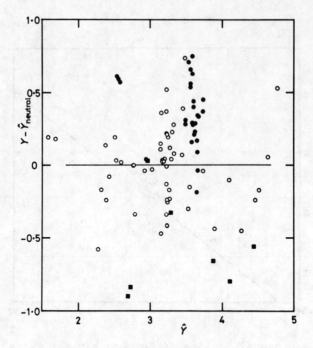

Fig. 8. Residual analysis for data shown in Fig. 7 (o) or
         bases (●) or acids (■) (see text).

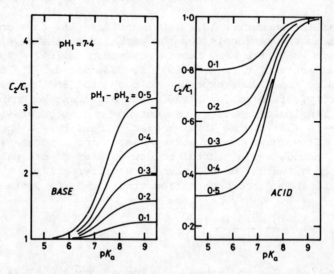

Fig. 9. Concentration gradients induced by a pH differential
         across a membrane permeable to uncharged molecules.

These functions are drawn in Fig. 9 for pH_1 = 7.4 and pH_2 = 6.9 to 7.3.   If we suggest, e.g., that at the site of action the pH is decreased relative to the bulk pH of 7.4, then a pH differential of 0.3 will induce a concentration effect for bases with pK > 8 by about a factor of 2, and a dilution effect by a similar factor for acids with pK < 6.   Whether this explanation is correct, the data appear to be reasonably well explained by such an analysis.   A factor 2 would give a mean residual of ca. $\pm$ 0.3, and if as an illustration we use pH_1 = 7.4, pH_2 = 7.1, we can describe the behaviour of 90 compounds, neutral, acids and bases (P > 0.1) by the equation :

$$-\log \left(C_{1.6} \left[C_2/C_1 \right] \right) = (6.81 \pm 0.20) + (9.15 \pm 0.51) \, E \qquad (28)$$

with R^2 = 0.787 and s = 0.291.   It is interesting to speculate that nitro compounds may act as uncouplers of oxidative phosphorylation and hence themselves induce a pH gradient by stimulating a 'proton pump' (62).   Of firmer foundation is the likelihood that tumour/ plasma ratios greater than unity for basic compounds arise from a decreased pH in the tumour mass (22,63).   Although equation (27) will not describe adequately the dynamic situation in animal experiments, it is sufficient in itself to justify further work in this area.

Cytotoxicity and Lipophilicity

Much of the foregoing discussion of neutral compounds is also applicable to the extended data file of measurements of the chronic aerobic cytotoxicity (5).   An interesting comparison of cytotoxicity and sensitization behaviour for bases can be made.   Defining $\hat{Y}_n$ as before, obtained from 51 neutral compounds   ($|\log P| > 1$) with an equation (5) :

$$-\log C_c = (6.77 \pm 0.34) + (8.69 \pm 0.85) \, E \qquad (29)$$

then regression of residuals $(Y-\hat{Y}_n)$ for 16 bases with pK > 8.2 (any concentration effect having "levelled off", see Fig. 9) yields :

$$(Y-\hat{Y}_n) = (-0.22 \pm 0.07) + (0.29 \pm 0.06) \log P \qquad (30)$$

with R^2 = 0.655, s = 0.225 and F = 26.5 (critical F (1,14,0.99) = 8.86).   For the compounds covered (mean log P = 0.8) the mean value of $(Y-\hat{Y}_n)$ is close to zero, in contrast to radiosensitization, and there is a significant effect of log P.   The difference in protein binding characteristics of neutral and basic compounds of similar high P may be noted (32,43).

Adams et al. (6,64) reported different effects of increasing the alkyl chain length in (2-nitro-1-imidazolyl) alkylamines upon sensitization or cytotoxicity.   These observations can now probably be rationalized in terms of the above discussion, although the

interrelationships between E, pK and log P in these series greatly
complicate the problem.

"THIRD-GENERATION" (22) RADIOSENSITIZERS :   NON-NITRO COMPOUNDS

The problem of identifying alternatives to the nitro group as
electron-affinic (9) radiosensitizers was discussed briefly by
Wardman et al. (22).   We might add two pertinent notes.   Firstly,
the usefulness of the substituent constant approach advocated may
be questioned from a fundamental standpoint.   Wardman et al. (22)
demonstrated a Hammett relationship for the ionization of the N-1
proton (i.e. acidic) in 2-substituted imidazoles :

$$pK = (14.19 \pm 0.32) - (9.48 \pm 0.68) \sigma_m \qquad\qquad (31)$$

and suggested this pK as a guide to relative electron affinity
caused by multiple substitution.   Of course, the N-1 unsubstituted
series would be unsuitable for QSARs because of the several effects
of acidic ionization, and protonation of the imidazolyl N can no
longer be neglected (65).   In spite of the attraction of these
concepts, and the proposed extension to factoring the substituent
constants (22), the definition itself of such constants implies
observation of the effects of the substituent on another reaction
centre.   It is not a fundamental property of the substituent itself,
which would be expected to be the reaction centre in "electron-
affinic" sensitization.

A second problem is that several non-nitrosubstituents may also
be good "leaving groups" upon nucleophilic attack and may sensitize
in part by a different mechanism.   Some possible examples have
been discussed (64,66).   Obviously compounds sensitizing by quite
different mechanisms cannot be included in the same QSAR, whether
by multiple regression or indicator variable (13,14,34,54) techniques.

CONCLUSION

In 1977 we drew attention (2) to the need to measure the effect
of lipophilicity upon the radiosensitization and pharmacological
properties of potential radiosensitization in vivo.   Recent work in
mouse (61) and man (60) illustrates the much greater effects of P
on such properties, compared to the studies in vitro outlined in
this paper.   A diversity of biological responses for radiosensitizers are now being measured in vivo and it is hoped that this
discussion of the techniques useful for multivariate analysis will
help in identifying optimal structures.   Reviewing QSAR in cancer
chemotherapy, Hansch (15) noted that the first QSAR in this field
was established 27 years after the first patient had been treated
with a nitrogen mustard (ironically, also dinitrobenzenes and
therefore radiosensitizers).   A quantitative structure-activity

relationship for nitroaryl radiosensitizers was published (10)
4 years after the first report (67) of the activity of a nitro
compound in vitro and before the first patient was treated with a
nitroimidazole as a potential radiosensitizer.

ACKNOWLEDGEMENTS

This work is supported by the Cancer Research Campaign. I am
grateful to Professor Breccia for the invitation to participate in
this Study Institute.   The work described in this paper would not
have been possible without the expertise and effort of colleagues
in the Gray Laboratory, Brunel University, and Roche Products Ltd
and I am indebted to all my colleagues and to Professor Adams for
their continuing advice, help and encouragement.

REFERENCES

1.   A. Spinks, The changing role of chemistry in product innovation,
     Chem. Ind. (London) 885 (1973).
2.   P. Wardman, E. D. Clarke, I. R. Flockhart, and R. G. Wallace,
     The rationale for the development of improved hypoxic cell
     radiosensitizers, Br. J. Cancer 37:1 (1978).
3.   P. Wardman, The chemical basis for the development of hypoxic
     cell radiosensitizers, in: "Radiosensitizers of Hypoxic
     Cells", A. Breccia, C. Rimondi, and G. E. Adams, eds.,
     Elsevier, Amsterdam (1979).
4.   G. E. Adams, E. D. Clarke, I. R. Flockhart, R. S. Jacobs,
     D. S. Sehmi, I. J. Stratford, P. Wardman, M. E. Watts,
     J. Parrick, R. G. Wallace, and C. E. Smithen, Structure-
     activity relationships in the development of hypoxic cell
     radiosensitizers. I. Sensitization efficiency, Int. J.
     Radiat. Biol. 35:133 (1979).
5.   G. E. Adams, E. D. Clarke, P. Gray, R. S. Jacobs,
     I. J. Stratford, P. Wardman, M. E. Watts, J. Parrick,
     R. G. Wallace, and C. E. Smithen, Structure-activity
     relationships in the development of hypoxic cell radio-
     sensitizers. II. Cytotoxicity and therapeutic ratio, Int.
     J. Radiat. Biol., 35:151 (1979).
6.   G. E. Adams, I. Ahmed, E. D. Clarke, P. O'Neill, J. Parrick,
     I. J. Stratford, R. G. Wallace, P. Wardman, and M. E. Watts,
     Structure-activity relationships in the development of
     hypoxic cell radiosensitizers. III. Effect of basic sub-
     stituents in nitroimidazole sidechains, Int. J. Radiat.
     Biol., in the press (1980).
7.   R. F. Anderson, and K. B. Patel, Effect of lipophilicity of
     nitroimidazoles on radiosensitization of hypoxic bacterial
     cells in vitro, Br. J. Cancer 39:705 (1979).
8.   G. E. Adams, I. J. Stratford, R. G. Wallace, P. Wardman and
     M. E. Watts, The toxicity of nitro compounds towards hypoxic
     mammalian cells in vitro: dependence on reduction potential,
     J. Natl. Cancer Inst. 64:555 (1980).

9.   G. E. Adams, and M. S. Cooke, Electron-affinic sensitization.
     I. A structural basis for chemical radiosensitizers in
     bacteria, Int. J. Radiat. Biol. 15:457 (1969).

10. J. A. Raleigh, J. D. Chapman, J. Borsa, W. Kremers, and
     A. P. Reuvers, Radiosensitization of mammalian cells by
     p-nitroacetophenone. III. Effectiveness of nitrobenzene
     analogues, Int. J. Radiat. Biol. 23:377 (1973).

11. M. Simic, and E. L. Powers, Correlation of the efficiencies of
     some radiation sensitizers and their redox potentials,
     Int. J. Radiat. Biol. 26:87 (1974).

12. N. R. Draper, and H. Smith, "Applied Regression Analysis",
     Wiley, New York (1966).

13. C. Hansch, Recent advances in biochemical QSAR, in: "Correla-
     tion Analysis in Chemistry. Recent Advances", N. B. Chapman
     and J. Shorter eds., Plenum, New York (1978).

14. J. A. Keverling Guisman, ed., "Biological Activity and Chemical
     Structure," Elsevier, Amsterdam (1977).

15. C. Hansch, QSAR in cancer chemotherapy, Il. Farmaco - Ed. Sc.
     34:89 (1979).

16. P. Wardman, The use of nitroarometic compounds as hypoxic cell
     radiosensitizers, Curr. Top. Radiat. Res. Quart. 11:347
     (1977).

17. P. Wardman, Application of pulse radiolysis methods to study
     the reactions and structure of biomolecules, Rep. Prog.
     Phys. 41:259 (1978).

18. S. Arai, and L. M. Dorfman, Rate constants and equilibrium
     constants for electron transfer reactions of aromatic mole-
     cules in solution, Adv. Chem. Ser. 82:378 (1968).

19. K. B. Patel, and R. L. Willson, Semiquinone free radicals and
     oxygen. Pulse radiolysis study of one electron transfer
     equilibria, J.C.S. Faraday I 69:814 (1973).

20. D. Meisel, and P. Neta, One-electron redox potentials of nitro
     compounds and radiosensitizers. Correlation with spin
     densities of their radical anions, J. Amer. Chem. Soc. 97:
     5198 (1975).

21. P. Wardman, and E. D. Clarke, One-electron reduction potentials
     of substituted nitroimidazoles measured by pulse radiolysis,
     J.C.S. Faraday I 72:1377 (1976).

22. P. Wardman, E. D. Clarke, R. S. Jacobs, A. Minchinton,
     M. R. L. Stratford, M. E. Watts, M. Woodcock, M. Moazzam,
     J. Parrick, R. G. Wallace and C. E. Smithen, The development
     of hypoxic cell radiosensitizers: the second and third
     generations, in: "Radiation Sensitizers: Their Use in the
     Clinical Management of Cancer," L. W. Brady ed., Masson,
     New York (1980).

23. J. C. Asquith, M. E. Watts, K. B. Patel, C. E. Smithen, and
     G. E. Adams, Electron-affinic sensitization. V. Radio-
     sensitization of hypoxic bacteria and mammalian cells in
     vitro by some nitroimidazoles and nitropyrazoles, Radiat.
     Res. 60:108 (1974).

24. I. V. Khudyakov, V. B. Kuzhkov, and V. A. Kuz'min, Redox
    potentials of radical anions of nitrofuran derivatives,
    Doklady Phys. Chem. 246:424 (1979) (Engl. transl. of
    Dokl. Acad. Nauk, SSSR, 246:397 (1979)).

25. A. Breccia, G. Berrilli, and S. Roffia, Chemical radiosensi-
    tization of hypoxic cells and redox potentials. Correlation
    of voltammetric results with pulse radiolysis data of nitro
    compounds and radiosensitizers, Int. J. Radiat. Biol. 36:
    89 (1979).

26. P. L. Olive, Inhibition of DNA synthesis by nitroheterocycles.
    I. Correlation with half-wave reduction potential, Br. J.
    Cancer 40:89 (1979).

27. P. L. Olive, Correlation between metabolic reduction rates and
    electron affinity of nitroheterocycles, Cancer Res. 39:
    4512 (1979).

28. P. L. Olive, Mechanisms of the in vitro toxicity of nitrohetero-
    cycles, including Flagyl and metronidazole, in: "Radiation
    Sensitizers: Their Use in the Clinical Management of Cancer",
    L. W. Brady, ed., Masson, New York (1980).

29. C. Hansch, and A. J. Leo, "Substituent Constants for Correlation
    Analysis in Chemistry and Biology," Wiley, New York (1979).

30. A. Leo, C. Hansch, and D. Elkins, Partition coefficients and
    their uses, Chem. Revs. 71:525 (1971).

31. G. E. Adams, I. R. Flockhart, C. E. Smithen, I. J. Stratford,
    P. Wardman, and M. E. Watts, Electron-affinic sensitization.
    VII. A correlation between structures, one-electron reduc-
    tion potentials and efficiencies of nitroimidazoles as
    hypoxic cell radiosensitizers, Radiat. Res. 67:9 (1976).

32. M. E. Watts, R. F. Anderson, R. S. Jacobs, K. B. Patel,
    P. Wardman, M. Woodcock, C. E. Smithen, M. Moazzam,
    J. Parrick, and R. G. Wallace, Evaluation of novel hypoxic
    cell radiosensitizers in vitro: the value of studies in
    single-cell systems, in: "Radiation Sensitizers: Their Use
    in the Clinical Management of Cancer," L. W. Brady, ed.,
    Masson, New York (1980).

33. B. N. La Du, H. G. Mandel, and E. L. Way, "Fundamentals of
    Drug Metabolism and Drug Disposition", Williams and
    Wilkins, Baltimore (1971).

34. Y. C. Martin, "Quantitative Drug Design. A Critical Introduc-
    tion", Dekker, New York (1978).

35. G. G. Gallo, C. R. Pasqualucci, P. Radaeilli, and G. C. Lancini,
    The ionization constants of some imidazoles, J. Org. Chem.
    29:862 (1964).

36. C. E. Smithen, E. D. Clarke, J. A. Dale, R. S. Jacobs, P.
    Wardman, M. E. Watts and M. Woodcock, Novel (nitro-1-
    imidazolyl) alkanolamines as potential radiosensitizers
    with improved therapeutic properties, in: "Radiation
    Sensitizers: Their Use in the Clinical Management of
    Cancer," L. W. Brady, ed., Masson, New York (1980).

37. B. Cavalleri, G. Volpe, and R. Pallanza, 1-Alkyl-2-nitro-imidazol-5-yl derivatives, I. Arzneim.-Forsch.(Drug Res.) 25:148 (1975).

38. J. W. Bridges, and A. G. E. Wilson, Drug-serum protein inter-actions and their biological significance, in: "Progress in Drug Metabolism, vol. 1", J. W. Bridges and L. F. Chausseaud, eds., Wiley, New York (1976).

39. J. M. Vandenbilt, C. Hansch, and C. Church, Binding of apolar molecules by serum albumin, J. Med. Chem. 15:787 (1972).

40. D. R. Sanvordeker, Y. W. Chein, T. K. Lin, and H. J. Lambert, Binding of metronidazole and its derivatives to plasma proteins: an assessment of drug binding phenomenon, J. Pharm. Sci. 64:1797 (1975).

41. L. P. Hammett, "Physical Organic Chemistry. Reaction Rates, Equilibria, and Mechanisms", 2nd edn., McGraw-Hill Kogakusha, Tokyo (1970).

42. T. Fujita, J. Iwasa, and C. Hansch, A new substituent constant, π, derived from partition coefficients, J. Amer. Chem. Soc. 86:5175 (1964).

43. E. D. Clarke, and P. Wardman, unpublished measurements.

44. P. Neta, M. G. Simic, and M. Z. Hoffman, Pulse radiolysis and electron spin resonance studies of nitroarometic radical anions. Optical absorption spectra, kinetics and one-electron redox potentials, J. Phys. Chem. 80:2018 (1976).

45. L. Sjöberg and T. W. Erikson, Nitrobenzenes: a comparison of pulse radiolytically determined one-electron reduction potentials and calculated electron affinities, J.C.S. Faraday I 76:1402 (1980).

46. R. F. Rekker, "The Hydrophobic Fragmental Constant", Elsevier, New York (1977).

47. W. M. Clark, "Oxidation-Reduction Potentials of Organic Systems", Williams and Wilkins, Baltimore (1960).

48. P. Wardman, Oxygen-like radiosensitizing drugs: the importance of free-energy relationships, in: "Proc. Int. Conf. on Oxygen and Oxy-Radicals in Chemistry and Biology," E. L. Powers and M. A. J. Rodgers, eds., Academic Press, New York (1981).

49. J. E. Biaglow, and R. E. Durand, The effects of nitrobenzene derivatives on oxygen utilization and radiation response of an in vitro tumour model, Radiat. Res. 65:529 (1976).

50. R. L. Willson, W. A. Cramp, and R. M. J. Ings, Metronidazole ("Flagyl"): mechanisms of radiosensitization, Int. J. Radiat. Biol. 26:557 (1974).

51. G. W. Snedecor, and W. G. Cochrane, "Statistical Methods", 6th edn., Iowa State Univ. Press, Ames (1967).

52. W. P. Purcell, G. E. Bass, and J. M. Clayton, "Strategy of Drug Design: A Guide to Biological Activity", Wiley, New York (1973).

53. J. E. Overall, and C. J. Klett, "Applied Multivariate Analysis", McGraw-Hill, New York (1972).

54. A. J. Stuper, W. E. Brügger, and P. C. Jurs, "Computer Assisted Studies of Chemical Structure and Biological Function", Wiley, New York (1979).

55. W. H. Davies, Jr., and W. A. Pryor, Measures of Goodness of Fit in Linear Free Energy Relationships, J. Chem. Educ. 53:285 (1976).

56. R. F. Anderson, and K. B. Patel, unpublished data.

57. H. Kubinyi, Lipophilicity and biological activity, Arzneim.-Forsch.(Drug Res.) 29:1067 (1979).

58. R. M. Hyde, Relationships between the biological and physico-chemical properties of series of compounds, J. Med. Chem. 18:231 (1975).

59. G. F. Whitmore, S. Gulyas, and A. J. Varghese, Studies on the radiation-sensitizing action of NDPP, a sensitizer of hypoxic cells, Radiat. Res. 61:325 (1975).

60. S. Dische, J. F. Fowler, M. I. Saunders, M. R. L. Stratford, P. Anderson, A. I. Minchinton, and M. E. Lee, A drug for improved radiosensitization in radiotherapy, Br. J. Cancer 42:in the press (1980).

61. J. M. Brown, and P. Workman, Partition coefficient as a guide to the development of radiosensitizers which are less toxic than misonidazole, Radiat. Res. 82:171 (1980).

62. B. Chance, and M. Montal, Ion-translocation in energy-conserving membrane systems, Curr. Topics Membranes and Transport 2:99 (1971).

63. M. R. L. Stratford, A. I. Minchinton, F. A. Stewart, and V. S. Randhawa, Pharmacokinetic studies on some novel (2-nitro-1-imidazolyl)propanolamine radiosensitizers, in: "Proc. Conf. on Nitroimidazoles, Cesenatico, Italy", in the press (1980).

64. G. E. Adams, I. Ahmed, E. M. Fielden, P. O'Neill, and I. J. Stratford, The development of some nitroimidazoles as hypoxic cell sensitizers, Cancer Clin. Trials 3:37 (1980).

65. M. Charton, Electrical effects of ortho substituents in imidazoles and benzimidazoles, J. Org. Chem. 30:3346 (1965).

66. E. D. Clarke, and P. Wardman, Are ortho-substituted 4-nitro-imidazoles a new generation of radiation-induced arylating agents? Int. J. Radiat. Biol. 37:463 (1980).

67. G. E. Adams, J. C. Asquith, and R. L. Willson, in: "British Empire Cancer Campaign for Research, 47th Annual Report", pp.167, 168 (1969).

PHYSICO-CHEMICAL METHODS FOR INVESTIGATING MECHANISMS OF

RADIOSENSITIZATION

F. Busi and A. Breccia

University of Bologna
Bologna
Italy

INTRODUCTION

We will examine the techniques most commonly used for the study
of the physico-chemical properties of compounds which are important
for application in radiosensitization experiments.

Firstly, we will consider the reactivity of the drug with the
radiation-induced transients and the identification of the stable
products formed during radiolysis. The technique used for the
study of fast reactions induced by radiation is pulse radiolysis
which employs various detection methods: optical spectroscopy, ESR,
NMR, conductivity. The stable products produced in the radiolysis
of solutions are analysed by conventional analytical methods:
chromatography (paper chromatography, thin-layer chromatography,
gas chromatography, high pressure liquid chromatography), spectroscopy and polarography. The same analytical techniques are often
used for the identification of the products of metabolism.

The redox properties of compounds can be investigated by
electrochemical techniques such as polarography, linear sweep voltammetry, potential controlled electrolysis and coulometry. The
redox properties of the transients produced in irradiated systems
are studied by pulse radiolysis using optical spectroscopy or
polarography as detection methods.

INTERACTION OF IONIZING RADIATIONS WITH CHEMICAL AND BIOLOGICAL
SYSTEMS

Radiotherapy involves the interaction of high energy radiation
with matter. Radiolysis of a chemical or biological system is a

complex series of processes which follow the primary act of energy
transfer from the radiation to the molecules of the absorbing system.
The primary processes are ionization and excitation of molecules.
The primary species - excited molecules, molecular ions, ejected
electrons and radicals - undergo fast secondary reactions which
ultimately lead to the formation of the stable end-products of radiolysis.   The process important in radiotherapy is the radiation-
killing of cells.

In mammalian cells the exponential region of a plot of the
logarithm of the surviving fraction of cells against radiation dose
shows a non-exponential region.   The slope of the linear portion of
the plot is a measure of the sensitivity of the system to radiation.

The modification of cellular radiosensitivity due to physical
or chemical changes of the internal or external environment of the
cell, before, during, or after irradiation occurs by changes in the
mechanism of the overall radiolysis of the system.   In particular,
chemical radiosensitization occurs through the interaction of the
sensitizer with free radicals, or other transient species, produced
during the radiolysis of the cell.   Mammalian cells are highly
concentrated aqueous mixtures and water radiolysis is, therefore,
the major process involved in the interaction of ionizing radiation
with cells.   However, the energy which the incident radiation
transfers to the various components of the interacting system depends
upon their relative electron fractions.   Therefore the overall
radiobiological effect probably is due to reactions of the products
of water radiolysis with biological molecules and to direct interaction of radiation with biological target molecules.   The complexity of the internal structure of the cell requires the application of matrix isolation techniques to the study of model systems.
Dilute aqueous solutions are a convenient matrix in which to study
the reactions of intermediates from water radiolysis with biomolecules.   Direct irradiation of biological material in the pure state
gives information concerning, for example, the formation of
biological free radicals and properties such as long range energy
and charge migration in biological molecules.

RADIOLYSIS OF AQUEOUS SOLUTIONS

Methods used for the study of the radiolysis of any system are
steady-state irradiation and pulse radiolysis.   The steady-state
irradiation method gives information about the stable end-products
of radiolysis and their yields, which are necessary in order to
evaluate the radiation chemical mechanism.   In steady-state experiments, the dose rate (i.e. the energy transferred to the system per
unit time) is low and the irradiation time is generally much longer
than the life-time of the unstable primary and secondary species
which initiate and propagate the radiolysis process.   Therefore,
the stationary steady-state concentration of the transients during

the experiment is far too low for direct observation and the role of these species in the radiolysis mechanism must be interpolated from the analysis of the stable end-products.

The radiolysis of water is generally represented by Equation 1.

1) $\quad H_2O \xrightarrow{\quad\quad} H_3O^+, OH^-, e^-_{aq}, OH, H, H_2, H_2O_2$

$\quad G = 3.3, 0.6, 2.7, 2.8, 0.55, 0.45, 0.70.$

where G is the yield of a product expressed as the number of molecules, ions, radicals or atoms produced or destroyed for each 100 eV of energy absorbed by the system. The mechanism of the radiolysis can be represented by the following reactions :

a) $\quad H_3O^+ + e^-_{aq} \longrightarrow H + H_2O$

b) $\quad OH + OH \longrightarrow H_2O_2$

c) $\quad OH + H \longrightarrow H_2O$

d) $\quad H + H \longrightarrow H_2$

Equation 1 shows that during water radiolysis, transients are produced with high reducing properties, i.e., H and e^-_{aq}, and with oxidizing properties, i.e., OH. Suitable solutes present at convenient concentrations can rapidly convert the reducing species to oxidizing species or vice versa. Therefore, it is possible to study the reducing and oxidizing processes separately.

The radiolysis of saturated solutions of nitrous oxide can be represented by Equation 2.

2) $\quad H_2O \xrightarrow{\quad N_2O\ saturated\quad} H_3O^+, OH^-, H, OH, H_2O_2, H_2$

$\quad G = 3.3, 0.6, 0.55, 5.9, 0.70, 0.45$

Equation 2 shows that the presence of N_2O in the irradiated system converts e^-_{aq} into the OH radical.

The radiolysis of aqueous solutions containing formate or isopropanol can be represented by Equation 3.

3) $\quad H_2O \xrightarrow{\quad HCO_2^-\ or\ (CH_3)_2CHOH\quad} H_3O^+, OH^-, CO_2^-\ (or\ (CH_3)_2COH),$
$\quad\quad\quad\quad\quad\quad\quad\quad\quad\quad\quad\quad e^-_{aq}, H_2, H_2O_2$

$\quad G = 3.3, 0.6, 3.3, 2.7, 0.45, 0.70$

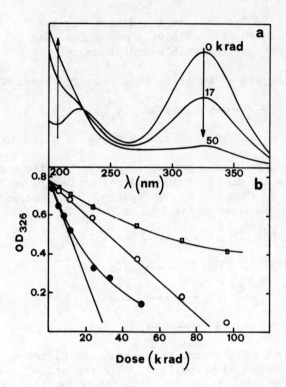

Fig. 1. a) Change of optical absorption in N_2O-saturated irradiated
         solutions of misonidazole irradiated by ^{60}Co γ rays.
         b) Rate of destruction of misonidazole chromophore at
         326 nm with dose in $10^{-4}M$ solution.
         o N_2O-saturated; o N_2-saturated with 0.2 M t.butanol;
            N_2-saturated with 0.2 M 2-propanol (from ref. 1).

The CO_2^- and $(CH_3)_2COH$ radicals can often transfer an electron
to a solute S to yield the radical S^- which is the same as that
produced in the reaction with e_{aq}^-.

The stationary-state γ-radiolysis of solutions containing compounds which are potential radiosensitizers, i.e. nitroimidazole
compounds, has been reported (1,2). The common effect of ionizing
radiation on these systems is the production of permanent changes in
the optical absorption spectra of the solutions irradiated under
different conditions.

The yield of the destruction of the different compounds can be
calculated from the molar extinction coefficients of the solutes.
The changes in optical absorption, at the peak, are not always linear
with the dose for all compounds indicating that permanently absorbing
products are formed. The G-values are calculated from the initial

Table 1.

Compound	G (calculated from ref. 2)
Metronidazole (Flagyl)	2.2 ± 0.2
Misonidazole	2.2 ± 0.2
(5-nitro) CM 54020	1.2 ± 0.1
Desmethylmisonidazole	0.8 ± 0.1
(5-nitro) DA 3838	1.6 ± 0.2
(5-nitro) DA 3829	2.4 ± 0.2

slope of the plots of OD (optical density) vs. dose.

Table 1 reports G-values obtained from irradiated argon-saturated solutions (2) where the radicals present, which can react with the solutes, are OH, e_{aq}^- and H.

In the γ-radiolysis of N_2O-saturated solutions of these compounds, the radicals formed which can react with the solutes are OH and H.   The G-values obtained for the destruction of the compounds are given in Table 2.

In the γ-radiolysis of deaerated solutions in the presence of 0.2 M 2-propanol, where the radicals which can react with the solute are e_{aq}^- and $(CH_3)_2COH$, the G-values obtained for the solute destruction are given in Table 3.

Table 2.

Compound	G	
Metronidazole	2.6[1]	2.8[3]
Misonidazole	2.8[1]	

Table 3.

Compound	G
Metronidazole	1.6[1]
Misonidazole	1.0[1]

Table 4.

Compound	$G\ (NO_2^-)$
Metronidazole	2.2 ± 0.2
Misonidazole	0.8 ± 0.1
CM 54020	1.1 ± 0.2
Desmethylmisonidazole	0.3 ± 0.1

The pulse radiolysis experiments described below show that the $(CH_3)_2COH$ radical rapidly reduces the solutes via a one electron transfer reaction to form the same radical-ion produced in the reaction of the corresponding solute with e_{aq}^-. On the basis of the results reported, it is impossible to deduce a common mechanism for solute destruction. We can only suggest that secondary reactions, which depend on the experimental conditions and on the solutes, play an important role in the γ-radiolysis of nitroimidazoles.

The complete analysis of the radiolysis products of nitroimidazole solutions has not been reported. However, in a recent study the yields of nitrite formed from a number of compounds have been determined. Table 4 reports $G(NO_2^-)$ values obtained from radiolysis of argon-saturated solutions.

Comparison of the results of Tables 1 and 4 shows that the destruction of different compounds follows different mechanisms. Metronidazole destruction yields nitrite with fairly high efficiency; the other compounds undergo radiation-induced destruction via processes which have different probabilities.

In pulse radiolysis experiments, the system to be studied is perturbed by a short and intense pulse of high energy radiation. Its relaxation to equilibrium is followed by observing the variation with time of physico-chemical properties associated with relaxation processes. The radiation pulse must be short compared to the lifetime of the process under investigation and its intensity sufficient to produce concentrations of intermediates high enough to be detected by fast physico-chemical techniques. The radiation pulse is obtained from an electron accelerator. The detection methods most commonly used in pulse radiolysis experiments for investigation of the properties of transient chemical species include optical and electrochemical techniques and electron spin resonance spectroscopy.

Pulse irradiation of deaerated solutions of nitroimidazoles shows changes in the OD in the spectral region 350-500 nm. These changes are due to loss of some of the absorption of the ground state and to the formation of transient absorption spectra. Under

Table 5.

Compound	k
Metronidazole [1]	$5.5 \pm 0.2 \times 10^9$ M^{-1} s^{-1}
Misonidazole [2]	$7.1 \pm 0.2 \times 10^9$ M^{-1} s^{-1}
DA 3838 [3]	$4.0 \pm 0.2 \times 10^9$ M^{-1} s^{-1}
DA 3804 [3]	$3.0 \pm 0.2 \times 10^9$ M^{-1} s^{-1}

these conditions, the transient absorptions are due to the products
of the reactions of the solutes with all the radicals present, i.e.
OH, H and e_{aq}^-. The pulse radiolysis of nitroimidazole solutions
saturated with N_2O, where the radicals present are almost entirely
OH, shows a transient absorption due to the product of the reaction

4)   NI + OH $\longrightarrow$ NIOH

Rate constants for reaction 4 have been calculated from the analysis
of the formation of the transient absorption at different solute
concentrations and the values obtained are reported in Table 5.
The transient spectrum observed in deaerated solutions containing
0.2 M t-butanol is the same as that from deaerated solutions containing 0.2 M 2-propanol and the yields in the different conditions
are in the ratio of the expected G-values, i.e.,

$$G(e_{aq}^-) \Big/ G(e_{aq}^-) + G((CH_3)_2\dot{C}OH).$$

The results indicate that there is no fast oxidation of t-butanol
radicals by the solutes and that the 2-propanol radical reduces the
solutes by one-electron transfer. The rate constants of the reaction

5)   NI + e_{aq}^- $\longrightarrow$ NI^-

calculated from the decay of the absorption of the solvated electron
at 625 nm at different solute concentrations, are reported in Table 6.

Table 6.

Compound	k
Metronidazole [1]	$3.0 \pm 0.3 \times 10^{10}$ M^{-1} s^{-1}
Misonidazole [1]	$3.0 \pm 0.3 \times 10^{10}$ M^{-1} s^{-1}
DA 3838 [3]	$2.6 \pm 0.2 \times 10^{10}$ M^{-1} s^{-1}
DA 3804 [3]	$1.8 \pm 0.2 \times 10^{10}$ M^{-1} s^{-1}

The products of reaction 1 disappear in 0.2 M 2-propanol solutions by a second order reaction.

The electron affinity of the compounds is an important property with respect to their sensitization ability. The electron-affinity of a compound is related to its mono-electron redox-potential. The nitroimidazole radical-anions are unstable and in water undergo fast protonation. Therefore the conventional method for measuring the redox potential of the couple

6) $NI^- \rightleftharpoons NI + e^-$

cannot be used. For these systems, the redox potential has been determined by the measurement of the equilibrium constant

7) $NI^- + Q \rightleftharpoons NI + Q^-$

where Q is a redox reference compound such as quinone and Q^- is its reduced form. If equilibrium (7) is attained much faster than the rate of disappearance of the NI^- radical and one of the reactants or products has an optical absorption, then the equilibrium constant can be measured by pulse radiolysis with the optical detection technique. The fast electro-chemical method, such as cyclic voltammetry has also been used for the determination of the mono-electron redox potential as is described below.

Another method of considerable radiation chemical and biological interest is the study, using polarography of current at a mercury electrode caused by electrochemical reactions involving species produced by the interaction of a pulse of ionizing radiation with the system (3). The electrochemical behaviour of the products of reaction 8 for metronidazole and misonidazole has been studied, in 0.5 M Na_2SO_4, using this technique (4). The metronidazole radical-anion, produced in 0.5 M Na_2SO_4, 0.2 M HCOONa argon-saturated solution, is oxidized at the DME until the potential becomes more negative than -0.45 V vs. SCE. At more negative potential, the observed signal is strongly distorted by the electrode surface. The behaviour of the misonidazole radical-anion is similar but the potential range available for measurement is limited to -0.3 V vs. SCE. The species produced in N_2O-saturated solution is reduced in the same range of potential where the radical-anion is oxidized for both nitroimidazoles. The results indicate that in argon-saturated solution two radicals are present, i.e. the nitroimidazole radical-anion and the imidazolyl radical.

8) $NI + e^- \longrightarrow NI^-$

                                                         (argon)

       $\longrightarrow I + NO_2^-$

9)   NI   +   OH $\longrightarrow$ NIOH

(Nw)

10)   NIOH   +   NI$^-$ $\longrightarrow$ 2 NI   +   OH$^-$

STABLE PRODUCTS AND METABOLITE ANALYSIS

Conventional analytical methods are used to investigate the
stable derivatives of nitroimidazoles produced by irradiation or by
biological processes.   Many analytical techniques are available
for the quantitative evaluation of these compounds and their derivatives such as polarography, UV spectrometry and chromatography.
The first two techniques are fast and sensitive but the resolution,
for example, for misonidazole and its derivatives in biological media,
is not satisfactory.   The resolution can be better achieved by
chromatographic methods of which HPLC and reversed phase HPTLC are
the most suitable for routine analyses.   With both the methods, ten
samples of biological fluids, urine or serum, can be analysed in
about two hours, with a high resolution for separation of dismethyl-
misonidazole, misonidazole and other nitroimidazolyl-derivatives.

STUDY OF REDOX REACTIONS AND IONS LINKAGE IN BIOLOGICAL MEDIA

Three kinds of processes may be considered to be the main
biological processes undergone by nitroimidazoles during hypoxic cell
radiosensitization :

- reduction or oxidation by radiation or by enzyme action;
- reaction with ions or biological molecules;
- diffusion in hypoxic tissues and penetration into cells.

The mechanism of diffusion in tissues and of penetration into cells
is not known and is difficult to study because of the lack of
knowledge of the factors involved.   Lipophilicity, studied by
partition coefficient measurements and determination of the values
of the pKa of the drugs may give information on the efficiency of
penetration into cells and tissues.   In Table 7 values of P for a
few nitroimidazoles are given together with values of the half-lives
in the sera of dogs and humans.

Electrochemical methods seem to be the most suitable for the
study of redox processes for correlation with radiolysis studies.
The main electrochemical techniques useful for radiosensitization
studies are summarized below.

Table 7.

| Compounds | P (pH 7.4) | Half life (hrs) | |
		dog	patients
Ro 05-9963	0.11	2 - 3	5 - 6
Misonidazole	0.43	4 - 5.2	8 - 11
Metronidazole	0.086	5 - 6	8 - 12
DA 3829	0.044	4 - 6	-

- Polarography   - $E_{\frac{1}{2}}$; E' with surface active substances
                           (Tylose)

- Cyclic Voltammetry   - electron reaction reversibility;

                         - $E_{\frac{1}{2}}$ in aprotic systems;

                         - reaction mechanism of catalytic
                           processes;

- Coulometry   - n_{app} (number of electrons per mole of
                           reduced compound)

- Controlled potential   - n_{app} for large quantities;
                         - reduced derivatives production.

Interesting results can be obtained using polarography with surface
active substances or with organic solvents.   Nitro groups are
reduced at different potentials according to the nature of the side
chain or the substituent groups in the imidazole molecule.   The
electrochemical reduction of nitroimidazoles proceeds in the
adsorbed state.   Addition of 0.1 % of a surface active substance,
i.e. tylose, leads to the partial desorption of nitrocompounds.
In Table 8, the $E_{\frac{1}{2}}$ of various nitroimidazoles obtained in the presence of tylose using the polarographic technique, are reported.
Cyclic voltammetry is particularly suitable for the study of the
reversibility of the electron reaction with nitrocompounds mostly
in aprotic solutions (dimethylformamide with tetralkylammonium
salts) and for calculating the first cathodic potential for correlation with the enhancement ratio of the drugs.

In figure 2 are shown examples of a polarographic and cyclic
voltammetric curve for a 5-nitroimidazole in aprotic solution.

Table 8.

Compounds	$E_{\frac{1}{2}}'$	$E_{\frac{1}{2}}''$	$E_{\frac{1}{2}}'''$	$E_{\frac{1}{2}}$ without tylose
Metronidazole (5-nitro)	-700	-1055	-1470	-750
Misonidazole (2-nitro)	-615	-1295		-580
CM 54020 (5-nitro)	-315	- 445	- 515	-727
DA 3838 (5-nitro)	-860	-1155	-1580	-546

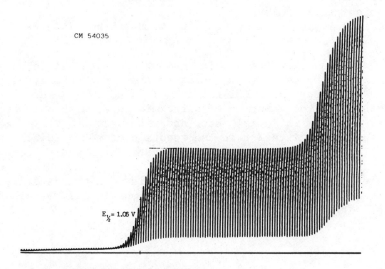

CM 54035

$E_{\frac{1}{2}} = 1.05$ V

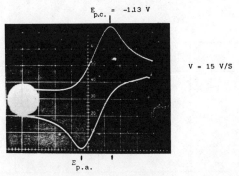

$E_{p.c.} = -1.13$ V

$V = 15$ V/S

$E_{p.a.}'$

Fig. 2. (a) Polarographic curve of a 5-nitroimidazole. (b) Cyclic
voltammetry curve of the compound in dimethylformamide
(aprotic solution).
Structure :

Table 9.

Compounds	$E_{\frac{1}{2}}$		$E_{\frac{1}{2}}$ Fe^{3+}		$E_{\frac{1}{2}}$ Fe^{2+}
Misonidazole	-725	-1470	-445	-1235	-625
Metronidazole	-786		-545	-1275	-575
Ro 05-9963	-665	-1510	-465	-1300	
Ions (alone)			-1315	-1570	-1325

$V_i = -50$; $V_f = -1850$.

Technique of differential polarography.
Pulse height 20 mV.
Concentration of compounds 10^{-4} M in ethanol (95%)/KCl
0.1 M, 1:1

    The compound shows an anodic peak with a 60 mV difference between the two peaks. This indicates the reversibility of the reaction with electrons. Polarography is also a good method for investigation of the reaction of nitroimidazoles with cations such as $Fe^{++}/^{+++}$, Co^{++}, Zn^{++}, Mg^{++} etc. and with drugs. It is known that these cations interact in the reaction of metronidazole with biological molecules such as cystine, cysteine, proteins, etc.

    Table 9 shows the reduction potentials of new derivatives formed from misonidazole with various cations in dilute, ethanolic solutions (6).

Table 10.

Compounds	$E_{\frac{1}{2}}$ Zn^{2+}			$E_{\frac{1}{2}}$ Co^{2+}		$E_{\frac{1}{2}}$ Cu^{2+}		$E_{\frac{1}{2}}$ Mg^{2+}	
Misonidazole	-540	-1450	-475	-630	-1235	-180	-690	-695	-1450
Misonidazole in serum	-615	-1390	-660		-1340				
Ions (alone)		-1005		-1265			-175	no reduction potential	

$V_i = -50$; $V_f = -1850$

Technique of differential polarography.
Pulse height 20 mV
Concentration of compounds 10^{-4} M in ethanol (95%)/KCl 0.1M, 1:1.

In dilute serum solutions, only cobalt and tin ions give new derivatives as is shown in Table 10.   It is possible that this type of reaction could participate in the mechanism of neurotoxicity of hypoxic cell radiosensitizers.

REFERENCES

1.   D. W. Whillans, G. E. Adams, and P. Neta, Electron-affinic sensitization: vi. A pulse radiolysis and ESR comparison of some 2- and 5-nitroimidazoles, Radiat. Res., 62:407 (1975).
2.   A. Breccia, S. Roffia, E. Gattavechia, and A. Borgatti, Studi elettrochimici e di radiolisi γ sulla radiosensibilizzazione delle cellule in stata ipassico, La Chimica e l'Industria, 62:258 (1980).
3.   A. Breccia, and F. Busi, work in progress.
4.   F. Barigelletti, F. Busi, M. Ciano, V. Concialini, O. Tubertini, and G. C. Barker, J. Electroanal. Chem. 97: 127 (1979).
5.   E. Gattavechia, D. Tonelli, and A. Breccia, Determination of metronidazole, misonidazole and its metabolite in serum and urine by reversed phase high-performance thin-layer chromatography, J. Anal. Biochem. (1981) (in press).
6.   A. Breccia, S. Roffia, E. Gattavecchia, A. Grassi, R. Balducci, and G. Stagni, work in progress.
7.   D. Bahnemann, H. Basaga, J. R. Dunlop, A. J. F. Searle, and R. L. Willson, Metronidazole (Flagyl), Misonidazole (Ro 07-0582), Iron, Zinc, and Sulphur Compounds in Cancer Therapy, Br. J. Cancer 37:Suppl.III:16 (1978).

ACKNOWLEDGEMENTS

We are obliged to Drs R. Balducci, G. Stagni, E. Gattavecchia and O. Tubertini for their help in performing the experimental part cited in this paper.

Financial support was provided by CNR through the finalized project "Controllo della crescita neoplastica", research contract N. 80.01486.96.

RADIATION-INDUCED AND METABOLISM-INDUCED REACTIONS OF HYPOXIC SENSITIZERS WITH CELLULAR MOLECULES

J.D. Chapman, J. Ngan-Lee, C.C. Stobbe and B.E. Meeker

Department of Radiation Oncology, Cross Cancer Institute
and Department of Radiology, University of Alberta
Edmonton, Alberta, Canada T6G 1Z2

INTRODUCTION

Several nitroaromatic compounds have been shown to selectively radiosensitize hypoxic mammalian cells and various mechanisms have been proposed to account for this effect (1,2). Most studies show that a component of the sensitizing action of these drugs is mimetic of the sensitizing action of molecular oxygen and a rapid free radical mechanism is indicated. Another component of their radio-sensitizing action is dependent upon metabolism of the drugs by hypoxic cells (3) and can be resolved by studies which vary both temperature and exposure time (4). The molecular processes associated with this "metabolism-dependent" component of radio-sensitization may also be responsible for the hypoxic cell cyto-toxicity produced by the same drugs. Various "radiation-induced" and "metabolism-induced" reactions of hypoxic cell sensitizers with cellular molecules are reviewed. Addition products consisting of sensitizer and cellular macromolecules are generated by both radiation-induced and metabolism-induced reactions and could be responsible for the various biological effects of these drugs.

SOME BIOLOGICAL EFFECTS OF MISONIDAZOLE

Misonidazole [1-(2-hydroxy-3-methoxypropyl)2-nitroimidazole] (MISO) was found to be an effective radiosensitizer of hypoxic cells in vitro (5) and in vivo (6-8). Several clinical trials are in progress to determine if MISO can effect an improved radio-response of some cancers. Consequently, this drug has become the standard sensitizer with which the effect of new sensitizers should be compared. Figure 1 shows the effect of various concentrations of MISO on the radiation sensitivity of hypoxic Chinese hamster V79

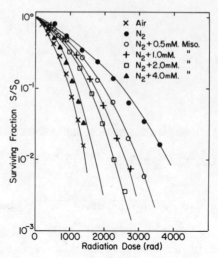

Fig. 1.   The radiation sensitivity of aerobic and hypoxic Chinese
hamster V79 cells and the radiosensitizing effect of
various concentrations of misonidazole.

cells at 37°C.   These concentrations of the drug did not alter
the radiation sensitivity of air-saturated cells treated in like
manner.   This direct radiation sensitization of resistant hypoxic
cells was the initial rationale for drug selection and application
in cancer therapy.   The MISO was in contact with the cells for 60
minutes prior to irradiation.   If these cells are exposed to MISO
in hypoxia at 37°C for longer times prior to irradiation, an
increase in radiosensitizing effect is observed.   The radiation
sensitivity of hypoxic cells exposed to 2mM MISO for 60 and 180
minutes is shown in Figure 2.   This increase in radiosensitizing
effectiveness is dependent upon both time and temperature, suggesting that a metabolism-related mechanism is involved.   A novel
feature of the data in Figure 2 is that the radiation sensitivity
of hypoxic cells exposed to 2mM MISO for 180 minutes is significantly greater than the sensitivity of normal oxygenated cells.   Several
experiments were performed with cells exposed to concentrations of
MISO for various times and at various temperatures.   Sensitizer
enhancement ratios for radiation doses required to reduce cell
survival to 0.10 ($SER_{10\%}$) are plotted in Figure 3 and are seen to
depend upon drug concentration, time, and temperature.   At room
and lower temperatures the time-dependent mechanism of MISO radiosensitization is almost negligible but at 37°C this mechanism
dominates after 120 minutes of incubation.   It should be noted that
the plating efficiency of cells exposed to 2mM MISO (the highest
concentration used in these studies) for 180 minutes was always
greater than 0.80 and was not different from 1.00 for the other drug
treatments.   Consequently, the enhanced radiosensitizing effect
after hypoxic metabolism of the drug cannot be explained as a
toxicity which adds to the radiation effect observed at lower
temperatures.

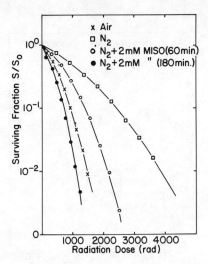

Fig. 2. The effect of 1 and 3 hour incubation of misonidazole with Chinese hamster V79 cells on hypoxic cell radio-sensitivity.

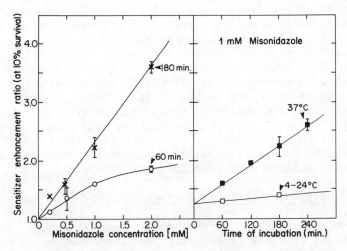

Fig. 3. Left panel – The sensitizer enhancement ratios (at 10% survival) of various concentrations of misonidazole after 1 and 3 hour incubations with Chinese hamster V79 cells at 37°C.

Right panel – The sensitizer enhancement ratios (at 10% survival) of 1 mM misonidazole as a function of time of incubation at 37°C and at room temperature and lower (4-24°C).

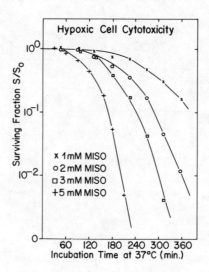

Fig. 4. The toxic effect of various concentrations of misonidazole
         exposed to Chinese hamster V79 cells for various times.

MISO was shown to be selectively cytotoxic to hypoxic Chinese
hamster cells (9,10).   Figure 4 shows the concentration and time
dependency of this effect on the cell line used in these studies.
There is little or no cell killing after a 60 minutes exposure to
5mM MISO or a 240 minute exposure to 1mM MISO.   After a characteristic threshold time, each of the concentrations tested resulted in
significant cell death.   These kinetics of cell inactivation are
indicative of a mechanism which involves some sublethal process
preceding and contributing to the ultimate lethal event.   It is
quite likely that the sublethal events within hypoxic cells that
precede MISO toxicity could be interactive with radiation-induced
cellular lesions and potentiate radiation inactivation.   Several
effects of MISO on specific cellular biochemistry and functions have
been reported and are discussed later.

Radiation-Induced Sensitizer Reactions

The radiobiological target within a mammalian cell most
readily linked with its reproductive death is the nucleoprotein.
Radiation induces numerous lesions in cellular nucleoprotein of
which unrepaired DNA strand-breaks and DNA cross-links might be
most critical for this cell function (11).   Nitroaromatic drugs
mimic molecular oxygen by enhancing the rates of radiation-induced
DNA strand breakage in hypoxic cells (12,13) and by rapidly
oxidizing free radicals generated in DNA by ionizing radiation (14,
15).

RADIATION-INDUCED REACTIONS OF HYPOXIC SENSITIZERS
WITH CELLULAR MOLECULES

DIRECT EFFECT OF RADIATION ON TARGET

$$\text{\Lightning} + NP \longrightarrow NP^{+}\cdot \longrightarrow NP^{\cdot} + H^{+}$$

$$NP^{\cdot} + S \longrightarrow NP\text{-}S^{\cdot} \text{ AND } NP^{+} + S^{\mp}$$

$$NP^{\cdot} + P \longrightarrow NP + P^{\cdot}$$

INDIRECT EFFECT OF RADIATION ON TARGET

$$\text{\Lightning} + H_2O \longrightarrow e^{-}_{aq}, OH^{\cdot}, H^{\cdot}, H_2, H_2O_2$$

$$e^{-}_{aq} + NP \longrightarrow NP^{\mp}$$

$$OH^{\cdot} + NP \longrightarrow NP\text{-}OH^{\cdot} \text{ AND } NP^{\cdot} + H_2O$$

$$H^{\cdot} + NP \longrightarrow NP\text{-}H^{\cdot} \text{ AND } NP^{\cdot} + H_2$$

$$NP^{\cdot} + S \longrightarrow NP\text{-}S^{\cdot} \text{ AND } NP^{+} + S^{\mp}$$

$$NP^{\cdot} + P \longrightarrow NP + P^{\cdot}$$

$$NP^{\overline{\cdot}} + S \longrightarrow NP + S^{\mp}$$

NP = NUCLEOPROTEIN,   S = SENSITIZER,   P = PROTECTOR

Fig. 5. Some radiation chemical processes initiated in mammalian
        cells by ionizing radiation which can result in
        "sensitizer-cellular molecule" adducts.

A process of target radical oxidation by molecular oxygen was
postulated as the potentially lethal chemical event within cells in
competition with a free radical repair process by hydrogen donation
from endogenous sulfhydryls (16-18).   The process of molecular
radical oxidation by nitroaromatic drugs and molecular oxygen com-
petes within cells with a process of molecular radical reduction by
endogenous reducing species (19,20).   Figure 5 shows a sequence of
radiation chemical reactions which likely occurs within cells,
whereby, DNA radicals can be oxidized or reduced by diffusible
chemicals.   A major component of hypoxic cells radiosensitization
by misonidazole could involve its interaction with transient DNA
radicals and consequently the drug must be present at the time of
irradiation.   This radiation-chemical process of direct radiosensitization accounts for most of the misonidazole effect observed
at lower temperatures and/or immediately after the addition of the
drug to cells at 37°C.   It should be noted that most of the
structure-activity studies with nitroaromatic drugs reported to date
have characterized only this "radiation-chemical" mechanism, that is,
experiments were performed at room temperature or lower (21-23).

When hypoxic solutions of macromolecules are irradiated with
^{14}C-misonidazole, a significant number of addition products are
formed.   Figure 6 shows the amount of ^{14}C-misonidazole covalently
bound to calf thymus DNA as a function of radiation dose and sensitizer concentration.   Previous studies with nitrofuran derivatives
had shown that addition products arose from reactions between

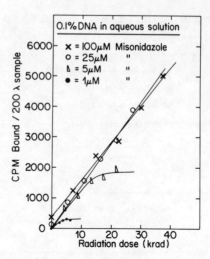

Fig. 6.   The amount of ^{14}C-misonidazole bound to calf thymus DNA
          irradiated in hypoxic solutions as a function of drug
          concentration and radiation dose.

sensitizer and DNA radicals generated by the indirect action of
OH· (14).   The initial rate of misonidazole binding in this
reaction mixture is relatively constant over the range of sensitizer concnetrations studied.   These data support the previous
observation that misonidazole-DNA adducts can be produced by
radiation-induced processes but cannot be extended directly to a
cellular system since an important component of the cellular
target environment, the competing radical reducing species, were
not present in the reaction mixtures.   Several radical reducing
molecules have been found to compete in such radiation-chemical
reactions and lower the yield of addition products (14,15).
Unfortunately an in vitro mixture of DNA, radical oxidizing species,
and radical reducing species which closely mimics the cellular
target environment has not, as yet, been devised.

The detailed chemistry of the radiation-induced sensitizer-DNA
addition products remains to be defined.   Consequently, it is too
early to speculate about the details of how such lesions might
potentiate radiation-induced cell killing.

Metabolism-Induced Effects of Sensitizers

The nitroimidazole drugs in current clinical trials as hypoxic
cell radiosensitizers were originally developed as antibacterial and
antitrichomonal agents.   There is a wealth of literature on the
pharmacology and metabolism of nitroimidazoles, nitrofurans, nitro-
thiazoles, and other electron-affinic nitro-compounds.   This latent

application of an established class of drug has benefited from these previous studies. The radiobiological and cytotoxic effects of nitroimidazoles on mammalian cells requires, in general, higher concentrations of drug and more extreme hypoxia than had previously been investigated. Several metabolism related effects of sensitizers have been described.

Production of lesions in cellular DNA. Olive and McCalla (24) reported that the exposure of several mammalian cell lines to various nitrofuran derivatives resulted in damage to cellular DNA as measured by an alkaline sucrose gradient technique. Additional studies which utilized two different techniques for assaying damage to DNA (25,26) confirmed that DNA damaging effects of several nitro-furans were accelerated several-fold by hypoxia. When the oxygen concentration was varied, a correlation was observed between the rate of reduction of nitrofurazone by mouse L cells, the rate of single-strand break production in cellular DNA, and the rate of cell killing. Tonomura and Sasaki (27) had previously reported un-scheduled DNA repair and induction of chromatid aberrations in cultured human lymphocytes after exposure to several different nitrofurans. The evidence for hypoxic cell metabolism of nitro-furans leading to damage in cellular DNA is quite convincing and has been recently reviewed (28). A correlation has also been observed between cell inactivation and DNA damage in cells (as measured by an alkaline sucrose quadient technique) exposed to misonidazole in hypoxia (29).

Mitochondrial swelling and cytoplasm disruption. Roizin-Towle et al. (30) reported that hypoxic Chinese hamster cells incubated with 5mM MISO for 4 hours showed damage to cellular structures in both cytoplasm and nucleus, the majority of damage occurring in the cytoplasm. Several alterations were observed in the structure of mitochondria, the rough endoplasmic reticulum, and ribosomes and it was suggested that the cellular target for MISO cytotoxicity was cytoplasmic. Mitochondrial alterations have also been observed in Amoeba proteus cells incubated aerobically for several hours in the presence of 10-20 mM MISO (31). These treatments induced no detectable changes in nuclear morphology and this result supports the suggestion that the cellular target for MISO cytotoxicity is cytoplasmic, and possibly involves the disruption of normal mito-chondrial activity.

Modification of cell respiration. Biaglow and Durand (32) have shown that several nitroaromatic drugs can inhibit cellular oxygen utilization and that the consequent reoxygenation of hypoxic cells in multicellular spheroids might account for part of a compound's radiosensitizing effect. Further studies with a wider selection of drugs identified some that could stimulate, that had no effect, and that inhibited oxygen utilization in Ehrlich tumor and Chinese hamster cells (33). In fact, misonidazole at

1 mM concentration had no effect on oxygen utilization and at 5 mM produced a 20% inhibition.   This observed effect on cells could be involved in the mechanism of misonidazole cytotoxicity in oxygenated cells.   The compounds which have the greatest thera- peutic effect as hypoxic cell radiosensitizers in animals are those which least inferfere with cell respiration.   Whether or not these studies relate to mechanisms of misonidazole toxicity in hypoxic cells remains to be seen.

   Production of toxic reduction products.   Intermediates (possibly free radicals) of intracellular reduction of nitroaromatic drugs have been postulated as the toxic species associated with their antibacterial activity (34).   Several cellular enzyme systems are known to reduce the nitro group of various drugs (35-37). Wong et al. (3) suggested that the increase in toxicity and the increase in radiosensitizing effectiveness of misonidazole after prolonged incubation under hypoxic conditions are related to the formation of metabolites which accumulate in cells.   Radio- sensitizers are likely to effect cellular toxicity by interacting in electron transfer processes within cells (Fig. 7) (38).   Under hypoxic conditions, such reactions could lead to the depletion of the cellular pool of reductants and/or to nitroso and hydroxylamino products.   Under aerobic conditions such reactions could lead to depletion of the pool of reductants and the formation of peroxide (39).   That intracellular reduction of nitroaromatic drugs is a prerequisite for drug action and toxicity is widely held by researchers investigating drug mechanisms.   Unfortunately, the

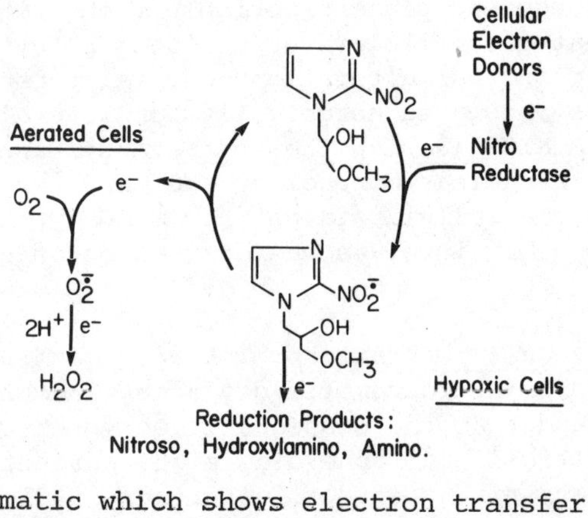

Fig. 7.   A schematic which shows electron transfer processes which can lead to the reduction of misonidazole within aerobic and hypoxic cells.

details of specific biochemical and chemical mechanisms associated with misonidazole cytotoxicity and metabolism-dependent radiosensitization are not known.

Microsomal electron-transfer stimulation.   Studies with in vitro microsomal preparations have shown that nitroaromatic drugs can stimulate electron transfer in this system (40,41).   The electron-donating systems of the cellular microsomes are a logical candidate for the intracellular reduction of misonidazole by hypoxic cells because of their known role in drug detoxification. In vitro results depend upon several factors including the level of reducing equivalents and cannot be immediately extrapolated to the whole cell situation.   Consequently, whether or not the stimulation of microsomal electron transfer processes within cells can account for the biological effects of MISO remains to be demonstrated.

Depletion of non-protein thiols.   Varnes et al. (42) have reported that the levels of non-protein sulfhydryls in Chinese hamster (CHO) and mouse (ET) cells are lowered by incubation in hypoxia in the presence of MISO.   Cells were incubated in phosphate buffer without glucose to demonstrate the effect, although it was suggested that the rates of thiol loss were similar in cells suspended in tissue culture media and in glucose-containing buffer. We have been unable to observe a comparable reduction in the level of cellular non-protein sulphydryl in Chinese hamster V79 cells exposed to MISO at concentrations up to 5 mM in hypoxia for up to 5 hours.   These same cells exposed to MISO in the same hypoxic chamber show cytotoxicity (Fig. 4) and enhanced radiosensitization (Fig. 2).   The most commonly occurring non-protein sulphydryl in cells is reduced glutathione (43) but the radiation sensitivity of cells does not always correlate with the redox state of this molecule (44).   Nevertheless, the depletion of non-protein sulphydryls in cells could be indicative of the redox state of the, as yet, unidentified cellular reducing species which are intimately involved in the rapid free radical processes at the cellular target. Other nitroaromatic compounds are known to deplete mammalian cells of reducing equivalents (45).

Sensitizer adducts to cellular macromolecules.   Sensitizer adducts to cellular macromolecules are a significant product of radiation-induced reactions and have been implicated as important in the mechanism of hypoxic cell radiosensitization (14).   Sensitizer adducts to the macromolecules of hypoxic cells are also a significant product of metabolism-induced reactions as shown in Fig. 8.   The amount of ^{14}C-MISO bound to the acid insoluble fraction of hypoxic Chinese hamster V79 cells is shown as a function of sensitizer concentration and time of incubation.   Some ^{14}C-MISO is bound to aerobic cells and to hypoxic cells immediately after the

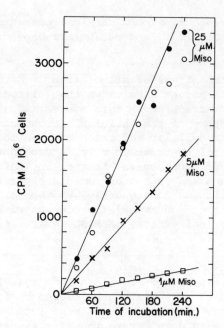

Fig. 8.   The amount of ^{14}C-misonidazole bound to the
           macromolecules of hypoxic Chinese hamster V79
           cells as a function of drug concentration and
           time at 37°C.

addition of drug but no increase in bound MISO was observed upon
incubation of cells aerobically at 37°C.   This background of
bound drug has been subtracted from the data presented in Fig. 8
to emphasize the metabolism-induced component of binding.   With
a concentration of 50μM ^{14}C-MISO the amount of labelled drug
bound to hypoxic cells after three hours' incubation is at least
12X that bound to aerobic cells.   This metabolism-dependent binding of misonidazole to hypoxic cells is dependent upon drug concentration (Fig. 8), cell line (46), and time and temperature and
has been suggested as a possible mechanism for misonidazole cytotoxicity and metabolism-dependent radiosensitization (47).   The
detection of sensitizer adducts using radioactively-labelled drug
is a relatively easy matter but details of the specific biochemistry
of the binding process and the chemical structure of the addition
products are not known.   In this regard, Raleigh et al. (48) have
shown that a nitrobenzene radiosensitizer can bind to a lipid
molecule as a consequence of reduction by cytochrome C reductase.
The reactive reduction intermediate is presumably the nitrosobenzene product since the nitroxyl radical formed as final product
in the reaction is indistinguishable from the product formed when
pure nitrosobenzene reacts with the same lipid molecule.   In the
case of misonidazole, addition products might be expected to form
through carbon atoms on the ring as well as through the nitro group.

Research into the specific chemistry of the sensitizer addition reactions could prove useful in elucidating mechanisms of sensitizer action in cells. It should be noted that the level of misonidazole bound to cells in the experiments shown in Fig. 8 does not cause cytotoxicity or hypoxic cell radiosensitization. As well we have shown that cells labelled for 3 hours with ^{14}C-MISO (50μM) are capable of subsequent proliferation. Studies are in progress to determine the site or sites within mammalian cells where the drug is bound.

A novel application of this information on metabolism-induced adduct formation has been our ability to label viable hypoxic cells in animal tumors with ^{14}C-MISO and visualize the location of hypoxic cells in histological preparations of animal tumors by autoradiography (49,50). Sensitizers will undoubtedly serve as a marker for hypoxic cells in studies of animal tumor biology and tumor cell kinetics and might have a role in cancer diagnosis (51).

CONCLUSIONS

Although several radiation-induced and metabolism-induced reactions of nitroaromatic sensitizers with cellular molecules have been identified, the details of the molecular mechanisms of hypoxic cell radiosensitization and hypoxic and aerobic cell toxicity remain to be identified. Biological effectiveness of these compounds is a strong function of their electrophilicity and redox processes are strongly implicated. Studies into the details of adduct formation between MISO and cellular molecules are needed to determine the potential role of such products in radiation and toxic drug mechanisms.

ACKNOWLEDGEMENTS

This research was supported by the Alberta Heritage Savings and Trust Fund - Applied Cancer Research and the National Cancer Institute of Canada. The skilful assistance of Gail Page, Karl Liesner and Frank LoCicero in preparing this manuscript is appreciated.

REFERENCES

1. G. E. Adams, Adv. Radiat. Chem. 3: 125 (1972).
2. J. D. Chapman, A.P. Reuvers, J. Borsa, J.S. Henderson and R.D. Migliore, Cancer Chemother. Rep., Part 1, 58:559 (1974).
3. T. W. Wong, G. F. Whitmore and S. Gulyas, Radiat. Res. 75: 541 (1978).
4. J. D. Chapman, J. Ngan-Lee and B.E. Meeker, in: "Molecular Action and Targets for Cancer Chemotherapeutic Agents",

A. Sartorelli, ed., Academic Press, New York, p.419 (1980).

5. J. S. Asquith, M.E. Watts, K. Patel, C. E. Smithen and G. E. Adams, Radiat. Res., 60:108 (1974).

6. A. M. Rauth, and K. Kaufman, Brit. J. Radiol., 48:209 (1975).

7. J. Denekamp and S. R. Harris, Radiat. Res., 61:191 (1975).

8. J. M. Brown, Radiat. Res., 64:633 (1975).

9. E. J. Hall and L. Roizin-Towle, Radiology, 117:453 (1975).

10. J. K. Mohindra and A. M. Rauth, Cancer Res., 36:930 (1976).

11. A. Cole, R. E. Meyn, R. Chen, P. M. Corry and W. Hittelman, in: "Radiation Biology in Cancer Research", R. E. Meyn and H. R. Withers, eds., Raven Press, New York, p.33 (1980).

12. D. L. Dugle, J. D. Chapman, C. J. Gillespie, J. Borsa, R. G. Webb, B. E. Meeker and A. P. Reuvers, Int. J. Radiat. Biol., 22:545 (1972).

13. J. D. Chapman, D. L. Dugle, A. P. Reuvers, C. J. Gillespie and J. Borsa, in: "Radiation Research - Biomedical, Chemical, and Physical Perspectives", O. F. Nygaard, H. I. Adler and W. K. Sinclair, eds., Academic Press, New York, p.752 (1975).

14. J. D. Chapman, C. L. Greenstock, A. P. Reuvers, E. McDonald and I. Dunlop, Radiat. Res., 53:190 (1973).

15. C. L. Greenstock, J. D. Chapman, J.A. Raleigh, E. Shierman and A. P. Reuvers, Radiat. Res., 59:556 (1974).

16. T. Alper, Radiat. Res., 5:573 (1956).

17. P. Howard-Flanders, Adv. Biol. Med. Phys., 5: 533 (1958).

18. P. Alexander, Trans. N.Y. Acad. Sci., 24:721 (1961).

19. J. D. Chapman, A. P. Reuvers, J. Borsa and C. L. Greenstock, Radiat. Res., 56:291 (1973).

20. J. S. Asquith, J. L. Foster, R. L. Willson, R. Ings and J. A. McFadzean, Brit. J. Radiol., 47:474 (1974).

21. J. D. Chapman, J. A. Raleigh, J. Borsa, R. G. Webb and R. Whitehouse, Int. J. Radiat. Biol., 21:475 (1972).

22. J. A. Raleigh, J. D. Chapman, J. Borsa, W. Kremers and A. P. Reuvers, Int. J. Radiat. Biol., 23:377 (1973).

23. G. E. Adams, E. D. Clarke, I. R. Flockhart, R. S. Jacobs, D. S. Sehmi, I. J. Stratford, P. Wardman, M. E. Watts, J. Parrick, R. G. Wallace and C.E. Smithen, Int. J. Radiat. Biol., 35: 133 (1979).

24. P. L. Olive and D. R. McCalla, Cancer Res., 35, 781 (1975).

25. D. R. McCalla, P. L. Olive and Y. Tu, in: "Fundamentals in Cancer Prevention", P. N. Magee, ed., Univ. Press, Baltimore, p.229 (1976).

26. P. L. Olive and D. R. McCalla, Chem. Biol. Interact., 16:223 (1977).

27. A. Tonomura and M. S. Sasaki, Jpn. J. Genet., 48:291 (1973).

28. P. L. Olive, in: "Nitrofurans: Chemistry, Metabolism, Mutagenesis and Carcinogenics", G. T. Bryan, ed., Raven Press, New York, p.131 (1979).

29. B. Palcic and L. D. Skarsgard, Brit. J. Cancer 37, Suppl.III, 54 (1978).

30. L. Roizin-Towle, L. Roizen, E. J. Hall and J. C. Liu, abstract
    Radiat. Res., 74:471 (1978).
31. R. A. Smith, Brit. J. Cancer, 41:305 (1980).
32. J. E. Biaglow and R. E. Durand, Radiat. Res., 65:529 (1976).
33. J. E. Biaglow, Pharmacol. and Therapeutics, 10:283 (1980).
34. D. R. McCalla, A. Reuvers and C. Kaiser, J. Bacteriol.,104:
    1126 (1970).
35. M. Morita, D. R. Feller and J. R. Gillette, Biochem. Pharmacol.
    20:217 (1971).
36. C. H. Wong, B. C. Behrens, M. Ichikawa and G. T. Bryan,
    Biochem. Pharmacol., 23:3395 (1974).
37. K. Tatsumi, S. Kitamura, H. Yoshimura and Y. Kawazol, Chem.
    Pharmacol. Bull., 26:1713 (1978).
38. J. D. Chapman, J. A. Raleigh, J. E. Pedersen, J. Ngan, F. Y.
    Shum, B. E. Meeker and R. C. Urtasun, in: "Radiation
    Research", S. Okada, M. Imamura, T. Terashima, H.
    Yamaguchi, eds., Jap. Assoc. Radiat. Res., Tokyo, p.885
    (1979).
39. E. Perez-Reyes, B. Kalyanaraman and R. P. Mason, Mol.
    Pharmacol., 17:239 (1980).
40. J. E. Biaglow, M. E. Varnes, C. J. Koch and R. Sridhar, in:
    "Free Radicals and Cancer", R. Floyd, ed., Marcel-Dekker
    (1981) in press.
41. J. E. Biaglow, Radiat. Res. (1981) in press.
42. M. E. Varnes, J. E. Biaglow, C. J. Koch and E. J. Hall, in:
    Proceedings of "Combined Modality Cancer Treatment:
    Radiation Sensitizers and Protectors" Conference, Key
    Biscayne, Florida, Oct. 1979 (1981) in press.
43. P. S. Jocelyn, in: "Biochemistry of the SH Group", Academic
    Press, London, p.10 (1972).
44. J. W. Harris and J. A. Power, Radiat. Res., 56:97 (1973).
45. L. F. Chasseaud, Adv. Cancer Res., 29:175 (1979).
46. Y. C. Taylor and A. M. Rauth, Cancer Res., 38:2745 (1978).
47. A. J. Vanghese and G. F. Whitmore, Cancer Res., 40:2165 (1980).
48. J. A. Raleigh, F. Y. Shum and S. F. Lui, Biochem. Pharmacol.
    (1981) in press.
49. J. D. Chapman, A. J. Franko and J. Sharplin, Brit. J. Cancer
    (1981) in press.
50. J. D. Chapman, A. J. Franko and C. J. Koch, in: "Biological
    Bases and Clinical Implications of Tumor Radioresistance",
    G. H. Fletcher, C. Nervi and H. R. Withers, eds., Masson
    Publ. (1981) in press.
51. J. D. Chapman, New Engl. J. Med., 301:1429 (1979).

RADIATION-INDUCED CELLULAR DNA DAMAGE AND REPAIR, AND THE EFFECT

OF HYPOXIC CELL RADIOSENSITIZERS

E. Martin Fielden[*] and O. Sapora[**]

[*] Radiobiology Unit, Institute of Cancer Research
Sutton, Surrey, UK.

[**]Istituto Superiore di Sanità, Viale Regina Elena
Rome, Italy

DNA AS A TARGET

Chromosomal deoxyribonucleic acid (DNA) is accepted as an important target for radiochemical damage in biological systems following ultraviolet and ionizing irradiation. Several types of experimental data support this hypothesis for numerous biological systems including both mammalian and bacterial cells. The isolation and consequent studies on several mutant strains of Escherichia coli of differing DNA repair capabilities (1,2) have helped to clarify the role of DNA as a primary target and has revealed the significance of post-irradiation cellular repair activity (Table 1).

IONIZING RADIATION DAMAGE TO DNA

Ionizing radiation is known to produce several different types of physicochemical damage in the DNA macromolecule such as:

1) breaks in the sugar-phosphate backbone of one of the poly-nucleotide strand (single strand breaks)

2) adjacent or near adjacent single strand breaks in both poly-nucleotide strands (double strand breaks)

3) intra and intermolecular cross-links between DNA or DNA and protein

4) base alterations

105

Table 1. List of genes affecting radiation sensitivity in E.coli

---

Rec genes: deficient mutations reduce recombinant formation,
    confer differing degrees of sensitivity to ionizing and UV-
    irradiation.

Uvr genes: deficient mutations confer sensitivity to UV-
    irradiation and other agents.

Dna genes: deficient mutations confer a conditional block in DNA
    synthesis and sensitivity to ionizing and UV-irradiation.

Pol genes: polymerase deficiency confers sensitivity to ionizing
    and UV-irradiation.

Lex gene: a regulatory gene involved in controlling the
    expression of recA and other genes.

Lig gene: structural gene for DNA ligase.

Lon gene: deficiency leads to UV sensitivity and radiation
    induced filament formation.

Sbc B gene: structural gene for exonuclease I.

Xth A gene: structural gene for exonuclease III.

Exr A gene: similar to Lex A gene.

---

5) rupture of hydrogen bonds leading to permanent deformation of
    the DNA structure.

DNA REPAIR BY BIOCHEMICAL PROCESSES

    Repair of DNA damage is connected with DNA replication and
several enzymes and binding proteins involved in replication are
essential for repair. DNA replication itself is coordinated with
growth and cell division (3-7).

    In general, DNA repair appears to fall into two categories:
repair that results in the removal of damage and in the restor-
ation of the normal DNA structure (error-free repairs); and
tolerance responses that enhance the capacity of the cell to
survive in spite of unrepaired damage (error-prone repair).

    Various classification schemes for DNA damage and repair
enzymes have been proposed. One of the most popular classifies
according to the repair pathways that act on lesions:-

1) Repair pathways that can act in non-growth conditions. The
    enzymes involved are constitutive and they can repair thymidine
    dimers by photoreactivation or by excision, single strand
    breaks, and some types of base damage.

2) Repair pathways that only act in growth conditions.   The
   enzymes are induced and synthesised ex novo.   These pathways
   are described as post-replication repair and SOS repair (4,5).
   The various repair processes are described below in more detail.

Repair of missing, incorrect or altered bases

     Base loss may occur spontaneously following radiation damage
and can be restored directly by reinsertion using the
complementary base as the template.   However, a more general
repair mechanism is the excision repair initiated by an
Apurinic-endonuclease.   Several AP-endonucleases have now been
characterized from a variety of bacterial sources.   Any damaged
or incorrect bases that can be removed leaving an AP-active site,
would provide the substrate for excision repair.   The general
principle of this repair is very simple: the damage is recognized,
a phosphodiester strand scission is made (incision), the lesion is
excised along with adjacent nucleotides (excision), the deleted
strand is reconstituted utilizing the intact complementary strand
as template (synthesis and joining) (Fig.1).

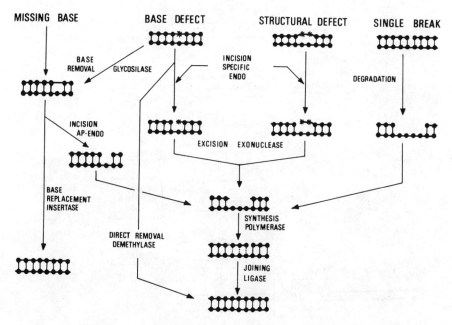

Fig. 1.   Repair pathways for radiation-induced DNA damage by
          constitutive-enzymes.

Incorrect bases, such as uracil or deaminated cytosine,
adenine or guanine, can be removed by specific glycosilases
leaving an AP site.   An alternative mechanism for the removal
may be the excision repair initiated by endonuclease.   Since
all the incorrect bases are, by definition, wrongly paired, they
may be subject to mismatch repair if they are not promptly
excised.   This can be an important source of mutation events.

Post-replication repair

A recombinational process, generally known as post-
replication repair, is also necessary for the replication of
damaged DNA, probably when the amount of remaining damage is not
too large.   Replication is arrested at each lesion, but re-
initiated a few hundred bases further, leaving a large gap in the
newly synthesized daughter strand.   These gaps are filled by a
displaced parental strand of similar polarity.   This mechanism
will provide two DNA molecules, the first one intact and correct,
the second one containing the original damage (Fig. 2).

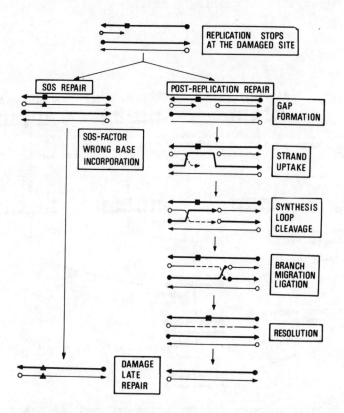

Fig. 2.   Post-replication and SOS repair pathways active under
          growth conditions.

SOS repair

This repair is induced when damage has not been eliminated or overcome by one of the above processes. It is triggered by a block in DNA synthesis which can result not only from a DNA lesion but also by starvation of the cell for an important DNA precursor, such as thymidine. It is probably dependent on poly- merase III, necessary for replication. The lesion which consti- tutes a "non coding" template will accept any base for incorpora- tion but this base will be subsequently removed by the 3'-5' edit- ing site of the enzyme, since any base opposite the lesion consti- tutes a mispair (Fig. 2). The SOS trigger signal induces the synthesis of new proteins, necessary to suppress the editing function of polymerase III and thus permitting the permanent inclusion of an incorrect base.

Two important genes, the RecA and the LexA, are essential for the induction of SOS repair which has a transient effect (8). The fact that only a small portion of cells are repaired by this process suggests that most cells which survive have had their DNA repaired by the other processes before or during replication.

METHODS FOR DNA DAMAGE AND REPAIR EVALUATION

1) Rapid-lysis technique

This technique is based on the use of an electron pulse generator able to deliver pulses of electrons of short duration. Typically a 30 krad dose is delivered by six pulses, with 15 msec total irradiation time. At a selected time after irradiation, 0.5 ml of a lysis solution, in a 5 ml syringe, is pushed by an electrically activated ram into the cell suspension in the irradiated vessel. The signal for addition of lysis solution is controlled by an electronic timer system. The total time required to add 0.5 ml of lysis solution is 250 msec (Fig. 3) (9).

One of the advantages of the rapid lysis technique is the possibility of measuring the initial number of "radiation produced" breaks by lysing the cells at times less than 1 sec after irradiation, before the various enzymatic systems, present in the cell, can act on the damaged DNA, producing new, enzymatically-induced breaks or repairing the breaks (Fig. 4). The estimation of the damage is then made by the sedimentation technique.

2) Sedimentation technique

Since McGrath and Williams first published the sedimentation technique (10) it has been widely used. The principle is simple.

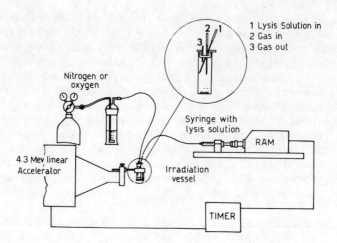

Fig. 3. Schematic diagram of the rapid-lysis apparatus.

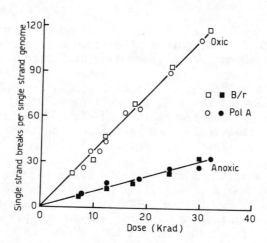

Fig. 4. Yield of single strand breaks per single strand genome
         as a function of radiation dose for two strains of
         E.coli, B/r and Pol.A⁻.   Open and closed symbols are
         for cells irradiated oxically and anoxically respectively
         with lysis at 0.2 sec after irradiation.

Cells labelled with tritiated thymidine are carefully placed on the type of an alkaline sucrose density gradient, lysed and centrifuged. At the end of the run the gradients are fractionated and the fractions collected and counted for the radioactivity incorporated into the DNA. In the rapid-lysis method the cells are lysed with a NaOH, EDTA and sarkosyl solution and then carefully transferred to the top of the gradient (9).

The molecular weight of the DNA can be calculated from the sedimentation profile. Several methods are available; however, the one most used involves the calculation of the number average molecular weight

$$Mn = \Sigma W_i / \Sigma (W_i / M_i)$$

where W_i is the weight of DNA proportional to the radioactivity in fraction i and M_i is the molecular weight calculated using Studier's relationship (11).

The derivation of the number of ssb can be made with increased accuracy from the experimental profile using a computer fit method described by Fox (12). The computer fit method is much less sensitive to any residual activity in the first few fractions.

3) Enzyme techniques

Both bacterial and mammalian cells may remove, as outlined in the previous section, various sorts of damage from their DNA. These processes can be detected in different ways. For example, Hariharan and Cerutti developed a sensitive radiochemical assay for monitoring the appearance in the medium of two derivatives of thymine released from the DNA of irradiated Micrococcus Radiodurans (13).

The initial step of the excision repair process is mediated by an endonuclease specific for ionizing radiation damage. Data from several independent investigators indicate that extracts of M. Luteus contain such characteristics. Wilkins (14) has demonstrated such a repair process in E.coli by monitoring their DNA for the disappearance of sites which are sensitive to the endonucleolitic action of M. Luteus extract (Fig. 5). After irradiation, bacteria are incubated in growth medium for various periods and then lysed. Each sample is divided into two portions, one of which is treated with the extract. Both lysates are then centrifuged on an alkaline gradient to assay the DNA for ssb. The DNA in the untreated sample contains additional breaks produced by endonuclease action. As few as one or two of these additional breaks, which represent endonuclease sensitive sites,

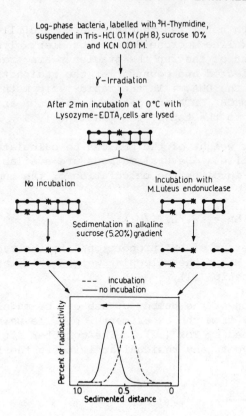

Fig. 5. Assay of DNA for endonuclease sensitive sites.

can be detected per 10^8 Mw of DNA.   Between two and three endonuclease sensitive sites are produced in the DNA for every direct
single strand break.   These sites largely disappear after
incubation in medium or in buffer at 37°C.   In fact, after five
minutes the DNA is no longer susceptible to endonuclease action.

4) Hydroxyapatite technique

An alternative to sedimentation, for detecting ssb has been
developed (15).   The method is based on the principle that ssb
and dsb serve as unwinding points during strand separation in
mildly alkaline solution (Fig. 6), and that DNA is transformed
into the single stranded form in proportion to the number of breaks
present initially.   After neutralization, followed by a short
treatment with ultrasound to fragment the DNA, single and double
stranded DNA are separated by hydroxyapatite chromatography.   The
rate of strand separation is influenced by temperature and ionic
strength during the unwinding process (16).   By varying these
two parameters, the effect of irradiation may be conveniently
studied in the dose range 1 Gy to 200 Gy.   In fact, at 20°C and

high ionic strength (NaCl 1M) the kinetics of strand separation
are so strongly accelerated that the effect of doses as low as
0.1 Gy can be detected.

Against this method is the fact that the characteristics of
the hydroxyapatite can drastically change between one batch and
another and the cell lysis interferes with the unwinding process.
Also the method is not absolute and requires calibration to give
the number of breaks.

EFFECTS OF RADIOSENSITIZERS

Not all of the above techniques have yet been applied to
study the effect of hypoxic cell radiosensitizers on DNA damage.
The nitroaromatic sensitizers, e.g. misonidazole, have been
investigated using the rapid lysis technique and the time scale
of ssb production and repair compared to that found for oxygen.
As this method involves lysis under strongly alkaline conditions
the ssb yields measured must necessarily include all alkali-
labile sites on the damaged DNA.

The initial yield of ssb in bacteria remains constant over
the time scale 10 msec to 1 sec after irradiation (17,18) and only
chemical interaction with the irradiated DNA, e.g. by oxygen,
sensitizers and sulphydryl compounds, can influence these yields
(17).   After 1-2 seconds the repair enzymes act, repairing
breaks or introducing new gaps to remove base alterations (9,19,
20) as described in Fig. 1.   Using mutants lacking in polymerase
I or ligase activity, it was possible to reveal the base-damage
excision repair and the polymerase I dependent repair (17,19).
This data is summarized in Fig. 7 which also includes the effects
of post-replication repair (e.g. rec dependent).   This latter
process can only be observed if the cells are held in growth conditions rather than buffer.   The results are in agreement with
data obtained by other or similar techniques (21,22,23).

When nitroaromatic sensitizers (PNAP, misonidazole) are
present at the time of irradiation under hypoxic conditions, the
initial yield of ssb was found to be identical to that found under
oxic conditions in both bacterial and mammalian cells (9,20,24).
In contrast, however, the nitroxyl sensitizers did not enhance
the initial yield of ssb (9,20,24) but there was evidence that
subsequent repair was inhibited so that the residual yield of
breaks at the end of the polymerase-dependent repair process was
the same for both PNAP and the nitroxyl NPPN (20).   Although
PNAP and misonidazole were as effective as oxygen in enhancing the
yield of ssb's they were not as effective as oxygen in enhancing
cell killing.   Using bacterial mutants deficient in repair
proficiency, evidence was produced that the nitroaromatic sensi-

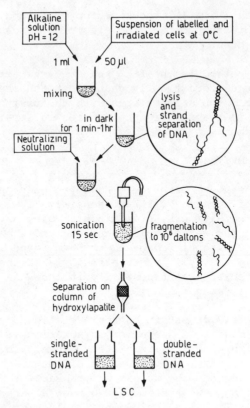

Fig. 6.   Assay of DNA strand breaks by the hydroxy-apatite
          method.

tizers did not enhance endonuclease sensitive base damage to the
same extent as oxygen (20).

    In an investigation of the hypoxic cell cytotoxicity of miso-
nidazole (25) it was reported that DNA ssb, detected by the
alkaline sucrose gradient technique, were induced before the onset
of toxicity.   Thus a 30 minute hypoxic incubation of Chinese
hamster cells with 15 mM misonidazole produced no cell killing
but a significant decrease in the molecular weight of the DNA if
assayed promptly after the treatment.   Incubation for 24 hours
before measuring the DNA molecular weight, however, showed complete repair (25).   Similar experiments using the hydroxyapatite
technique (26) did not show this effect except at much longer
cell-drug contact time.   It was suggested (26) that the apparent
discrepancy could be due to the very different lysing conditions
used in the two methods.

    In the same work, the radiation-induced oxygen enhancement
ratio for DNA damage, assessed by hydroxyapatite chromatography,

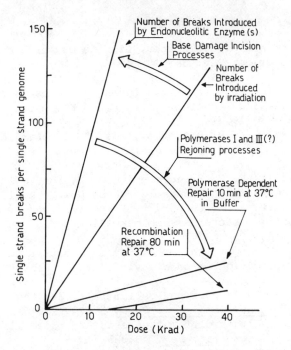

Fig. 7. Composite diagram showing the time course of ssb in
irradiated E.coli using the rapid lysis technique
(data from refs. 18,19). In order to see the effects
of recombination repair (lowest line) growth medium
was added to the suspending buffer, 10 minutes after
irradiation when the polymerase dependent repair was
complete.

compared well (2.7:2.8) with the OER for radiation cell killing
(26). Using misonidazole (5 mM in hypoxia) a good agreement was
also obtained for the increased DNA damage compared to cell
lethality (26). Possible complications due to variable amounts
of repair were avoided by irradiating and washing the cells before
assay in ice-cold P.B.S.

It is apparent that it will be necessary to use a variety of
techniques, as described above, to fully define the mode of action
of hypoxic cell radiosensitizers on DNA damage and its relation to
cell killing.

REFERENCES

1. A. L. Taylor and C. D. Trotter, Linkage map of E.coli strain
    K12, Bacteriol. Rev. 36:504 (1972).
2. O. Sapora, E. M. Fielden and P. S. Loverock, A comparative
    study of the effects of two types of radiosensitizers on
    the survival of several E.coli B and K12 mutants, Radiat.
    Res. 69:293 (1977).
3. P. C. Hanawalt and R. B. Setlow, eds. "Molecular Mechanisms
    for Repair of DNA, parts A and B", Plenum Press, New York
    (1975).
4. P. C. Hanawalt, E. C. Friedberg and C. F. Fox, eds. "DNA
    Repair Mechanisms", Academic Press, New York (1978).
5. P. C. Hanawalt, P. K. Cooper, A. K. Genesan and C. A. Smith,
    DNA repair in bacterial and mammalian cells, Ann. Rev.
    Biochem. 48:783 (1979).
6. M. Errera, DNA repair and mutagenesis in bacterial systems and
    their implication in oncology.   Int. J. Radiat. Onc. Biol.
    Phys. 5:1077 (1979).
7. M. M. Elkind, DNA repair and cell repair: are they correlated?
    Int. J. Radiat. Onc. Biol. Phys. 5:1089 (1976).
8. E. M. Witkin, Ultraviolet mutagenesis and inducible DNA repair
    in E.coli, Bacteriol. Rev. 40:869 (1976).
9. O. Sapora, E. M. Fielden and P. S. Loverock, The application
    of rapid lysis technique in radiobiology: I. The effect of
    oxygen and radiosensitizers on DNA strand break production
    and repair in E.coli B/r, Radiat. Res. 64:431 (1975).
10. R. A. McGrath and R. W. Williams, Reconstruction in vivo of
    irradiated E.coli deoxyribonucleir acid: the rejoining of
    broken pieces, Nature (London) 212:534 (1966).
11. U. K. Ehmann and J. T. Lett, Review and evaluation of molecular
    weight calculations from the sedimentation profiles of
    irradiated DNA, Radiat. Res. 54:152 (1973).
12. R. A. Fox, The analysis of single strand breaks in E.coli
    using a curve fitting procedure, Int. J. Radiat. Biol. 30:
    67 (1976).
13. P. V. Hariharan and P. A. Cerutti, Formation and repair of
    gamma-ray induced thymidine damage in Micrococcus
    radiofurans, J. Molec. Biol. 66:65 (1972).
14. R. J. Wilkins, Does the E.coli possess a DNA excision repair
    for gamma-ray damage? Nature New Biology, 244:269 (1973).
15. G. Ahnstron and K. Erixon, Radiation induced strand breakage
    in DNA from mammalian cells: strand separation in alkaline
    solution, Int. J. Radiat. Biol. 23:285 (1973).
16. B. Rydbert, The rate of strand separation in alkali of DNA
    of irradiated mammalian cells, Radiat. Res. 61:274 (1975).
17. O. Sapora, P. S. Loverock and E. M. Fielden, The role of
    radiation chemical and enzymatic processes on single
    strand breaks at short time after irradiation, Int. J.
    Radiat. Biol. 30:385 (1976).

18. R. A. Fox, E. M. Fielden and O. Sapora, Yield of single strand breaks in the DNA of E.coli 10 msec after irradiation, <u>Int. J. Radiat. Biol</u>. 29:391 (1976).

19. O. Sapora, E. M. Fielden and P. S. Loverock, The application of rapid lysis techniques in radiobiology: II. The time course of the repair of DNA fixed damage and single strand breaks in E.coli mutants, <u>Radiat. Res</u>. 72:308 (1977).

20. E. M. Fielden, O. Sapora and P. S. Loverock, The application of rapid lysis techniques in radiobiology: III. The effect of radiosensitizers on the production of DNA damage and the time course of its repair, <u>Radiat. Res</u>. 75:54 (1978).

21. N. V. Tomilin, Repair of gamma-ray induced lesions in E.coli cells deficient in DNA polymerase I and having thermo-sensitive DNA polymerase III, <u>Molec. Gen. Genet</u>. 129:97 (1974).

22. R. J. Wilkins, Endonuclease-sensitive sites in the DNA of irradiated bacteria: a rapid and sensitive assay, <u>Biochem. Biophys. Acta</u> 312:33 (1973).

23. E. Boye, I. Johansen and T. Brustad, Time scale for rejoining of bacteriophage deoxyribonucleic acid molecules in super-infected Pol[+] and PolA strains of E.coli after exposure to 4 MeV electrons, <u>J. Bacteriol</u>. 119:522 (1974).

24. B. C. Millar, E. M. Fielden and J. J. Steele, Effect of oxygen-radiosensitizer mixtures on the radiation response of Chinese hamster cells: II. Determination of the initial yield of ssb in the cellular DNA using a rapid-lysis technique, <u>Radiat. Res</u>. 83:57 (1980).

25. B. Palcic and L. D. Skarsgard, Cytotoxicity of misonidazole and DNA damage in hypoxic mammalian cells, <u>Br. J. Cancer</u> 37, Suppl.III:54 (1978).

26. S. Rajaratnam, The interaction of hyperthermia with the cytotoxicity of electron-affinic radiosensitizers <u>in vitro</u>, Ph.D. Thesis, London University (1980).

BIOLOGICAL METHODS FOR STUDYING RADIOSENSITIZATION

Juliana Denekamp

Gray Laboratory of the Cancer Research Campaign
Mount Vernon Hospital, Northwood, Middlesex HA6 2RN
England

Many aspects of research in radiobiology and radiotherapy depend upon the belief that hypoxic cells exist in human tumours, and that these radioresistant cells determine whether or not the tumour will be cured or will recur after radiotherapy.   Hypoxic cells are believed to develop because of the imbalance between tumour cell production and the growth of blood vessels to provide nutrients, including oxygen (1,2).   A corded structure similar to that shown in Figure 1 was first demonstrated by Thomlinson and Gray in human lung tumours (3).   They postulated that necrosis at 100-150 μm resulted from severe hypoxia and that a rim of hypoxic cells which were about to die existed at the boundary between the viable and dead tissue.

Cells at the boundary between viable and necrotic layers would be protected against X-rays by their hypoxia; and consequently the tumours would be radioresistant.   However, these cells would only be important in determining the outcome of therapy if they were rescued from their imminent hypoxic death by an improved nutritional supply.   This has been termed "reoxygenation" (4) and has been demonstrated experimentally in several types of tumour (for review see ref.5).

Hypoxic, radioresistant cells have now been demonstrated in a wide variety of animal tumour, and the recent use of radiosensitizers in the clinic has shown them to exist in human tumours too (Table 1). Many of these values are in the range 10-20% and are consistent with the predictions of Thomlinson and Gray (3).

119

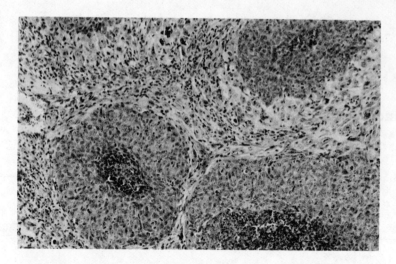

Fig. 1. Photomicrograph of a mouse mammary carcinoma (x 130).
        Central necrosis can be observed in the tumour cords, at
        a distance of about 100 μm from the capillaries in the
        surrounding connective tissue.

    Thus hypoxic cells appear to be important; methods of eliminat-
ing them must be developed and quantitatively compared so that the
most effective treatments can be rapidly adopted in clinical
practice.   Any technique for measuring tumour response that yields
dose response curves can be used for such quantitative evaluations.

    The experimental techniques in common use are illustrated in
Figure 2. They include assays that can be made on tumours left in
situ, which most closely relate to the clinical situation.   More
accurate quantitation can sometimes be obtained by excising the
tumour cells after treatment and assaying for surviving fraction.
However, the cells are then removed from their original environment
and this may rescue (or kill) the hypoxic cells in which we are
interested (11).   All of these techniques have been used to demonstrate the existence of hypoxic cells and the benefits of misonidazole (see ref. 10).

    One of the commonly used techniques (regrowth delay) is illustr-
ated in Figure 3 for a mouse fibrosarcoma.   When radiation kills
tumour cells, the tumour ceases to grow, or even shrinks.   It
fails to grow again until the survivors have replenished the original
population.   Thus cell depletion can be assessed from the induced
delay in growth of the tumours, from treatment size to a specified
larger size.   This technique usually results in biphasic curves for
tumours irradiated in air-breathing animals (e.g. Figure 3).   At low

Table 1. Proportion of Hypoxic Cells in Experimental Tumours

Tumour Identification	Hypoxic Cells	Reference
CBA Sarcoma F	> 50	Hewitt and Wilson, 61.
Gardner Lymphosarcoma	1	Powers and Tolmach, 63.
Adenocarcinoma MTG-B	21	Clifton et al., 66.
C3H Sarcoma KHT	14	van Putten and Kallman, 68.
Rhabdomyosarcoma BA1112	15	Reinhold, 66.
Squamous Carcinoma D	18	Hewitt, 67.
C3H Mammary (250 mm^3)	> 20	Suit and Maeda, 67.
Carcinoma (0.6 mm^3)	O.2	" " "
C3H Mammary Carcinoma	7	Howes, 69.
Osteosarcoma C22LR	14	van Putten, 68.
Fibrosarcoma RIB5	17	Thomlinson, 71.
Fibrosarcoma KHT	12	Hill et al,, 71.
Carcinoma KHJJ	19	Kallman, 74.
Sarcoma EMT 6	35	Kallman, 74.
C3H Mammary (females)	1	Fowler et al., 75.
Carcinoma (males)	17	" "
CBA Sarcoma F (in situ)	< 10	McNally, 75.
(excised)	50	"
Squamous (intradermal)	< 1	Peters, 76.
Carcinoma G (subcutaneous)	> 46	"
WHT Anaplastic (in situ)	> 80	McNally and Sheldon, 77.
'MT' (excised)	5	" " "
Carcinoma DC	10-30	Denekamp et al.)
Carcinoma RH	2-25	" ")
CBA Carcinoma NT	7-18	" ")
Sarcoma S	< 0.01	" ") ref. 6.
" " (fast variants)	1-30	" ")
Sarcoma FA	30-70	" ")
Sarcoma BS 2b	5-25	" ")
Human Tumour Nodules*	12-20	Thomlinson et al. ref. 7.
Human Tumour Nodules*	1-80	Ash et al. ref. 8

* These values have been calculated from the published SER data
  using the method described by Denekamp et al. (ref. 9).

All other references taken from ref. 10.

TUMOUR ASSAYS

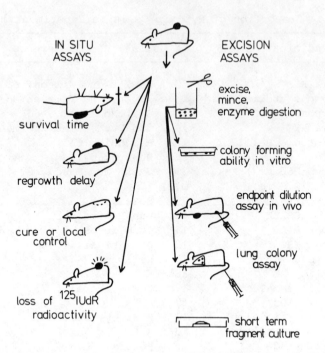

IN SITU
ASSAYS

EXCISION
ASSAYS

survival time

excise,
mince,
enzyme digestion

regrowth delay

colony forming
ability in vitro

cure or local
control

endpoint dilution
assay in vivo

loss of ^{125}IUdR
radioactivity

lung colony
assay

short term
fragment culture

Fig. 2.   Schematic representation of the different methods in
          common use for assessing the response of rodent tumours
          to irradiation (ref. 12).

doses the cell killing of the 80-90% of sensitive, well-oxygenated
cells dominates the response and it is only at higher doses that the
hypoxic cells which are approximately three times more resistant
become significant.   It is therefore only at the higher doses that
radiosensitization becomes more marked.   The upper points have
upward arrows indicating that some tumours never regrew, i.e. they
were cured.   It is a natural extension of this assay to score the
percent of locally controlled tumours over a more limited (and high)
dose range, as in Figure 4.

From any pair of dose response curves the sensitizer enhancement ratio can be derived from the doses to produce equivalent
effects.   The observed (SER') will be smaller than the full effect
on a purely hypoxic population (SER) because of the "masking effect"
of the well-oxygenated tumour cells, especially at low doses, as
shown in Figure 3.   This masking effect is less apparent at higher
and higher doses; hence the maximum values of SER' will be obtained
in experiments using large radiation doses, e.g. local control, high

levels of regrowth delay, or from the ratio of slopes on survival
curves.   Figure 5 shows the measured enhancement ratios (SER′) for
a wide variety of mouse tumours that have been tested using several
different doses of the electron affinic radiosensitizer misonidazole.
These experiments were all performed using single doses of both drug
and radiation.   They demonstrate that significant enhancement
ratios are obtainable, even with doses of 0.1 mg/g or lower.   This
large body of experimental data forms the foundation of the present
clinical studies of misonidazole as a radiosensitizer.

In clinical studies, however, large single doses of drug and of
radiation will <u>not</u> be used, except perhaps for palliative treatments.
Thus the influence of drug dose, radiation dose and of reoxygenation
between successive fractions must all be considered.   The number
of experimental studies of fractionated treatments are fewer; these
are listed in Table 2.   In all cases the enhancement ratio is
diminished with fractionation, but a significant effect is still
seen in most tumours, even with 10 or 20 fractions.

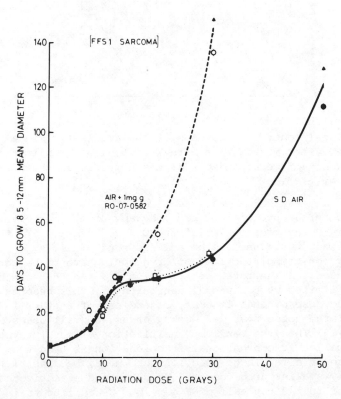

Fig. 3.   The response of a mouse fibrosarcoma to X-rays alone
          (solid line), with misonidazole administered 15 minutes
          before irradiation (dashed line), or 5 minutes after
          irradiation (dotted line).

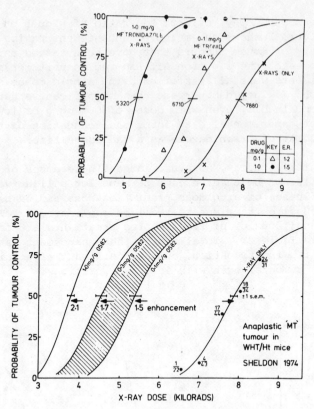

Fig. 4.   Local control at 80 days of the anaplastic mouse tumour
          MT after irradiation with X-rays alone or with different
          doses of metronidazole or misonidazole (redrawn from
          ref. 13).

The clinical practice of radiotherapy usually involves many
small daily X-ray treatments (often 30 x 200 rads).   In this case
the sensitizer would need to be administered 30 times.   Unless it
is totally non-toxic, the dose of drug would have to be correspondingly reduced.   The total dose of misonidazole that can be administered is limited by peripheral neuropathy.   This becomes serious
if the drug dose exceeds 12 g/m^2, regardless of whether it is given
in a few large doses over 2-3 weeks, or as 30 small doses over 6
weeks (14).   Thus the maximum sensitization of purely hypoxic cells
will be smaller if conventional fractionation is used than if a
single dose or a few large fractions are used, because of the
necessarily smaller drug doses.   This reduced effectiveness is
illustrated in the top half of Figure 6.   According to in vitro
data for V79 cells, and the measured serum concentrations in patients,
an SER of 1.34 can be expected with 30 fractions and of 1.73 of 6
fractions.   However, this SER will be further reduced by the
presence of some oxic cells in the tumour.   The bottom panel shows

Table 2. Sensitizer Enhancement Ratios for Fractionated Irradiations in Mice

Tumour	Drug dose per fraction (mg/g)	Single dose	2F	3F	5F	10 or 20F	Reference
Misonidazole							
CBA Ca NT	0.67	2.1	1.6	—	1.3	—	Denekamp and Harris, 76b.
C3H Ca Mam.	0.67–1.0	1.8	—	1.1	1.2	—	Sheldon et al., 75.
	0.67 (5F/9d)	—	—	1.1	—	—	Fowler et al., 76.
WHT MT	0.3 (5F/4d)	1.7	—	—	1.5	—	Sheldon et al., 77.
WHT MT	Any 2 out of 5F	—	—	—	1.3	—	Sheldon et al., 77.
WHT MT	All 5 + 2 inj after each	—	—	—	1.6	—	Sheldon and Fowler, 78.
WHT MT	0.2 x 20	1.7	1.6	—	—	1.3 (20F)	Sheldon and Fowler, 78.
WHT Bone Sa 2	0.67	1.9	—	—	—	—	Denekamp and Stewart, 78.
WHT Fibro Sa a	0.67	1.9	—	—	<1.1	—	Denekamp and Stewart, 78.
WGT Fibro Sa b	0.67 1st two	—	—	—	1.1	—	Denekamp and Stewart, 78.
WHT Fibro Sa	0.67 last two	—	—	—	1.0	—	Denekamp and Stewart, 78.
MDAH/M Ca 4	0.3	>1.8	—	—	—	—	Suit and Brown, 79.
	1.0	2.3	—	—	—	—	Suit and Brown, 79.
MDAH/M Ca 4	0.3	—	—	—	—	1.4 (10F)	Suit (pers. comm.)
Metronidazole							
C3H Ca Mam.	0.1	1.2	—	—	1.1	—	Stone, 76.
(MDAH-MCa-4)	1.0	1.5	—	—	1.3	—	Stone, 76.
WHT Fibro Sa	0.67	—	—	—	1.0	—	Denekamp and Stewart, 78.

For details of references see ref. 10.

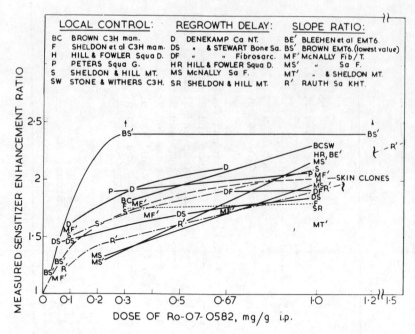

Fig. 5.   SER′ values for a wide variety of different mouse tumours.
These were obtained from pairs of dose response curves
using the three types of assay listed (from ref. 10).

the magnitude of the <u>observed</u> SER′ for a single dose of 200 or 600
rads given to a population containing 90% oxic and 10% hypoxic cells.
Clearly the sensitization will be very small if there are only 10%
of hypoxic cells present at each irradiation, with radiation doses
of these sizes.

The cell kill with a fractionated series of doses is illustrated in Figure 7, for 6, 9, 20 or 30 X-ray fractions of the size that
are proposed for clinical use.   The calculation is based on a
population characterised by an oxic D_O of 135 rads, a hypoxic D_O of
365 rads and extrapolation numbers (n) of 2, 20 or 215, as indicated
at the top of each panel.   If reoxygenation is sufficiently
extensive to return the hypoxic fraction to 10% for each dose, there
would clearly be little benefit from adding misonidazole.   The
cause of any radioresistance would then be some other parameter of
the radiation response (e.g. the size of the extrapolation number)
and not the oxygenation state of the cells.

Figure 8 shows the other extreme, in which no reoxygenation has
been assumed.   Here the SER′ would still be largest with a few

large drug doses, but <u>all</u> the sensitizer treatments would be much
better than the use of X-rays alone (15).

    We do not have any information about the reoxygenation patterns
of human tumours, but this factor clearly will be critical in determining how much clinical benefit can be expected from the use of
radiosensitizers.   The results from Urtasun et al. (16), Thomlinson
et al. (7) and from Ash et al. (8) are encouraging, but the critical
test is whether any multifraction treatment with a sensitizer will
be better than the conventional 30 fractions of X-rays alone.   If
there is no net gain, then sensitizers, hyperbaric oxygen and high

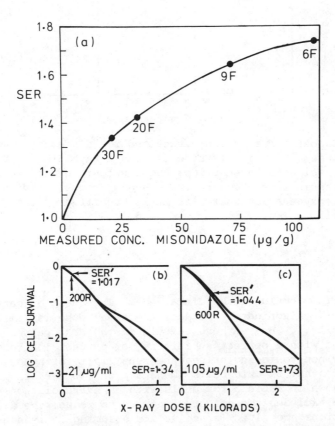

Fig. 6.   Upper panel.   SER values for V79 cells in culture.   The
          likely values achievable for the hypoxic cells in a tumour
          at appropriate serum concentrations for 30, 20, 9 or 6
          fractions are indicated (assuming total misonidazole dose
          cannot exceed 12 g/m^2).
          Lower panels.   The observable SER values at 200 rads or
          600 rads are much lower than the maximum SER because of
          the presence of 90% oxic cells (from ref. 15).

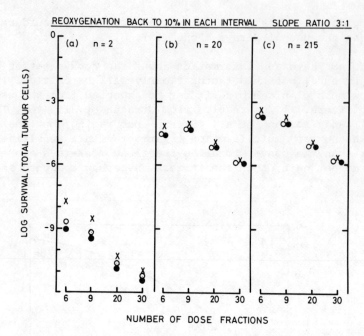

Fig. 7.   Calculated surviving fractions for different fractionation
schemes.   X = treatments with X-rays alone.   0 =
pessimestic assumptions about tumour levels.   ● = optimistic
assumptions about tumour concentrations.   With extensive
reoxygenation there is little benefit from the sensitizer
(15).

LET radiations could all be discarded!   The question cannot be
answered with misonidazole because the total dose is limited by
neurotoxicity.   But we have calculated the SER′ values that can
be expected with a <u>perfect</u> substitute for oxygen, i.e. one which is
completely non-toxic and brings the sensitivity of hypoxic cells
fully up to that of oxic cells (Denekamp and Joiner, in preparation).
This is shown in Table 3 for cells with an extrapolation number of 2.
This table excludes the effect of having to reduce the drug dose when
more fractions are given (since we are assuming it is non-toxic) and
simply demonstrates the effect of reoxygenation on the observed SER′.
With moderate or no reoxygenation the observed SER′ values remain
high.   However, with very effective reoxygenation (back to 10% at
each fraction), the SER′ would be reduced from 2.7 to 1.1 with 30
fractions.   Whilst this is a very disappointing conclusion, a 10%
gain in effective dose (SER′ = 1.1) would still be very useful in
clinical radiotherapy (Figure 9), if the dose response curves are as
steep as those obtained by Shukovsky (17).

Table 3.   Gain (SER') to be Expected from Brand X
           i.e. the Perfect Oxygen Substitute where SER = OER

Assumed Reoxygenation Pattern	30F x 192r in 6w.	20F x 255r in 4w.	9F x 440r in 3w.	6F x 599r in 3 w.
None	2.7	2.7	2.6	2.5
Moderate (20% per day)	1.6	1.7	1.9	1.8
Effective (Back to 10%)	1.1	1.1	1.2	1.3

Assumptions: $D_O = 135r$, $D_S/D_O = 3$, $n = 2$

OER = 2.7,   SER = 2.7,   No Toxicity

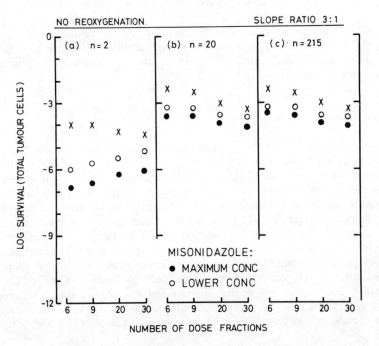

Fig. 8.   Surviving fractions calculated for 4 different fractionation
          schemes for a tumour in which no reoxygenation occurs.
          Very little cell kill is achieved with X-rays alone, and
          there is a large gain with misonidazole (15).

The fractionation schemes and doses are those proposed or in
current use in clinical trials (Denekamp and Joiner, unpublished).

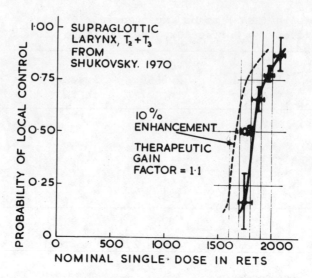

Fig. 9.   Clinical data from Shukovsky for local control of T_2 and
T_3 tumours of the supraglottic larynx, showing the benefit
that might be expected from a 10% increase in effective
dose to the tumour (17).

The search for a better sensitizer than misonidazole therefore
seems worthwhile; our recent experience with misonidazole should
enable us to know how to design efficient experiments in order to
find a better drug.   It is clear that pharmacology and toxicology
studies need to be undertaken in combination with the radiobiology
before a better compound will be identified.   A more useful
clinical compound would be one which has a greater therapeutic
index; this could be achieved by obtaining more sensitization for
the same degree of toxicity or less toxicity for the same degree of
sensitization.   It would also be useful to have a more efficacious
drug so that less grammes would be needed.   At present we seem to
be a long way from the ideal embodied in Brand X, i,e. the completely
non-toxic compound with an efficiency equal to that of oxygen.

Although misonidazole has been in experimental use now for more
than 6 years, we are still finding new aspects of its pharmacology.
Recent work by Workman (18) has shown that the half-life of the
compound in mice depends on the drug dose administered.   This is
attributed to the saturation of liver enzymes.   It can also be
influenced by the prior administration of other drugs, e.g.
barbiturates, presumably as a result of enzyme induction.   Another
factor which we have recently appreciated is the influence of the
strain and the weight of the mouse on the drug toxicity.   Heavy

mice of both the CBA and the WHT strain are much more susceptible to misonidazole toxicity, when dosed on a mg/kg basis. This is shown in Figure 10. The difference persists even if the dose is expressed on a mg/m^2 basis. It seems to result from a difference in the peak serum concentration, rather than from any change in the metabolic half-life. The differences cannot be accounted for simply on the basis of gross fat deposits and the twofold lower ability for misonidazole to be dissolved in lipids than in water (Denekamp, Minchinton, Stratford and Terry, unpublished). Figure 11 illustrates the toxicity and the blood concentrations. The LD$_{50}$ values and the drug dose needed to give 1000 μg/ml peak blood levels both differ by a factor of almost two over the range of mouse weights that have been tested. There is also a significant difference in the two strains.

Many other nitroimidazoles have been found to be better radiosensitizers <u>in vitro</u> than misonidazole (19, 20), but none of these has been definitely proven to be more clinically promising. In

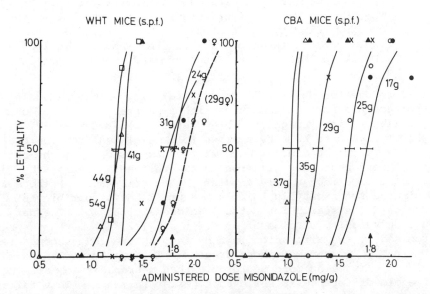

Fig. 10. Percentage of animals dead within 7 days after intraperitoneal injection of misonidazole. The heavy mice of each strain are more susceptible than the light mice (weight indicated against each line). There can be wide divergences from the published LD$_{50}$ value of 1.8 mg/g. (Denekamp and Terry, unpublished).

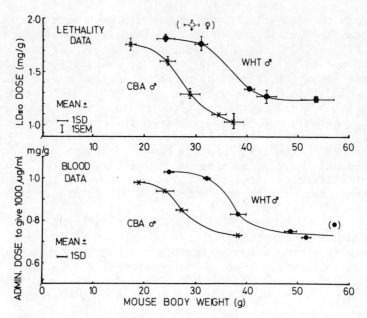

Fig. 11. LD$_{50}$ data and blood levels as a function of mouse weight
for the two mouse strains used at the Gray Laboratory.
The strains differ significantly, but both show an increased toxicity and a decreased dose needed to obtain
1000 μg/ml in the blood with increasing mouse weight.
(Denekamp, Minchinton, Stratford and Terry, unpublished).

order to reduce the dose-limiting neurotoxicity of misonidazole, it
has been postulated that compounds with a shorter half-life, or with
a lower lipophilicity might be more useful (21).   Certainly, less
lipophilic compounds have been shown to be excluded from the brain,
but it has yet to be demonstrated whether exclusion from the brain
or spinal cord bears any relation to the peripheral neuropathy which
seems to be an effect mainly on distal nerve fibres.   Methods for
assessing neurotoxicity in animals are still one of our biggest
handicaps in the search for better radiosensitizers.   The nerve
conduction velocity studies of Hirst et al. (22, 23) may have been
compromised by the alteration in body temperature that accompanies
administration of some of these drugs.   This assay failed to show
misonidazole as being more neurotoxic than metronidazole, although
a threefold difference is believed to exist in man.   This failure
may have been for technical reasons, or because nerve conduction
velocity, a motor nerve endpoint, is a poor measure of sensory nerve
alterations.   Alternatively, it may be that in this respect the
mouse is a poor model for man.   Other studies have involved
behavioural tests (e.g. swimming ability of goldfish, ability of
mice to stay on an accelerating rotating rod or to walk along a

narrowing plank, ability of chickens to walk up ladders, the degree
of foot splay when a mouse is suddenly dropped) and histological and
histochemical assessments of damage in nerve biopsies.   Of these
assays the histochemical assessment of lysosomal damage (24) and the
narrowing plank test (Sheldon, unpublished) seem to give the most
quantitative dose response data, but they have not yet been very
widely applied.

From the point of view of testing for radiosensitizing ability,
the in vivo skin clone system is still one of the most rapid and
highly quantitative techniques for looking at an artificially hypoxic
tissue.   Skin is made acutely hypoxic by giving the mice nitrogen to
breathe for 30 seconds before irradiation.   The survival of individual epidermal cells can be scored 12-21 days later when they appear
as macroscopic clones.   This system was used in the early sensitizer
studies of NDPP, metronidazole and misonidazole (25, 26) and is still
used as one of the first in vivo assays at the Gray Laboratory.   It
produces results within 3 weeks, allows sensitization to be measured
without any influence of hypoxic cell cytotoxicity, and allows many
different compounds or different drug doses to be intercompared within
one experiment.   Because 5 islands are scored on each mouse, five
mice give reasonable statistics and a dose response curve can be con-
structed using only 15-20 mice.   The data produced from one batch
of 160 mice (i.e. one experiment) is shown as an example in Figure
12.   It is obvious that all of the compounds tested can give sensitization of the anoxic skin at least half way towards the oxic sensitivity.   When trying to rank the compounds to select a more promising clinical alternative to misonidazole the difficulty arises in
deciding what toxicity to use to calculate a therapeutic index.
This is illustrated in Table 4 for seven compounds recently tested
using skin clone assay.

In the skin clone assay the timing of drug administration
relative to irradiation is probably not very critical because all
basal epidermal cells are close to the capillary bed;   irradiation
is therefore performed shortly after the peak drug concentration has
been achieved in blood (usually at about 10 minutes after intraperitoneal administration).   When we are interested in the hypoxic
cells in tumours, however, the optimum time interval may be longer
and will need to be determined for an appropriate intercomparison of
compounds to be possible.   Thus extensive radiobiology and pharmacology data of the kind shown in Figure 13 will be necessary.   The
time course of sensitization and the time course of the blood and
tumour concentrations have both been measured.   For drug concentrations the tumour is minced up and the drug extracted for HPLC determinations.   This is a measure of the concentration in the tumour
as a whole and may sometimes be a poor indication of the concentration in the critical 10-20% of hypoxic cells.   It is to be expected
that the concentration in these hypoxic cells may rise later than in

Table 4.   Ranking Order of some Compounds Tested as Hypoxic Cell
            Radiosensitizers using the Epidermal Clone Assay

Rank	Maximum SER Observed	SER Observed for 0.4 mg/g	SER at 200 ug/ml in blood	Therapeutic Ratio LD_{50} dose/dose to give SER = 1.6
1	Ro-03-8799	Ro-03-8799	Ro-03-8799	Ro-12-5272
2	Misonidazole	Misonidazole	Ro-12-5272	Ro-03-8800
3	Ro-12-5272	Ro-12-5272	Misonidazole	Ro-03-8799
4	Ro-03-8800	Ro-03-8800	Ro-03-8800	Misonidazole
5	Ro-05-9963	Ro-05-9963	Ro-05-9963	Ro-05-9963
6	Nimorazole	Nimorazole	Nimorazole	Nimorazole
7	Metronidazole	(Metronidazole)	Metronidazole	Metronidazole

For further details of the Roche compounds see refs. 19 and 27.

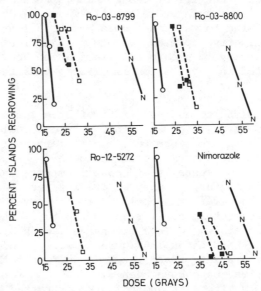

Fig. 12.   Epidermal clone regrowth after irradiation with X-rays
            alone or with 4 different radiosensitizers. O = irradiat-
            ions in oxygen. N = irradiations in nitrogen, without drug
            □ = irradiations in nitrogen after 0.4 mg/g of each drug.
            ■ = irradiations in nitrogen after administering half the
            LD_{50} dose. (Denekamp, unpublished).

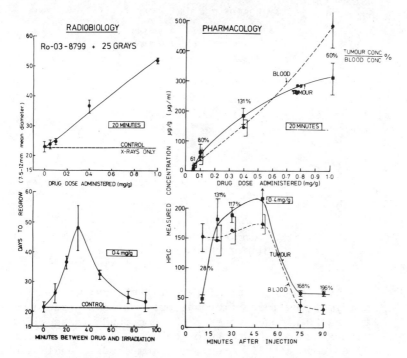

Fig. 13. The response of a mouse fibrosarcoma to Ro-03 8799 plus
         2500 rads (25Gy), as a function of dose or time interval
         between injection and irradiation.   Blood and tumour
         concentrations measured by HPLC are indicated in the
         right-hand panels.   Although tumour levels stay high
         for 50 minutes the maximum sensitization is observed at
         30 minutes (Randhawa, Denekamp, Stewart, Stratford and
         Michinton, unpublished).

the tumour bulk since they lie at a greater diffusion distance from
the blood vessels.   However, the extent of this delay is un-
predictable and will vary with lipophilicity and with the packing
fraction of cells in the particular tumour (i.e. the ratio of cell
mass to intercellular fluid).

    Even when the enhancement ratios have been determined for
several drug dose levels in a tumour, it is difficult to know how
to intercompare these.   It can be done as a function of the drug
dose administered, either on a micromolar basis or in relation to
the acute LD_{50}, as shown in Figure 14, or on the basis of the
tumour concentration that is achieved as shown in Figure 15.   When
compared in terms of administered dose or measured tumour concentration, the four compounds appeared similarly effective, although all
three new compounds had been predicted to give a greater therapeutic
index in vitro (27).   When related to the acute LD_{50} values for
single doses, the three newer Roche compounds all appeared to be less
effective than misonidazole.   It is obvious that the acute 7 day

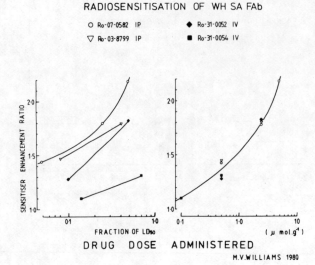

RADIOSENSITISATION OF WH SA FAb

○ Ro-07-0582 IP   ◆ Ro-31-0052 IV
▽ Ro-03-8799 IP   ■ Ro-31-0054 IV

M.V.WILLIAMS 1980

Fig. 14. SER values for four different drugs tested using regrowth
          delay of the mouse fibrosarcoma.   When plotted relative
          to the LD_{50} dose, none of the compounds is as efficient as
          misonidazole.   When plotted as a function of molarity
          (i.e. dose administered), the compounds are all similar in
          effectiveness. (Williams and Denekamp, unpublished).

LD_{50} will not be the appropriate clinical toxicity for such an intercomparison of data, but at present a more appropriate set of toxicity
data is not available for these compounds.

     Another aspect of radiosensitizers that has recently become of
great interest is their specific hypoxic cell cytotoxicity in the
absence of radiation (28, 29, 30).   This cytotoxicity cannot readily
be demonstrated in mouse tumours by simply giving a dose of the
appropriate drug;   even if it killed every cell in the hypoxic 10% of
the population, the tumour would continue to grow from the unaffected
90% of oxic cells.   Thus in order to demonstrate cytotoxicity, the
drug is usually given shortly after irradiation, so that the oxic
cells are killed by the radiation and the hypoxic cells by the drug.
Figure 16 summarises the Gray Laboratory data using regrowth delay
as an assay for cytotoxicity.   The cytotoxic effect is apparent in
some tumours, but not all, and is always much smaller than the radiosensitizing effect, indicating that not all of the hypoxic cells are
being killed.

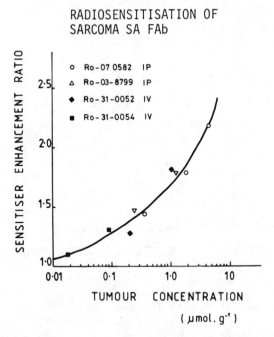

Fig. 15. SER values for four compounds expressed as a function of
the measured tumour concentrations.   All four appear
similar in effectiveness.   (Williams, Minchinton,
Randhawa, Stewart and Stratford, unpublished).

This poor result in mice could result from the rather short
drug exposure time in mice because of the short half-life of misonidazole (0.75 - 1.5 hours), or to the limited exposure under hypoxic
conditions because of hypoxic death, reoxygenation, or cyclic opening
and closing of blood vessels.

If such a direct cytotoxic action of misonidazole were more
effective in man (where the $T_{\frac{1}{2}}$ = 12–18 hours and there is therefore
a longer exposure time), then this would be of great clinical
significance.   The hypoxic cells in tumours are probably the same
as, or a subpopulation of, the chemoresistant cells that are in the
non-proliferative state because of nutrient depletion.   This
aspect of nitroimidazoles is being investigated in several labora-
tories at present.   Some recent results from the Gray Laboratory
for misonidazole used together with melphalan, adriamycin or
bleomycin, are illustrated in Figures 17 and 18.   With melphalan, a
large degree of additional tumour cell kill has been observed, as was

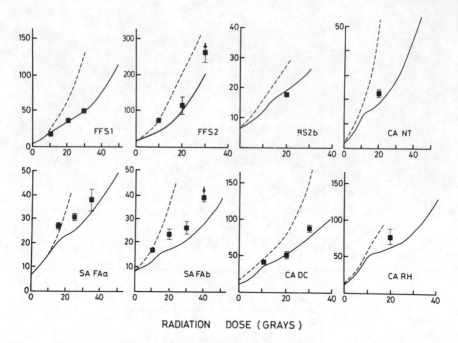

RADIATION   DOSE (GRAYS)

Fig. 16. Regrowth delay data for ten types of tumour irradiated
with X-rays alone (solid lines) or with X-rays after
misonidazole (dashed lines).   The data points shown
were obtained when misonidazole was given 5 minutes _after_
irradiation and illustrates the cytotoxic action of this
drug in some but not all of the tumours (6).

previously reported by Rose et al. (31).   With bleomycin and
adriamycin, no significant increase in tumour growth delay was
observed.   For cyclophosphamide (not shown), an intermediate,
moderate effect was observed (Randhawa and Denekamp, unpublished).

It now appears that misonidazole is a useful experimental tool
and first generation clinical radiosensitizer, but the search for
better compounds must continue.

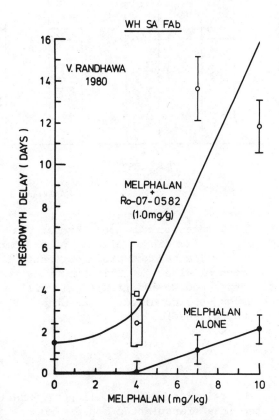

Fig. 17. Regrowth delay of a mouse fibrosarcoma treated with melphalan alone or in combination with misonidazole. Although the tumour is resistant to melphalan alone a large effect is seen with the combination (Randhawa, Stewart and Denekamp, unpublished).

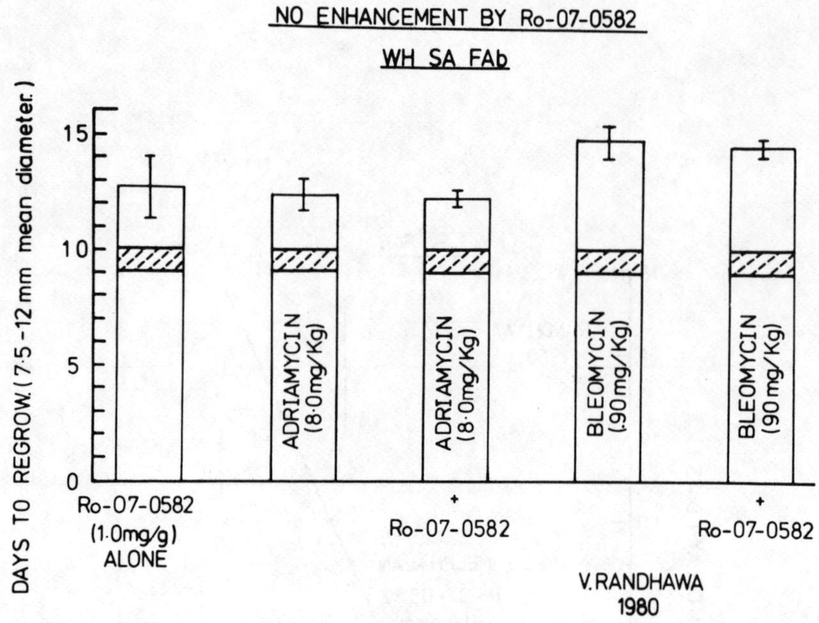

Fig. 18.   Regrowth delay data for a mouse fibrosarcoma treated with
           misonidazole, adriamycin or bleomycin, or combination of
           these drugs.   The hatched area represents the time for
           untreated control mice.   This tumour is resistant to
           all three drugs and no additional cell kill was observed
           when the drugs were combined.   (Randhawa, Stewart and
           Denekamp, unpublished).

REFERENCES

1. I. F. Tannock, The relation between cell proliferation and the
    vascular system in a transplanted mouse mammary tumour, Brit.
    J. Cancer 22:258 (1968).
2. D. G. Hirst, and J. Denekamp, Tumour cell proliferation in
    relation to the vasculature, Cell and Tissue Kinet. 12:31
    (1979).
3. R. H. Thomlinson, and L. H. Gray, The histological structure
    of some human lung cancers and the possible implications for
    radiotherapy, Brit. J. Cancer 9:539 (1955).
4. R. H. Thomlinson, Oxygen Therapy: Biological Considerations, in
    "Modern Trends in Radiotherapy", T. Deeley and C. P. Wood,
    eds., Butterworths (1967).
5. J. Denekamp, and J. F. Fowler, Cell proliferation kinetics and
    radiation therapy, in "Cancer: A Comprehensive Treatise",
    Vol. 6, ch. 4, F. F. Becker, ed., Plenum, New York and
    London (1977).

6. J. Denekamp, D. G. Hirst, F. A. Stewart, and N. H. A. Terry, Is tumour radiosensitization by misonidazole a general phenomenon? Brit. J. Cancer 41:1 (1980).

7. R. H. Thomlinson, S. Dische, A.J. Gray, and L. M. Errington, Clinical testing of the radiosensitizer Ro-07 0582. III. Response of tumours, Clinical Radiol. 27:167 (1976).

8. D. V. Ash, M. J. Peckham, and G. G. Steel, A quantitative study of human tumour response to radiation and misonidazole, Brit. J. Cancer 39:503 (1979).

9. J. Denekamp, J. F. Fowler, and S. Dische, The proportion of hypoxic cells in a human tumor, Int. J. Radiat. Oncol. Biol. Phys. 2:1227 (1977).

10. J. F. Fowler, and J. Denekamp, A review of hypoxic cell radio-sensitization in experimental tumors, Pharmacol. and Therap. 7:413 (1979).

11. J. Denekamp, Is any single in situ assay of tumour response adequate? Brit. J. Cancer 41:Suppl. IV, 56 (1980).

12. J. Denekamp, Experimental tumor systems: standardization of end-points, Int. J. Radiat. Oncol. Biol. Phys. 5:1175 (1979).

13. P. W. Sheldon and S.A. Hill, Hypoxic cell radiosensitizers and tumour control by X-ray of a transplanted tumour in mice, Brit. J. Cancer 35:795 (1977).

14. S. Dische, M. I. Saunders, M. E. Lee, G. E. Adams, and I. R. Flockhart, Clinical testing of the radiosensitizer Ro-07 0582: experience with multiple doses, Brit. J. Cancer 35:567 (1977).

15. J. Denekamp, N.J. McNally, J. F. Fowler, and M. C. Joiner, Misonidazole in fractionated radiotherapy: little and often? Brit. J. Radiol. (in press).

16. R. Urtasun, P. Band, J. D. Chapman, M. L. Feldstein, B. Mielke, and C. Fryer, Radiation and high dose metronidazole (Flagyl) in supratentorial glioblastomas, New England J. Med. 294: 1364 (1976).

17. L. J. Shukovsky, Dose, time, volume relationships in squamous cell carcinoma of the supraglottic larynx, Am. J. Roentgen 108:27 (1970).

18. P. Workman, Effects of pretreatment with phenobarbitone and phenotoin on the pharmacokinetics and toxicity of misoni-dazole, Brit. J. Cancer 40:335 (1979).

19, G.E. Adams, E. D. Clarke, I. R. Flockhart, R. S. Jacobs, D. S. Sehmi, I. J. Stratford, P. Wardman, M. E. Watts, J. Parrick, R. G. Wallace, and C. E. Smithen, Structure-activity relationships in the development of hypoxic cell radio-sensitizers. I. Sensitization efficiency, Int. J. Radiat. Biol. 35: 133 (1979).

20. P. Wardman, The use of nitroaromatic compounds as hypoxic cell radiosensitizers, Curr. Top. Radiat. Res. Quart. 11:347 (1977).

21. J. M. Brown, and P. Workman, Partition coefficient as a guide to the development of radiosensitizers which are less toxic than misonidazole, Radiat. Res. 82:171 (1980).

22. D. G. Hirst, B. Vojnovic, I. J. Stratford, and E. L. Travis, The effect of the radiosensitizer misonidazole on motor nerve conduction velocity in the mouse, Brit. J. Cancer 37 Suppl. III, 237 (1978).

23. D. G. Hirst, B. Vojnovic, and B. Hobson, Changes in nerve conduction velocity in the mouse after acute and chronic administration of nitroimidazoles, Brit. J. Cancer 39:159 (1979).

24. C. Clarke, K. B. Dawson, P. W. Sheldon, D. J. Chaplin, I. J. Stratford, and G. E. Adams, A quantitative cytochemical method for assessing the neurotoxicity of misonidazole, in "Radiation Sensitizers: Their use in the Clinical Management of Cancer", L. W. Brady, ed., Masson Publishing Inc., New York (1980).

25. J. Denekamp, and B.D. Michael, Preferential sensitization of hypoxic cells to radiation in vivo, Nature New Biol. 239: 21 (1972).

26. J. Denekamp, B. D. Michael, and S. R. Harris, Hypoxic cell radiosensitizers: comparative tests of some electron affinic compounds using epidermal cell survival in vivo, Radiat. Res. 60:119 (1974).

27. C. E. Smithen, E. D. Clarke, J. A. Dale, R. S. Jacobs, P. Wardman, M. E. Watts, and M. Woodcock, Novel (nitro-1-imidazolyl) alkanolamines as potential radio-sensitizers with improved therapeutic properties, Cancer Clin. Trials (in press).

28. N. M. Bleehen, D. Honess, and J. Morgan, The interaction of hyperthermia and the hypoxic cell sensitizer Ro-07 0582 on the EMT 6 mouse tumour, Brit. J. Cancer, 35:299 (1977).

29. G. E. Adams, J. F. Fowler, and P. Wardman, eds½. Hypoxic cell sensitizers in radiobiology and radiotherapy, Brit. J. Cancer 37, Suppl. III (1978).

30. I. J. Stratford, and G.E. Adams, The toxicity of the radio-sensitizer misonidazole towards hypoxic cells in vitro: a model for mouse and man, Brit. J. Radiol. 51:745 (1978).

31. C. M. Rose, J. L. Millar, J. H. Peacock, T. A. Phelps, and T. C. Stephens, Differential enhancement of melphalan cyto-toxicity in tumor and normal tissue by misonidazole, Cancer Clin. Trials (in press).

LIPOPHILICITY AND THE PHARMACOKINETICS OF NITROIMIDAZOLES

Paul Workman

MRC Clinical Oncology and Radiotherapeutics Unit
The Medical School, Hills Road
Cambridge CB2 2QH, England

INTRODUCTION

The processes of absorption, distribution and elimination are vitally important in all drug therapy, for collectively they determine the drug concentrations present at the sites of toxic and therapeutic effects. Pharmacokinetic considerations are especially critical for drugs with low therapeutic ratios, e.g. antineoplastic agents. The pharmacokinetics of nitroimidazole radiosensitizers have been reviewed recently [1]. Considerable evidence now shows that all aspects of the pharmacokinetics of nitroimidazoles (as for other drugs) are strongly influenced by lipophilicity. The aim in this paper is to discuss the pharmacokinetics of nitroimidazole drugs with particular emphasis on this important property.

LIPOPHILICITY AND PARTITION COEFFICIENT

The lipophilicity of a drug measures its relative solubility in water and lipid. It is assessed from the drug's partitioning properties between an aqueous phase (water or buffer) and an immiscible organic phase, usually octanol, which is a model for lipid [2] (Fig. 1). The drug is dissolved in one phase, the two phases are then shaken until equilibrium is reached, and finally the concentrations of the drug in the two phases are determined. The partition coefficient P is given by : $P = \dfrac{\text{concentration in octanol}}{\text{concentration in water}}$. Referring to Fig. 1, drug A favours the organic phase, has a large partition coefficient (P=100) and is said to be lipophilic. Drug B favours the aqueous phase, has a small partition coefficient (P=0.01) and is less lipophilic or more hydrophilic than A. Thus a series of drugs can be ranked for lipophilicity using P values.

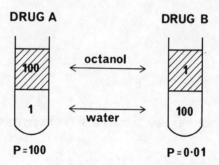

Fig. 1.   Measurement of lipophilicity by octanol/water partition
          coefficient. P = concentration in octanol/concentration in
          water (or buffer). Drug A is <u>lipophilic</u> (more affinity for
          lipid); drug B is <u>hydrophilic</u> (more affinity for water).

     The molecular bonding mechanisms responsible for partitioning
behaviour are complex and incompletely understood. A major factor
is the removal of the ordered sheath of water molecules which
surrounds lipophilic drugs in aqueous solution - the disordered
state has lower energy.   Hydrophilic drugs contain predominantly
groups which are polar and undergo hydrophilic interactions, such
as hydrogen bonding.   These include hydroxyl, carboxyl, amide and
amine groups.   In contrast, lipophilic drugs contain mainly non-
polar groups which participate in <u>hydrophobic</u> interactions. These
include alkyl (e.g. CH_3, C_2H_5) and aryl (e.g. phenyl) moieties.

     The structures and partition coefficients of selected nitro-
imidazoles are given in Table 1 with data for some other anticancer
agents for comparison. Misonidazole has a P value of O.43, indicating
a roughly two-fold greater affinity for the aqueous phase. P for
nitroimidazoles depends on the position of the nitro group (e.g.
5-nitroimidazoles are more lipophilic than equivalent 2-nitroimida-
zoles) and on the polarity of the ring substituents (8).   The
effects of ring substituents can be predicted accurately using the
substituent constant π_x (8).   For essentially unionised drugs P is
independent of the pH of the aqueous phase. For ionisable drugs
the pH is controlled to prevent ionisation and P is the value for the
unionised form. Another parameter is often quoted for ionised drugs,
P*.   This is given by P x the fraction unionised at pH 7.4 or is
determined experimentally at this pH.

MEMBRANE STRUCTURE

Why is lipophilicity so important in determining pharmacokinetic behaviour? This is best explained with a brief look at membrane structure (9). The precise composition varies with cell type, but in general mammalian cell memgranes consist of lipid (20-40% dry weight), protein (60-75%) and carbohydrate as glycolipid and glyco-protein (1-10%). About 20% of the total weight is bound water. Most of the lipid is phospholipid, such as phosphatidylcholine (lecithin) shown below.

$$CH_3-N^+-CH_2-CH_2-O-P-O-CH_2$$

with CH_3, CH_3 groups on nitrogen and O^-, O on phosphorus

$$CH-O-C-CH_2-CH_2-CH_2-CH_2-CH_2-CH_2-CH_2-CH=CH-CH_2$$
$$CH_2-O-CH=CH-CH_2-CH_2-CH_2-CH_2-CH_2-CH_2$$

Hydrophilic head

$$CH_3-CH_2-CH_2-CH_2-CH_2-CH_2-CH_2-CH_2-CH_2$$

Lipophilic tail

$$CH_2, CH_2, CH_2, CH_2$$
$$CH_3-CH_2-CH_2-CH_2$$

The hydrophilic head group and lipophilic hydrocarbon chain are characteristic.

Fig. 2 shows the widely accepted fluid mosaic model for cell membrane structure (10). The membrane is a fluid or dynamic mosaic structure consisting of globular proteins in a lipid bilayer matrix, with a thickness of about 100 Å.

LIPOPHILICITY AND MEMBRANE PERMEABILITY

Most drugs cross cell membranes by simple passive diffusion. This process follows first-order kinetics, i.e. the rate is propor-tional to the concentration gradient across the membrane. Classic studies have established that penetration rate is determined by partition coefficient, with lipophilic drugs penetrating faster than hydrophilic ones (11). For ionised drugs, the penetration rate is governed by the partition coefficient of the unionised form and P* is used in place of P. Thus for drug penetration, the rate-limiting feature is the lipophilic lipid bilayer which confers the property of selective permeability on the membrane.

Little information is available on the entry of nitroimidazoles into isolated cells, although the uptake of metronidazole by tricho-monads is by passive diffusion (12). However, there is evidence on their penetration through certain tissue boundaries which exhibit the selective permeability characteristics of lipoid cell membranes.

TABLE 1

Partition Coefficients of Radiosensitizers and Other Anticancer Agents

Data from refs. 3-7.

CLASS	COMPOUND	STRUCTURE	OCTANOL/AQUEOUS PARTITION COEFFICIENT P	P*
	Ro 07-1127	$R = CH_2CH(OH)CH_2O$⟨phenyl⟩	31	
	Ro 03-8799	$R = CH_2CH(OH)CH_2$⟨ring⟩	8.5	(0.14)
	Benznidazole (Ro 07-1051)	$R = CH_2CONHCH_2$⟨phenyl⟩	8.2	
	Ro 07-1052	$R = CH_2CH(OH)CH_2OCH(CH_3)_2$	3.2	
	Ro 07-0913	$R = CH_2CH(OH)CH_2OCH_2CH_3$	1.3	
2-nitroimidazoles	Misonidazole (Ro 07-0582)	$R = CH_2CH(OH)CH_2OCH_3$	0.43	
	Ro 07-0741	$R = CH_2CH(OH)CH_2F$	0.41	
	Desmethylmisonidazole (Ro 05-9963)	$R = CH_2CH(OH)CH_2OH$	0.13	
	SR-2508	$R = CH_2CONHCH_2CH_2OH$	0.046	
	SR-2555	$R = CH_2CON(CH_2CH_2OH)_2$	0.026	
	SR-2530	$R = CH_2CONHCH_2CH(OH)CH_2OH$	0.014	
5-nitroimidazoles	Metronidazole	$R_1 = CH_2CH_2OH; \quad R_2 = CH_3$	0.96	
	Nimorazole	$R_1 = CH_2CH_2N$⟨morpholine⟩$O, \quad R_2 = H$	1.4	

(Structures: 2-nitroimidazole ring with R substituent at N1 and NO_2 at C2; 5-nitroimidazole ring with R_1 at N1, R_2 at C2, and O_2N at C5.)

TABLE 1 (continued)

	Structure	Value	
4-Nitroacetophenone	O_2N—⟨benzene⟩—$COCH_3$	31	
CCNU		280-630	
BCNU		25	
Cyclophosphamide		4.3	
Cytotoxics Chlorambucil	Various (Non-nitro)	2.0	(0.049)
5-Fluorouracil		0.10	
Methotrexate		0.028	(0.003)
Arabinosylcytosine		0.0074	

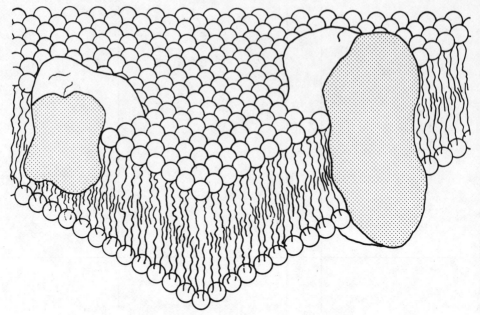

Fig. 2.   Cross-section of a cell membrane according to the fluid
          mosaic model (redrawn from Ref. 10). The phospholipids
          form a bilayer with the polar head groups facing the
          aqueous environment and the hydrophobic tails sequestered.
          Membrane proteins are also shown.

     Cell-cell junctions in vertebrates can be classified into two
broad categories (13). In one (adherens junction) the membranes of
adjacent cells are separated by a 150-350 Å space, which permits
diffusion between cells.   In the other (occludens junction) the
adjacent membranes are in direct contact.   The extreme form of the
latter is the tight junction (zonula occludens) in which a belt is
formed which entirely surrounds each cell.   Drug penetration across
a layer of such cells can only occur by diffusion through the cells,
and a selective permeability barrier is thereby formed.   Tight
junctions are found at important selective permeability barrier
sites (13,14); those of immediate interest are shown in Table 2.

     We can now illustrate how lipophilicity influences the penetra-
tion of nitroimidazoles through these barriers.   It is to be
emphasised that they are selective and not absolute permeability
barriers.

Blood-CSF barrier

     This is formed by the epithelial cells of the choroid plexus
in the brain. Fig. 3 shows data from White and co-workers (16-18)

TABLE 2.   Important Selective Permeability Barrier Sites in the
           Body (see Refs 6, 13-15).

Cells with tight junctions	Selective Permeability Barrier
Endothelium of cerebral capillaries	Blood-brain
Epithelium of choroid plexus	Blood-CSF
Endothelium of capillaries in endoneurium of peripheral nerves	Blood-peripheral nerves
Epithelium of gastro-intestinal tract	Surface of lumen
Peritoneal membrane	Surface of peritoneal cavity
Epithelium of renal tubules and bladder	Surface of lumen

for the penetration of neutral nitroimidazoles into CSF from plasma
in the dog.   The data are plotted so that the slopes give the rates
of penetration.   The most lipophilic, misonidazole, penetrates
CSF 20 times more rapidly than the most hydrophilic, SR-2555.   The
linearity of the plots indicates first-order kinetics.

Blood-brain barrier

     This is formed by the endothelial cells of the vascular
capillaries in the brain. Fig. 4 (closed circles) shows data for
the penetration of a number of neutral nitroimidazoles into mouse
brain as a function of partition coefficient (3,19). Data are
plotted as the brain/plasma ratios for the areas under the curves
(AUCs) of concentration x time, a measure of drug exposure. At P
values of 0.43 and greater, the ratios are constant at 80-100%.
There is no tendency to concentrate in brain even at quite high P
values.   However, at values < 0.43 a progressive exclusion is seen.
Thus, as for CSF, the more lipophilic nitroimidazoles penetrate the
brain more effectively than those more hydrophilic.   Similar results
were obtained in dogs (17,18) where, for example, brain AUCs for
desmethylmisonidazole and SR-2508 were lower than misonidazole by
factors of 2 and 5 respectively (after correction for differences
in plasma clearance).   The importance of lipophilicity for blood-
brain barrier penetration is known for other classes of drugs
(6,11).   For example, the highly lipophilic nitrosourea CCNU enters
the brain far more effectively than hydrophilic cytotoxic drugs such
as the antimetabolite methotrexate (P values, Table 1).

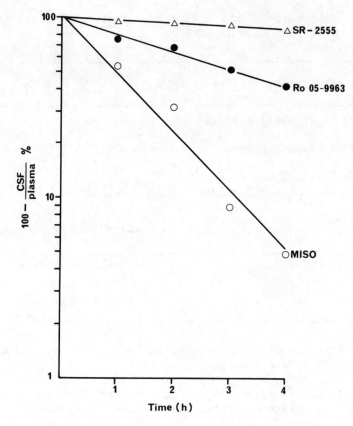

Fig. 3.   Penetration of nitroimidazoles into CSF from plasma in the
          dog.   Data from Refs 16-18.

Blood-peripheral nerve barrier

This is formed by the endothelial cells of the capillaries
supplying the endoneurium.   Peripheral nerves are also protected
by the outer layers of the perineurium.   Exclusion of hydrophilic
nitroimidazoles from peripheral nerves, similar to that seen for
brain, has been observed in dogs (17,18) and mice (Brown, J.M.,
personal communication).

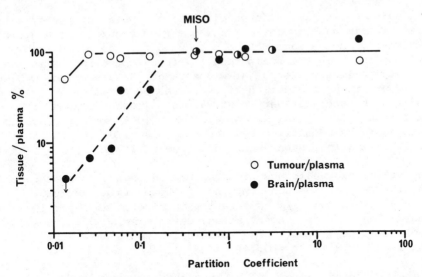

Fig. 4. Effect of lipophilicity on the penetration of nitroimidazoles into brain and EMT6 tumour in BALB/c mice. Data
from Refs 3 and 19.

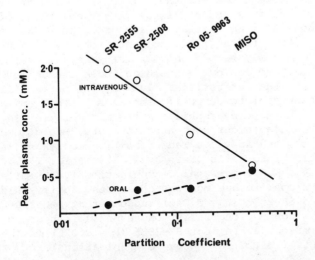

Fig. 5. Effect of lipophilicity on peak plasma nitroimidazoles after
oral and intravenous administration in the dog. Values
normalised to a dose of 0.5 mmoles/kg. Data from Refs 16-18.

Blood-tumour barrier

Also shown in Fig. 4 (open circles) are data for penetration of
neutral nitroimidazoles into EMT6 mammary adenocarcinomata grown
intradermally in the same BALB/c mice used for the brain study (3,
19).   Compared with the brain results, tumour penetration is independent of lipophilicity over a far wider range (P values from 0.026-
3.1).   There is an indication of decreased penetration at P values
< 0.026 and possibly at very high values.   Tumour/plasma ratios
equal to, or better than, misonidazole (80-100%) were also observed
with the more hydrophilic drugs desmethylmisonidazole, SR-2508 and
SR-2555 in various spontaneous dog tumours (17,18).

.Misonidazole analogues with basic side-chains have attracted
recent interest.   One such compound, the piperidine derivative
Ro 03-8799 gives tumour/plasma ratios in mice of at least 100%, with
an indication of some concentration, despite being 95% ionised at
physiological pH (19,20).   The unionised base is, however, very
lipophilic (P = 8.5; P* = 0.14).

The clear indication is that essentially no permeability
barrier exists for penetration of nitroimidazoles into the gross
tissue of tumours over a wide range of lipophilicity.   The blood
capillaries supplying the tumour, in common with non-barrier sites
in normal tissues (e.g. liver, kidney, muscle) have fenestrations
or perforations (i.e. they are 'leaky') allowing free diffusion
through spaces between the endothelial cells.   It should be remem-
bered, however, that assays of tissue levels do not discriminate
between intracellular and extracellular drug, but measure the tissue
as a whole.   Interstitial fluid accounts for 16% of the total body
weight in man, and may be much higher for some tumours.   Thus it
would be possible to achieve quite high whole tissue levels with a
drug confined to the interstitial fluid by the permeability barrier
imposed by individual tumour cell membranes.   This appears to happen
with SR-2530, the most hydrophilic nitroimidazole in Fig. 4 (P =
0.014).   The whole tumour concentrations are 2-fold lower than the
other analogues, and in vitro radiosensitization experiments suggest
poor penetration into cells (Refs 3,21; Stratford, I.J., Anderson,
R.F., and Patel, K.B., personal communications).   Similar studies
with other hydrophilic analogues such as desmethylmisonidazole
(P = 0.13) and SR-2508 (P = 0.046) suggest that penetration to
critical sites controlling radiation response in hypoxic cells is as
good as with misonidazole, but SR-2555 (P = 0.026) may be a border-
line case (Refs 3,21,22, and above communications).

Barrier at gastro-intestinal tract

Drugs administered orally are absorbed through the gastrointestinal tract, mainly the small intestine and stomach.   Hydrophilic nitroimidazoles are absorbed more slowly and less completely

than misonidazole (16-18). For example in the dog, the oral bioavailability (AUC oral(AUC i.v.) was 92% for misonidazole, 56% for
desmethylmisonidazole and only 19% for SR-2555. Peak plasma concentration is more important for radiosensitization than AUC, and
Fig. 5 shows that whereas i.v. peaks increase as lipophilicity is
reduced (see later) the oral peaks are considerably decreased.

Barrier at peritoneal membrane

The intraperitoneal route is widely used in small animal studies.
Absorption occurs across the large surface of the peritoneal membrane.
This also exhibits selective permeability barrier characteristics
with hydrophilic nitroimidazoles, such as SR-2555, absorbed much
more slowly and achieving lower peak plasma concentrations than
misonidazole (3).

Barrier at the renal tubules

Urinary excretion is an important route for drug elimination.
After filtration of plasma at the glomerulus, reabsorption into the
plasma occurs from the proximal and distal tubules, the epithelia
of which form a selective permeability barrier. Therefore,
reabsorption efficiency increases with lipophilicity. This is well
illustrated in Fig. 6, which shows the relationship between the%
the drug dose excreted unchanged in the urine of various species as
a function of partition coefficient. For the more lipophilic
(P 1.3) only 1% or less is excreted in this way. The amount
increases as lipophilicity decreases so that for the most hydrophilic,
SR-2555, (P = 0.046) 80-100% is excreted unchanged in the urine.
For misonidazole and metronidazole the figure is 5-20%.

LIPOPHILICITY AND METABOLISM

Virtually no administered nitroimidazole is recovered unchanged
in the faeces (26). As a result, the analogues whose lipophilicity
prevents efficient excretion by the kidneys are dependent on metabolism to more polar species for their elimination. Thus, Fig. 6
also illustrates the relationship between lipophilicity and the%
of the drug dose metabolised, which is estimated by subtracting
the % excreted unchanged in the urine from 100%.

The main metabolic routes for nitroimidazoles are oxidation,
conjugation and reduction. Most drug oxidations are catalysed by
hepatic microsomal mixed-function oxidases. For many drugs, the
processes of uptake into liver cells, binding to the hydrophobic
cytochrome P450 enzyme site located in the lipoid membrane of the
endoplasmic reticulum, and rate of metabolism are all dependent on
partition coefficient (28,29). This also appears to be true for
the metabolism of misonidazole analogues in vivo, the rate increasing
with increased lipophilicity (19). For example, in mice the

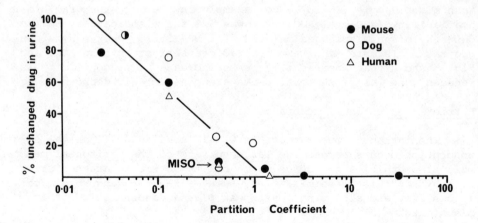

Fig. 6.   Effect of lipophilicity on the urinary excretion of
          unchanged nitroimidazoles.   mouse (data from refs
          19,23,24),   dog (refs 16-18, 25),   human (refs
          26,27, and Dische, S. et al., personal communication).

analogue Ro 07-0913 (O-ethyl-replacing O-methyl in the side chain;
P = 1.3) is metabolised about three times faster than misonidazole
(P = 0.43)(19).

     Drugs administered orally and intraperitoneally pass through
the portal circulation and the liver before reaching the systemic
circulation (15,30). For very lipophilic drugs with high hepatic
extraction ratios (rapid uptake and metabolism) systemic availability
can be severaly restricted by metabolism on the first-pass through
the liver (and gut for oral route)(30).   This is seen with certain
highly lipophilic nitroimidazoles (P > 10) (19).

     The metabolism of lipophilic nitroimidazoles, e.g. demethylation
of misonidazole, can be speeded up by pretreating animals or patients
with certain agents, notably phenobarbitone or phenytoin, which
increase the levels of hepatic microsomal enzymes (23,31).

LIPOPHILICITY AND SYSTEMIC PHARMACOKINETICS

     The sequence of steps between drug administration and biological
effect involves a series of membrane transitions (Fig. 7). In view
of the foregoing discussion, it is not surprising that lipophilicity
profoundly affects systemic pharmacokinetics.   Some important
effects of lipophilicity are summarised in Table 3.

     Systemic pharmacokinetic studies usually involve predictions
of tissue concentrations from blood or plasma concentrations.

TABLE 3.   Some Important Effects of Lipophilicity on Nitroimidazole
           Pharmacokinetics.
           (Changes in lipophilicity are made relative to misonida-
           zole as standard.)

Pharmacokinetic Property	Effect of Lipophilicity
Oral absorption	Rate and extent reduced with decreased lipophilicity. May also be reduced by poor aqueous solubility and first-pass metabolism of very lipophilic analogues.
Peak plasma concentration - oral	Reduced with decreased lipophilicity.
- intravenous	Increased with decreased lipophilicity.
Tumour/plasma ratios	Constant over a wide range.
Nervous tissue/plasma ratios	Reduced with decreased lipophilicity.
Metabolic clearance	Increased with increased lipophilicity.
Renal clearance	Increased with decreased lipophilicity.
Area under curve (plasma)	Reduced by increased or decreased lipophilicity.

Pharmacokinetic models for nitroimidazoles have been reviewed
previously (1).   Most nitroimidazoles follow the two-compartment
open model (Fig. 8A).   Here, after intravenous injection, the drug
distributes instantaneously in the central compartment, comprising
blood and well-perfused organs such as liver and kidney, from which
elimination occurs.   It distributes more slowly to peripheral
tissues in the distributive or α phase, which is followed by the
terminal, elimination, or β phase.   The plasma decay is
bi-exponential. Highly lipophilic drugs will penetrate tissue cells
so rapidly that blood flow becomes rate-limiting, whereas for
hydrophilic drugs penetration is limited by partition coefficient
(1).

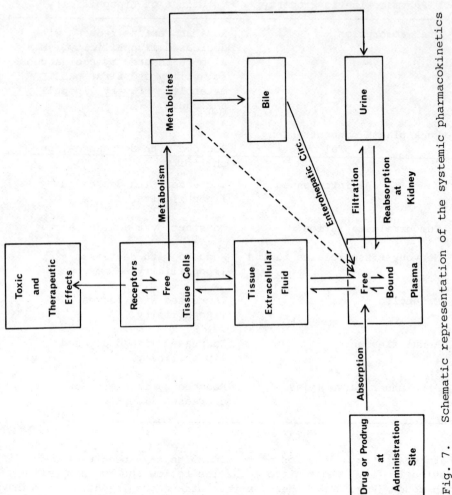

Fig. 7. Schematic representation of the systemic pharmacokinetics of nitroimidazoles.

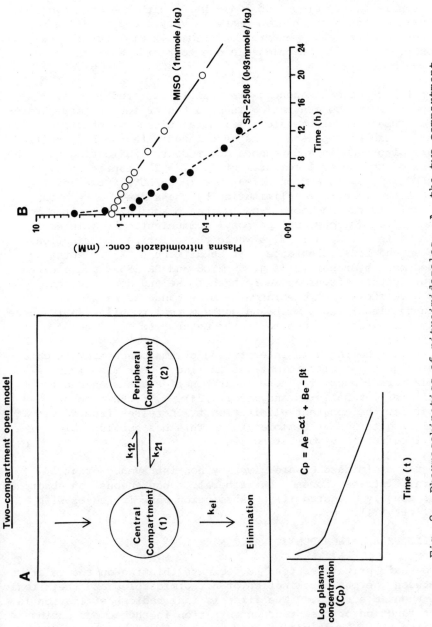

Fig. 8. Pharmacokinetics of nitroimidazoles. A, the two-compartment open model; B, pharmacokinetics of misonidazole and SR-2508 in the dog (18).

Fig. 8B shows data for intravenous misonidazole and SR-2508 in
the dog (18). For the more lipophilic misonidazole the distribution
phase is so rapid it is often undetectable ($t\frac{1}{2}\alpha$ < 2 min) whereas the
elimination is fairly slow ($t\frac{1}{2}\beta$ = 4-5 h). With the more hydrophilic SR-2508 the distributive phase is very pronounced due to
slower peripheral tissue penetration ($t\frac{1}{2}\alpha$ = 12 min) but the terminal
$t\frac{1}{2}$ is shorter than for misonidazole due to rapid renal clearance
($t\frac{1}{2}\beta$ = 2-3 h).

Two important consequences are well illustrated in Fig. 8B.
1) The peak plasma concentration is much higher for the more hydrophilic drug because of the slow peripheral tissue penetration.
Moreover, these high plasma peaks associated with the hydrophilic
drugs are also seen in spontaneous dog tumours, indicating that they
form part of the central compartment (18). 2) Despite this, the
plasma AUC is reduced and the clearance (dose/AUC) increased
because of the more rapid elimination by the kidney. Desmethylmisonidazole is cleared more rapidly than misonidazole in the dog
(17) and in man (Dische, S., personal communication). Interestingly, this is not seen in mice where the relative contributions of
metabolism and renal clearance must be different (19). Other
analogues more hydrophilic (e.g. SR-2508 and SR-2555) are cleared
more rapidly than misonidazole in both mouse and dog. Recent
studies have shown that clearance in mice can also be increased
compared to misonidazole with analogues more lipophilic (19). Here,
more rapid clearance is due to faster metabolism.

Care must be taken in interpreting plasma concentration data
after high doses of nitroimidazoles in mice. For misonidazole and
compounds more lipophilic, non-linear kinetics are seen due to
saturation of metabolising enzymes (19,24). In the case of
misonidazole, the apparent elimination $t\frac{1}{2}$ increases from 40 min at
0.5 mmoles/kg to 3 h at 5 mmoles/kg. This has considerable
implications for in vivo testing (24).

When nitroimidazoles are given by non-intravenous routes
(e.g. oral, intraperitoneal, intrathecal, subcutaneous) an absorption
phase is usually detected (1). Absorption rate increases with
lipophilicity (1).

LIPOPHILICITY AND THERAPEUTIC RATIO

Two basic principles tend to dominate thinking on the relationship between the pharmacokinetics of nitroimidazoles and their toxic
and therapeutic effects. The first is that radiosensitization is
a direct function of the drug concentration in the tumour during
irradiation (32). More recent studies (33) show that the maximum
radiosensitization of EMT6 mouse tumours occurs 30 min after the
peak tumour concentration for both misonidazole and SR-2555. This
suggests a 30 min delay between the whole tumour peak concentration

and the peak in the critical sites in the hypoxic cells. With this
modification the principle is useful, and to improve the therapeutic
ratio of sensitizers one aim should be to increase tumour concentration.

The second principle is that toxicity is related to plasma AUC.
This relationship is indicated for misonidazole acute lethality in
mice (23) and peripheral neuropathy in man (34).   The AUC in the
sites of dose-limiting toxicity, the nervous tissues, is probably
the most critical.   Thus a further aim should be to reduce exposure
to these sites.

With these considerations in mind, we can consider how modification of lipophilicity may influence toxicity, radiosensitization
and, most important of all, therapeutic ratio.

Lipophilicity and toxicity

In the mouse acute LD_{50}s for single doses are much higher for
hydrophilic analogues (e.g. SR-2508) than for misonidazole (3).
In the dog, desmethylmisonidazole is less toxic than misonidazole
after chronic dosage (17). These findings are explained by the
more rapid clearance of the hydrophilic drugs and their exclusion
from nervous tissue.

An alternative strategy towards reducing toxicity would be to
increase lipophilicity to exploit the more rapid metabolism.
Usually, the products of metabolism are more polar and less toxic
than the parent drug.   One example is desmethylmisonidazole compared to misonidazole.   More dramatically, the acute LD_{50} (with
95% confidence limits) for a single intravenous dose of
p-nitrophenol in C3H/He mice is 0.14 (0.11-0.15) mmoles/kg compared
with 2.12 (1.77-2.56) mmoles/kg for its principal metabolite, the
highly polar O-glucuronide conjugate (19).   This represents a
15-fold difference in toxicity.   On the other hand, if normal
tissue toxicity is caused by toxic metabolites, e.g. nitroreduction products (35,36), this may be less successful.

Clinical studies have shown that misonidazole neurotoxicity is
reduced in patients on the anticonvulsants phenobarbitone and
phenytoin and the steroid dexamethasone (31,37). The anticonvulsants
shorten the t½ and reduce the AUC for misonidazole in experimental
animals and in man by induction of demethylation (Fig. 9)(23,31,37).
In mice, the plasma and brain AUCs are reduced but not peak tumour
concentration (23).   Dexamethasone does not alter misonidazole
metabolism; but under certain conditions it reduces the brain AUC
by about 15%, possibly by reduced cerebrovascular permeability (38).
These studies suggest possible mechanisms for the protective
effects of the three agents.

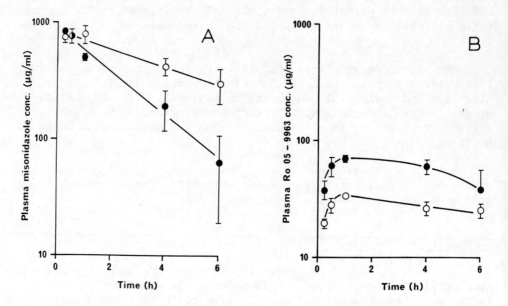

Fig. 9. Effect of phenobarbitone on the pharmacokinetics of
         misonidazole in mice (23).   A, misonidazole; B, metabolite
         Ro 05-9963.   O Control mice, ● Phenobarbitone pretreated.

LIPOPHILICITY, RADIOSENSITIZATION AND THERAPEUTIC RATIO

        There is now good evidence that the therapeutic ratio of nitro-
imidazole radiosensitizers can be improved in experimental systems
by altering lipophilicity (3).   Peak tumour concentrations are
increased with hydrophilic radiosensitizers, but i.v. administration
is required to maximise the benefit.   Alternatively, a lipophilic
prodrug would be well-absorbed and then metabolised rapidly to
release the hydrophilic drug.   The diacetate prodrug of desmethylmisonidazole provides higher peak desmethylmisonidazole concentrations after intraperitoneal injection in the mouse (39).

        There is likely to be a limit to which lipophilicity can be
usefully reduced, since extreme hydrophilicity will reduce penetration into tumour cells.   It is interesting to note (Table 1) that
the commonly used anti-neoplastic agents 5-Fluorouracil, methotrexate and arabinosylcytosine are all more hydrophilic than misonidazole and desmethylmisonidazole.   However, antimetabolites commonly
enter cells by utilising membrane transport mechanisms for natural

substances;   for example, methotrexate is taken up by the carrier
for reduced folates, and decreased active transport leads to drug
resistance (40).   It is not inconceivable that highly hydrophilic
nitroimidazoles could be designed to exploit similar transport
mechanisms.

Tumour levels comparable to misonidazole are obtained with analogues more lipophilic;   oral absorption is likely to be good, and
their rapid metabolic clearance may be advantageous.   However, with
highly lipophilic analogues, poor water solubility may restrict
absorption and first-pass metabolism can be a problem.   Plasma
protein-binding may also restrict tumour penetration of some lipophilic analogues.

We do not yet know whether hydrophilic analogues excluded from
normal brain will penetrate brain tumours.   The blood-brain barrier
is known to be defective in large but not small brain tumours (6,7,
41).   Nevertheless, lipophilic cytotoxic agents seem to be the most
effective for brain tumour chemotherapy (41).   A lipophilic nitroimidazole with a more rapid metabolic clearance than misonidazole
might be optimal.

The very broad structural requirements for radiosensitization
by nitroimidazoles in vitro, where redox properties predominate (5),
allows considerable scope for the pharmacological fine-tuning of this
type.   However, recent in vitro studies suggest that lipophilicity
may also be important in a way distinct from purely pharmacokinetic
considerations (42).   Enhanced radiosensitization efficiency considerably greater than that predicted from redox potential measurements was seen with neutral nitroimidazoles with P values > 3.5.
It is tempting to speculate that the interaction of nitroimidazoles
with 'receptors' critical for radiosensitivity (e.g. hydrophobic
regions in membranes or nucleoproteins) may also be dependent on
lipophilicity.

As well as the relative solubility in lipid and water, it is
likely that absolute solubility in these phases will be very
important.

CONCLUDING REMARKS

The aim of this review has been to highlight the importance
of lipophilicity for the pharmacokinetics and, in turn, the therapeutic ratio of nitroimidazoles.   An encouraging aspect from the
point of view of drug development is that the structure-pharmaco-
kinetic correlations of the type shown here allow some prediction of
pharmacokinetic behaviour on the basis of lipophilicity.   However,
this is not to say that other structural parameters should be
ignored.   The importance of lipophilicity is best studied when other
factors are held constant, as in most examples presented here.

But steric properties, ionisation and particularly redox potential
must all be taken into consideration in structural optimization
directed towards improved radiosensitizers for clinical use. Rapid
metabolism is probably responsible for fast clearance and poor tumour
levels of highly electron affinic radiosensitizers active _in vitro_
but less active and very toxic _in vivo_. In addition, different
structural and pharmacokinetic characteristics may be required to
optimize for properties such as antitumour cytotoxicity and beneficial
interactions with other cytotoxic agents.

1.   P. Workman, _Cancer Clin. Trials_ (in press)(1980).
2.   C. Hansch, and W. J. Dunn, _J. Pharm. Sci._ 61:1 (1972).
3.   J. M. Brown, and P. Workman, _Radiat. Res._ 82:171 (1980).
4.   G. E. Adams, I. R. Flockhart, C. E. Smithen, I. J. Stratford,
     P. Wardman, and M. E. Watts, _Radiat. Res._ 67:9 (1976).
5.   G. E. Adams, I. R. Flockhart, R. S. Jacobs, D. S. Sehmi,
     I. J. Stratford, P. Wardman, and M. E. Watts, _Int. J. Radiat._
     Biol. 35:133 (1979).
6.   S. I. Rapoport, _in_: "Blood-Brain Barrier in Physiology and
     Medicine", Raven, New York (1976).
7.   R. G. Blasberg (in press).
8.   P. Wardman, _in_: "Radiosensitizers of Hypoxic Cells",
     A. Breccia, C. Rimondi, and G. E. Adams, eds., Elsevier,
     Amsterdam (1979).
9.   R. Harrison and G. G. Lunt, _in_: "Biological Membranes", Blackie,
     Glasgow (1975).
10. S. J. Singer, and G. L. Nicolson, _Science_ 175:720 (1972).
11. B. B. Brodie, _in_: "Absorption and Distribution of Drugs",
     T. B. Binns ed., Livingstone, Edinburgh (1964) pp 16-48.
12. M. Muller, D. G. Lindmark, and J. McLaughlin, _in_:
     "Metronidazole", S. M. Finegold ed., Excerpta Medica,
     Amsterdam (1977) pp 12-19.
13. R. S. Weinstein, and N. S. McNutt, _New Engl. J. Med._, 286:521
     (1972).
14. M. G. Farquhar, and G. E. Palade, _J. Cell Biol._ 17:375 (1963).
15. G. L. Lukas, S. D. Brindle, and P. Greengard, _J. Pharm. Exp._
     Ther. 178:562 (1971).
16. R. A. S. White, P. Workman, L. N. Owen, and N. M. Bleehen,
     Br. J. Cancer 40:284 (1979).
17. R. A. S. White, and P. Workman, _Br. J. Cancer_ 41:268 (1980).
18. R. A. S. White, P. Workman, and J. M. Brown, _Radiat. Res._
     (in press) (1980).
19. P. Workman, unpublished (1980).
20. P. Wardman, E. D. Clarke, J. A. Dale, R. S. Jacobs, A.
     Minchinton, M. Stratford, M. E. Watts, M. Woodcock, M.
     Moazzam, J. Parrick, R. G. Wallace, C. E. Smithen, and
     D. Brown, _Cancer Clin. Trials_, (in press)(1980).

21.   J. M. Brown, and W. W. Lee, Cancer Clin. Trials (in press)
      (1980).
22.   I. R. Flockhart, P. W. Sheldon, I. J. Stratford, and M. E. Watts
      Int. J. Radiat. Biol. 34:91 (1978).
23.   P. Workman, Br. J. Cancer 40:335 (1979).
24.   P. Workman, Cancer Chemother. Pharmacol. (in press)(1980).
25.   R. M. Ings, J. A. McFadzean, and W. A. Ormerod, Xenobiotica
      5:223 (1975).
26.   I. R. Flockhart, P. Large, D. Troup, S. L. Malcom, and
      T. R. Marten, Xenobiotica 8:97 (1978).
27.   P. N. Giraldi, G. P. Tosolini, E. Dradi, G. Nannini, R. Longo,
      G. Meinardi, G. Monti, and I. De Carneri, Biochem. Pharmac.
      20:339 (1971).
28.   R. E. McMahon, J. Pharm. Sci. 55:457 (1966).
29.   H. P. A. Illing, Biochem. Pharmac. 29:999 (1980).
30.   D. Perrier, and D. Gibaldi, J. Pharm. Exp. Ther. 191:17 (1974).
31.   P. Workman, N. M. Bleehen, and C. R. Wiltshire, Br. J. Cancer
      41:302 (1980).
32.   N. J. McNally, J. Denekamp, P. W. Sheldon, I. R. Flockhart and
      F. A. Stewart, Radiat. Res. 73:568 (1978).
33.   J. M. Brown, and N. Y. Yu, submitted for publication (1980).
34.   S. Dische, M. I. Saunders, I. R. Flockhart, M. E. Lee and
      P. Anderson, Int. J. Radiat. Oncol. Biol. Phys., 5:851 (1979).
35.   A. J. Varghese, S. Gulyas, and J. K. Mohindra, Cancer Res.
      36:3761 (1976).
36.   Y. C. Taylor, and A. M. Rauth, Cancer Res. 38:2745 (1978).
37.   T. H. Wasserman, T. L. Phillips, G. Van Raalte, R. Urtasun,
      J. Partington, D. Koziol, J. G. Schwade, D. Gangji, and
      J. M. Strong, Br. J. Radiol. 53:172 (1980).
38.   P. Workman, Biochem. Pharmac. (in press)(1980).
39.   P. Workman, J. M. Brown and S. Zamvil, in preparation.
40.   K. R. Harrap, in: "Scientific Foundations on Oncology",
      T. Symington, and R. L. Carter, eds, Heineman, London,
      (1976) pp 641-654.
41.   V. A. Levin, C. S. Patlak, and H. D. Landahl, J. Pharmacokinet.
      Biopharm. (in press).
42.   R. F. Anderson, and K. B. Patel, Br. J. Cancer 39:705 (1979).

PHARMACOKINETIC STUDIES ON SOME NOVEL (2-NITRO-1-IMIDAZOLYL)

PROPANOLAMINE RADIOSENSITIZERS

M. R. L. Stratford, A. I. Minchinton, F. A. Stewart
and V. S. Randhawa

Cancer Research Campaign Gray Laboratory
Mount Vernon Hospital
Northwood, Middlesex HA6 2RN, England

One area of current interest in radiosensitizer development is
in the use of nitroimidazoles of a more polar nature than misonidazole, combining the benefits of a shorter half-life, and thus reduced
tissue exposure, which has been correlated with the neuropathy
observed with misonidazole (1), while also minimising brain penetration through the blood-brain barrier (2).   In the Gray Laboratory
development programme, one aim has been to attempt to combine the
advantages of a highly polar compound with an increased radiosensitizing efficiency by including basic functions in the 2-nitroimida-
zole side chain.   Preliminary data for one of these, the propanolamine Ro 03-8799, indicating favourable pharmacokinetic properties
following intraperitoneal administration have already been published
(3).

We present here some data on the comparative pharmacokinetics
of Ro 03-8799 and two other compounds in this class, Ro 31-0052 and
Ro 31-0054, together with misonidazole, following intravenous
administration to WH male mice bearing a fibrosarcoma, at a dose of
0.5 μmoles/g.   In addition to blood and tumour concentration
measurements, drug levels in brain were also determined as these
may be related to the neurotoxicity which limits the maximum dose
which can be administered to human patients.

The structures and some physicochemical properties of the four
drugs used are shown in Fig. 1.   The pK values indicate that all
three propanolamines will have a significant fraction in the
protonated form at physiological pH.

Drug	R	pK_a	P^a
Ro 07-0582 misonidazole	$-CH_2CHOHCH_2OCH_3$	-	0.43
Ro 03-8799	$-CH_2CHOHCH_2N$⟨hexane ring⟩ 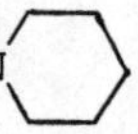	8.7	8.5
Ro 31-0052	$-CH_2CHOHCH_2N$⟨hexane ring⟩OH 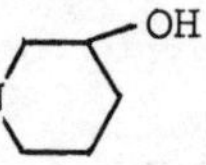	7.5	0.3
Ro 31-0054	$-CH_2CHOHCH_2NHCH_2$⟨benzene ring⟩OCH_3 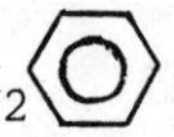	7.9	7.5

[a]Partition (oct.:H_2O) of free base, i.e. at pH (pK_a +2)

Fig. 1.   Structures and some physicochemical properties
of the drugs used.

The drugs were dissolved in saline prior to administration via
the tail vein and the animals sacrificed by decapitation under
anaesthesia at various times following dosing.   Drug levels were
determined by high performance liquid chromatography of deproteinised
whole blood and aqueous homogenates of tumour and brain.

RESULTS AND DISCUSSION

Blood levels declined exponentially over the time period
studied (5-180 mins), while gross tumour levels did not peak until
5-10 mins after administration.   Diffusion to the site of action
may take substantially longer.   The blood levels observed, together
with the tumour to brain ratios are shown in Table 1.   Brown and
Workman (2) have suggested that this ratio may be a useful way of
assessing the potential of a compound as a sensitizer, since tumour
concentrations relate to the sensitization which would be observed,
while brain levels may correlate with toxicity.   Thus, maximising
this ratio may yield a compound with an improved therapeutic index.
All the propanolamines look promising in this respect since they all
show some degree of concentration in tumour relative to blood, a
phenomenon not shown by misonidazole.   This could be related to the
slightly lower pH observed in tumours which would tend to trap the
charged form of the drug.   However, if this is an extracellular
effect it would act to inhibit the passage of drug into the cell,
and thus reduce the amount of radiosensitization observed.

Table 1. Blood levels and tumour/brain concentration (T/B) ratios after 0.5 μmoles/g.

Time (mins)	Misonidazole* Blood (μmoles/ml)	T/B	Ro 03-8799 Blood (μmoles/ml)	T/B	Ro 31-0052 Blood (μmoles/ml)	T/B	Ro 31-0054 Blood (μmoles/ml)	T/B
5	0.63	1.1	0.38	1.9	0.29	>66	–	–
10	0.59	1.3	0.33	1.8	0.17	30	0.10	1.5
15	–	–	0.26	2.2	0.19	>52	0.08	1.7
20	0.49	1.2	0.21	0.9	0.18	>51	0.07	1.5
30	0.42	1.7	0.16	1.9	0.08	>43	0.02	2.4
45	0.35	1.6	0.10	1.5	0.04	>30	0.01	1.1
60	0.33	2.0	0.06	0.9	0.03	>18	–	–

* Includes desmethylmisonidazole.

Table 2. Biological parameters of the drugs used.

Drug	LD_{50} mg/g	$t_{\frac{1}{2}}$ (min)	Partition x Fraction unionized
Misonidazole	1.34 $\pm$ 0.15	39 $\pm$ 1	0.43
Ro 03-8799	1.34 $\pm$ 0.04	22 $\pm$ 1	0.43
Ro 31-0052	3.1 $\pm$ 0.09	18 $\pm$ 1	0.13
Ro 31-0054	0.34 $\pm$ 0.03	11 $\pm$ 1	1.8

The ratio for misonidazole and desmethylmisonidazole shows a
gradual increase over the period studied. This is due to the
increasing proportion of the more polar metabolite. However, the
most striking feature in this table is the data for Ro 31-0052,
the large values being almost entirely due to its nearly complete
exclusion from the brain.

These results can be rationalised by reference to Table 2,
which shows the intraperitoneal (i.p.) LD_{50}, the half-life ($t_{\frac{1}{2}}$)
observed in this experiment, and the product of the partition
coefficient and the fraction unionized at pH 7.4 (PxF). The i.p.
LD_{50} is shown since the bases showed an atypical acute toxic response when given intravenously (i.v.). Death is almost instant-
aneous, and thus it was thought that this would bear little
relationship to their chronic toxicities. The PxF function would be
expected to relate to the neurotoxicity since it is the uncharged
fraction only which can cross the blood-brain barrier.

The toxicities of the propanolamines correlate fairly well with
PxF, with the most toxic Ro 31-0054 having the highest product,
while Ro 31-0052, which showed almost no brain penetration, is the
least toxic. Correlation is slightly better if account is taken of
the $t_{\frac{1}{2}}$ and thus total area under the curve (AUC). However, they
all appear more toxic than misonidazole on this basis. This may
be due to two different toxic responses acting together, in view of
the qualitative as well as quantitative differences in response
shown by the bases following i.v. and i.p. administration. This
would probably be less important in a fractionated dosing regime.

All three of the new drugs show an in vitro sensitizing ability
an order of magnitude better than misonidazole, and of these,
Ro 31-0052 looks to have the greatest potential in vivo, and further
radiosensitizing experiments on all three compounds are currently
in progress.

REFERENCES

1. S. Dische, M. I. Saunders, I. R. Flockhart, M. E. Lee, and
    P. Anderson, Misonidazole - A drug for trial in radiotherapy
    and oncology, Int. J. Rad. Oncol. Biol. Phys. 5:851 (1979).
2. J. M. Brown, and P. Workman, Partition coefficient as a guide
    to the development of radiosensitizers which are less toxic
    than misonidazole, Radiat. Res. 82:171 (1980).
3. J. Denekamp, Testing of hypoxic cell radiosensitizers in vivo,
    Cancer Clin. Trials 3:139 (1980).

THE EFFECT OF DEXAMETHASONE ON THE NEUROTOXICITY OF

NITROIMIDAZOLE COMPOUNDS

R. C. Urtasun*, H. Tanasichuk*, J. Partington*,
D. Koziol*, J. Allalunis and R. Turner.

Departments of Radiation and Medical Oncology
Cross Cancer Institute, University of Alberta
Edmonton, Alberta, Canada

ABSTRACT

A total of 300 patients have been entered in our Institution
to receive either Misonidazole or Metronidazole in order to study
the usefulness of these compounds as hypoxic cell sensitizers.
The present report deals with our attempts to reduce the toxicity
of these drugs.

Acute GI toxicity, although present in 30-40% of our patients
(pending on the total dose and type of drug), has not been our
dose limiting factor.   On the other hand, peripheral neuropathies
have been the major obstacle in reaching blood and tumour tissue
drug therapeutic levels.

Consequently we have explored the possible protective effect
of Dexamethasone against the neurotoxicity of Misonidazole.   A
preliminary analysis of our presently ongoing prospective study is
suggestive that Dexamethasone may exert a protective effect,
although we have found that unlike Phenytoin it does not appear to
alter the kinetics of Misonidazole in blood.

INTRODUCTION

A prospective phase I study of Misonidazole was completed one
year ago in our centre and the final results are analyzed in this
paper.

The acute drug toxicity observed with both Metronidazole
and Misonidazole consists mainly of nausea, anorexia, and vomiting

and peripheral as well as central nervous tissue damage.   The
incidence varies according to the total dose, the tissue exposure,
and to a lesser degree, the frequency of drug administration (1-5).
Bone marrow toxicity, although not demonstrable by routine peripheral blood counts, has been shown to occur in a group of patients
receiving Misonidazole which were submitted to bone marrow cultures
by the "in vitro" colony forming units technique.   This could be
of some relevance in the future use of these drugs, particularly
when combined with aggressive systemic chemotherapy and radiation
(6-11).   Because of the lower incidence of peripheral neuropathies
observed in patients receiving concommitantly Phenytoin Sodium and
Dexamethasone (12) a prospective randomized study was initiated
recently in our Institution in order to assess the effect of
Dexamethasone in reducing the incidence of Misonidazole neurotoxicity.   The pharmacokinetics of Misonidazole was studied in each
patient receiving Dexamethasone to determine any possible interaction of these two drugs.

MATERIALS AND METHODS

Misonidazole*

        Toxicity at different intermittent dose schedules.

        A total of 64 patients with different types of advanced
malignant solid tumours were entered on a controlled toxicity study
to assess different dose schedules in a step-wise controlled
increments while receiving a course of radiation (Table 1).   This
group includes 16 patients with the diagnosis of high grade
astrocytoma receiving Misonidazole at a dose of 1.25 g/m² and con-
commitant Dexamethasone with or without Phenytoin, and will be
analysed separately.   All patients had normal bone marrow, liver
and kidney functions before entering the study.   Their Karnofsky
functional status was 60% or over and they had no peripheral neuropathies.   All patients were restricted to liquids only, for 7
hours prior to drug administration and received 10 mg of proclor-
perazine as an antiemetic orally, 1 hour before drug ingestion.
All patients had baseline audiogram and neurological examination
performed prior to drug administration and repeated every 4 weeks
for the first three months.   Nerve conduction studies were performed
on those patients that developed peripheral neuropathies and
electronystagmogram (ENM) on those with abnormal audiograms.
Misonidazole was administered orally in capsule form of 500 mg
4 hours before radiation treatment.   Drug levels and blood and
urine were done using the High Performance Liquid Chromatography
assay (13).

_____
* Supplied by Hoffmann-La Roche, Montreal, Quebec, Canada.

Table 1. Phase I - Misonidazole multiple dose toxicity study.

Schedule		Mean Dose (g)	Mean Concentration (μM)	*Toxicity	No. of cases
1 g m²	2 wk/2 wk	7.5	228	0	2
2 "	2 wk/2 wk	14	364	1	2
2 "	2 wk/3 wk	11.5	479	1	3
.75 "	3 wk/2 wk	12	145	0	1
1 "	2 wk/2 wk	9	259	0	1
1.5 "	3 wk/2 wk	18	272	0	1
2 "	3 wk/2 wk	24	351	2	3
1 "	3 wk/3 wk	16.9	244	3	4
1.25"	3 wk/3 wk	18	251	5	22
1.5 "	3 wk/3 wk	19.3	285	1	2
2 "	3 wk/3 wk	23.3	389	2	4
2.5 "	1 wk/4 wk	17	512	1	4
3 "	1 wk/4 wk	22	556	3	4
4 "	1 wk/4 wk	25.2	815	3	4
2.5 "	1 wk/6 wk	26.2	373	1	5

* Toxicity = peripheral neuropathy, encephalopathy.

Table 2.   Immediate Toxicity

	Control	Metronidazole	Misonidazole
Anorexia Nausea/Vomiting	1/18	11/17	7/22
CNS*	8/18	12/17	5/22
Neuropathies	0/18	0/17	0/22
Dermatitis	1/18	2/17	3/22
Dose modifications	0/18	7/17	4/22
Treatment discontinued	0/18	0/17	0/22

*CNS symptoms : Dizziness, ataxia, seizures, drowsiness, intention tremors, shuffling gait.

Dexamethasone-Misonidazole Interaction

Eleven patients with different types of advanced malignant solid tumours undergoing palliative radiation, excluding brain tumour patients, were randomized to receive Misonidazole 1.25 g/m² three times a week for three weeks, or Misonidazole samd dose plus Dexamethasone (Decadron) at a dose of 2 mg three times a day for one week prior to and during the administration of Misonidazole. 24 Hour blood kinetic studies of Misonidazole were done before Decadron administration and repeated while receiving the drug combination.

Metronidazole*

In addition to our previously reported phase I toxicity study (1,2), this group includes 17 patients with malignant astrocytomas entered into a three-arm randomized study consisting of radiation only (control) radiation plus Metronidazole and radiation plus Misonidazole. All patients received Metronidazole 6 g/m² three times a week for three weeks, 4-6 hours before radiotherapy. All were on Decadron at different dosages for control of cerebral edema.

RESULTS

Metronidazole Toxicity

Eleven out of 17 patients with malignant brain tumours developed acute GI toxicity (Table 2) consisting of severe anorexia, nausea and vomiting, compared with 1/18 in the control group (radiation

_____

* Supplied by Poulenc, Montreal, Quebec, Canada.

Table 3.   Occurrence of Misonidazole Toxicities
(64 evaluable patients)

Effect	No. of cases	% Incidence	Minimum total drug dose (g)
Peripheral neuropathy	18	28	14
Dermatitis	2	3	12
Gastric toxicity	3	5	17.5
Encephalopathy	5	8	16
Ototoxicity	3	5	18

N.B. (1) 22 patients had astrocytomas and were treated with
Dexamethasone.
(2) Gastric toxicity: predominant at individual doses
25.5 g. Drug was well tolerated with anti-emetic
given prior to drug.

Grading of Neuropathies

O = none.
Grade 1 = no interference.
Grade 2 = some disability, difficulty in walking or
fastening buttons, paresthesia or pain.
Grade 3 = confining the patient to the house, requiring
strong analgesic, associated encephalopathies.

only) and 7/22 in the Misonidazole group.   12/17 Developed
shuffling gait, ataxia and dizziness suggestive of CNS toxicity.
CT scan and brain scan revealed the known tumour with the accompany-
ing edema but no evidence of normal brain tissue damage.   There
was no evidence of peripheral neuropathies in this group of
patients.

Misonidazole Toxicity at Multiple Intermittent Dose Schedules

A total of 64 patients were studied (22 were brain tumours
receiving Dexamethasone concommitantly for the purpose of controlling brain edema).   For total doses of Misonidazole from 12
to 35 g, the incidence of different toxicities are listed in
Table 3.   We have found that the dose-limiting neurotoxicity is
manifested by peripheral neuropathies, ototoxicity and encephalopathies.   As long as the dose was kept under 18 g, the incidence
of central and peripheral nervous system toxicity was acceptable
and the patients were able to be treated either over a three week

Table 4.   Number of Patients Developing Neurotoxicities
(includes patients receiving Dexamethasone)

Dose	Once or twice weekly			Thrice weekly		
	None	Gr. 1	Gr. 2 and 3	None	Gr. 1	Gr. 2 and 3
< 18 g	7	1	O	6	3	2
18 - 22 g	4	4	2	12	1	1
> 22 g	3	1	2	6	O	3

Table 5.   Number of Patients Developing Neurotoxicities
(excludes patients receiving Dexamethasone)

Dose	Once or twice weekly			Thrice weekly		
	None	Gr. 1	Gr. 2 and 3	None	Gr. 1	Gr. 2 and 3
< 18 g	7	1	O	5	3	2
18 - 22 g	4	4	2	1	1	1
> 22 g	3	1	2	2	O	3

Table 6.   % of Patients Developing Neuropathies Related
to Frequency of Drug Administration

	Once or twice weekly	Thrice weekly	
No neurotoxicity	58%	+70%	45%
Grade 1	25%	+12%	22%
Grades 2 and 3	17%	+18%	33%

(once or twice a week) schedule or over a four to six week (only once a week) schedule (Tables 4,5,6).   In cases where the total dose was below 18 g, there was a 20% incidence of Grade 2 and 3 neurotoxicities if treated three times a week compared to 0% incidence if treated once or twice weekly.   Above 18 g total dose (but less than or equal to 22 g) as many patients being treated once or twice weekly (40%) (Table 7) developed Grade 1 neuropathies, as did patients treated three times a week (33%).   However 13% more patients developed Grade 2 and 3 neuropathies in the latter group.

Of patients treated three times a week for a total dose greater than 22 g, 60% developed Grade 2 and 3 neuropathies. When considering the patients treated concommitantly with Decadron, the overall incidence of neurotoxicity in the three times a week schedule drops by 25%.   As well, patients receiving greater than 20 g total dose, the incidence of Grade 2 and 3 neuropathies is decreased by 23%.

Prospective Randomized Dexamethasone-Misonidazole Study

Of 11 patients entered into this study, 5 received Misonidazole alone, the other 6 received Dexamethasone as well as Misonidazole. Three out of the five patients receiving only Misonidazole developed sensory peripheral neuropathy, requiring analgesic medication for relief of their symptons.   Resolution of the neuropathies took from 6 weeks to 6 months.   Only 1 out of the 6 patients receiving Dexamethasone concommitantly with Misonidazole developed a Grade 1 peripheral neuropathy (Table 8).

Table 7.   % of Patients Developing Neuropathies Related to
          Total Dose and Frequency of Administration

Dose	Once or twice weekly		Thrice weekly			
	Gr. 1	Gr. 2 and 3	Gr 1		Gr. 2 and 3	
< 18 g	12%	0%	+27%	30%	+18%	20%
18 - 22 g	40%	20%	+ 7%	33%	+ 7%	33%
> 22 g	17%	33%	+ 0%	0%	+33%	60%

+   Data calculated including brain protocol patients
    treated with Dexamethasone.

Table 8. Decadron/Misonidazole Toxicity Study.

	N	G.I. Toxicity	CNS Symptoms* & Ototoxicity	Peripheral Neuropathy
Misonidazole - no Decadron	5	3/5	2/5	3/5
Misonidazole - plus Decadron	6	1/6	0/6	1/6

* CNS symptoms include dizziness, ataxia, drowsiness and shuffling gait.

Table 9. Decadron/Misonidazole Toxicity Study.
Pharmacokinetics : Arm I - No Decadron

0582	E.L.	R.G.	O.C.	F.E.	S.S.
Mean 4.5 hr conc. (NM)	174	194	157	144	
Hour to peak conc.	2.0 *0.5	2.5 3.0	1.0 2.0	1.0	1.0
T½ (hours)	13.0 *12.0	8.5 12.0	8.0 12.0	8.0 9.5	14.5
Area under curve	2388 *2885	2439 3916	2027 2532	1870 1727	2329
% recovery, urine	18.0 *26.0	29.6 34.0	36.4 40.9	44.3 84.7	

* Values repeated 1 week later under same conditions.

No significant differences were observed in the kinetics of Misonidazole in the blood of patients receiving Misonidazole with or without Decadron (Figures 1, 2, 3). When comparing the group of patients on Misonidazole alone, with the patients receiving Misonidazole and Decadron, there was no difference in the mean 4.5 hr drug blood levels, half-life of the drug, area under the curve, and percentage recovery in the urine (Tables 9 and 10).

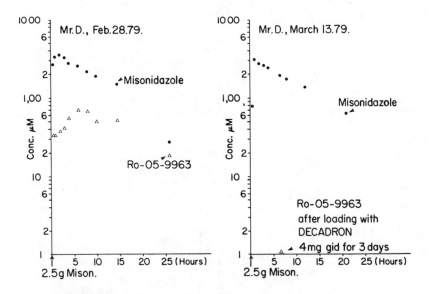

Figure 1

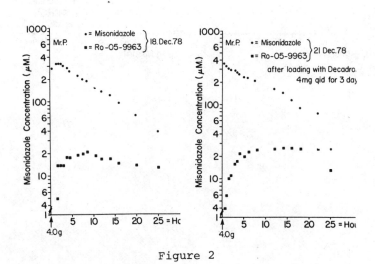

Figure 2

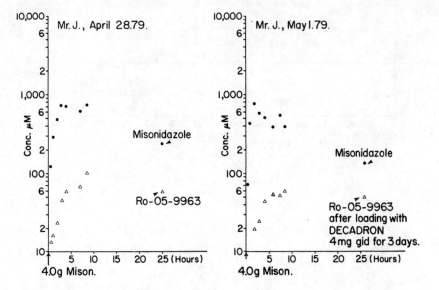

Figure 3

Table 10. Decadron/Misonidazole Toxicity Study.
Pharmacokinetics : Arm II - with Decadron

0582	J.D.	C.S.	F.G.	W.G.	A.R.	E.Z.
Mean 4.5 hr conc. (NM)	142	167	234	126	158	
Hour to peak conc.	1.25 *2	2.0 2.0	1.0 1.0	1.25		1.0
T½ (hours)	6.0 *7.0	8.0 9.5	13.0 10.0	9.0		9.0
Area under curve	1967 *2104	2287 1914	3764 3523	1685		2489
% recovery, urine	21.6 *24.0					

* Values repeated one week later, while on Decadron.
Previous values on Misonidazole alone.

Table 11. Maximum Tolerable Doses.

	Total dose	GI Toxicity	CNS Toxicity	Neuropathy
Metronidazole	53 g/m²	50%	25%	6%
Misonidazole	12 g/m²	18%	3%	25%
	12 g/m²	16%	8%	41%

CNS includes: dizziness, tremors, ataxia, confusion.

DISCUSSION

When Metronidazole and Misonidazole are administered at the
maximum tolerable dose, the incidence of peripheral neuropathies
appears to be less in the group of patients receiving Metronidazole
(Table 11).   However, in this group of patients there appear to
be more CNS symptoms, suggesting a possible encephalopathy.
Previous experience of higher incidence of acute GI toxicity on
patients receiving Metronidazole is confirmed with this selected
group.   Even at doses of Misonidazole over 12 g/m^2, the incidence
of CNS toxicity is much lower than patients receiving Metronidazole
at maximum tolerable levels of 53 g/m^2.   On the other hand, the
incidence of peripheral neuropathy is higher in the Misonidazole
group of patients and even higher when the dose is escalated to
over 12 g/m^2.   All in all, in our experience, we can say that when
Metronidazole is given at comparable maximum tolerable doses to
Misonidazole, it tends to show a clearly higher incidence of GI and
CNS toxicity while Misonidazole reveals a higher incidence of
peripheral neuropathies.

With regard to our toxicity study with multiple doses of
Misonidazole, we conclude that both frequency of administration and
total dose of the drug are influential in causing neurotoxicity.
It has been our observation that the total dose of the drug is the
most important determinant in the incidence of neuropathy; however,
in our experience there appears to be a relationship between the
frequency of drug administration and the occurrence of this toxicity.   This is particularly so when the total dose is over 18 g.
We found no relationship between the incidence of peripheral
neuropathies and the half-life of the drug.   The levels of zinc and
iron in blood appear to be unrelated to toxicity.

Our clinical experience with the Decadron-Misonidazole interaction tends to support the claim that Dexamethasone does in fact
have a protective effect in decreasing the incidence of peripheral
neuropathy.   Glucocorticoid administration has led to clinical
improvement in a wide variety of demyelinating diseases consistent
with a possible direct action on demyelinated nerve (7).

It has been established that the histopathological changes in
Misonidazole peripheral neurotoxicity in humans is segmental
demyelination (4).   The possible mechanism of action of Dexamethasone on demyelinated nerve is thought to be related to the
influence on the sodium and water movement out of cells, to
stabilization of cell membranes and to alteration of cell surface
properties (10).   It has been shown experimentally that hydro-
cortisone can restore the blood-nerve extracellular space barrier
and reduce the extracellular water content (10).   It is clear from
our data, and from previous studies done in animals (14) that
Dexamethasone does not change the pharmacokinetics of Misonidazole

in blood.   It is possible therefore that the effect of Dexamethasone in modifying the incidence of misonidazole toxicity could be
related to its action on nerve cell membranes.

REFERENCES

1.   R. C. Urtasun, J. Sturmwind, H. Rabin, P. R. Band, and
      J. D. Chapman, High dose Metronidazole: a preliminary
      pharmacological study prior to its investigational use in
      clinical radiotherapy trials, Brit. J. Radiol. 47:293
      (1974).
2.   R. C. Urtasun, J. D. Chapman, P. Band, H. Rabin, C. Fryer,
      and J. Sturmwind, Phase I study of high dose Metronidazole,
      an in vivo and in vitro specific radiosensitizer of hypoxic
      cells, Radiology 111:129 (1975).
3.   R. C. Urtasun, P. Band, J. D. Chapman, A. F. Wilson,
      B. Marynowski, and E. Starreveld, Misonidazole neuro-
      toxicity, New Engl. J. Med. 295:901 (1976).
4.   R. C. Urtasun, J. D. Chapman, M. L. Feldstein, P. R. Band,
      H. R. Rabin, A. F. Wilson, B. Marynowski, E. Starreveld,
      and T. Shnitka, Peripheral neuropathy related to misoni-
      dazole: incidence and pathology, Br. J. Cancer 37:
      Suppl.III:271 (1978).
5.   T. H. Wasserman, T. L. Phillips, R. J. Johnson, C. J. Gomer,
      A. G. Lawrence, W. Sadee, R. A. Marques, V. A. Levin, and
      G. VanRaalte, Initial clinical and pharmacologic evaluation
      of misonidazole (Ro-07-0582), a hypoxic cell radiosensitizer,
      Int. J. Radiat. Oncol. Biol. Phys. 5:775 (1979).
6.   J. M. Allalunis, R. A. Turner, J. P. Partington, and
      R. C. Urtasun, Effect of Misonidazole therapy on human
      granulopoietic stem cells, Cancer Treatment Reports
      64:1097 (1980).
7.   B. J. W. Arnason, and E. Chemilcka-Szorc, Peripheral nerve
      segmental demyelination induced by intraneural diphtheria
      toxin injection and the effect of hydrocortisone, Arch.
      Neurol. 30:157 (1974).
8.   S. Dische, M. I. Saunders, et al., Clinical testing of the
      radiosensitizer Ro-07-0582 - experience with multiple
      doses, Br. J. Cancer 35:567 (1977).
9.   S. Dische, M. I. Saunders, P. Anderson, R. C. Urtasun,
      K. H. Karcher, H. D. Kogelnik, T. Phillips and T. H. Wasser-
      man, The neurotoxicity of misonidazole: pooling of data
      from five centers, Brit. J. Radiol. 51:Lo23 (1978).
10.   V. A. Levin, E. Chemilcka-Szorc, and B. J. W. Arnason,
      Peripheral nerve segmental demyelination induced by intra-
      neural diphtheria toxin injection and the effect of hydro-
      cortisone, Arch. Neurol. 30:163 (1974).
11.   R. A. Turner, J. Allalunis, R. C. Urtasun et al., Cytotoxic and
      radiosensitizing effects of Misonidazole on haematopoiesis

in normal and tumor-bearing mice, <u>Int. J. Rad. Onc.</u> 6: 1157 (1980).

12. T. H. Wasserman, T. L. Phillips, G. VanRaalte, R. C. Urtasun, J. Partington, D. Koziol, J. G. Schwade, D. Gangji, and J. M. Strong, The neurotoxicity of misonidazole: potential modifying role of phenytoin sodium and dexamethasone, <u>Brit. J. Radiol.</u> 53:170 (1980).

13. C. R. Wiltshire, P. Workmsn, J. V. Watson, and N. M. Bleehen, Clinical studies with Misonidazole, <u>Br. J. Cancer</u> 37: Suppl.III:286 (1978).

14. P. Workman, Drug interactions with misonidazole: effects of dexamethasone and its derivatives on the pharmacokinetics and toxicity of misonidazole in mice, <u>Biochem. Pharmacol.</u> (1981) in press.

RADIOSENSITIZERS WITH HYPERFRACTIONATION IN RADIOTHERAPY

C. Rimondi

Department of Radiotherapy, Malpighi Hospital

Bologna, Italy

INTRODUCTION

The use of misonidazole in radiotherapy for the treatment of cancer confronts the therapist with the problem of choosing how to relate the administration schedules of the drug with the radiation schedule (1). He must decide whether it is advisable to keep the usual dose-fraction schedules - for which tolerance is well known - or whether these schedules can be changed in order to exploit in the best way possible the radiosensitizing effect of this drug on the hypoxic cells present in tumours.

Phase II clinical studies of misonidazole involve the use of the drug with both conventional and unconventional schedules of radiation fractionation. This is necessary before Phase III studies are initiated, designed to assess any real advantage of the combination of misonidazole and radiotherapy compared with the best schedule of radiation treatment alone.

This paper reviews various proposals for Phase II studies and discusses the radiobiological and clinical considerations from which such studies originate.

Firstly, some comments are necessary on the application of hyperbaric oxygen in X-ray therapy. This method represents the first approach in the attempt to achieve hypoxic cell radio-sensitization in the radiotherapy of cancer. Our comments are based on the general review by Glassburn et al. (2), on the results of 15-year trials carried out in Great Britain under the sponsorship of the Medical Research Council and on the discussion by Dische (3).

We agree with the remarks of Glassburn et al. (2) that it has not yet been possible to determine the full value of this method even after almost 25 years' experience with HPO involving hundreds of patients. This seems to be mainly due to the lack of prospective clinical studies with a sufficient number of cases for statistically reliable conclusions to be made. However, there is evidence for clinical benefit in some situations. The results of some of the MRC clinical trials (although limited to only a few disease sites) are highly relevant to the subject matter of this paper.

In carcinomas of the head and neck region and locally-advanced carcinoma of the cervix, a statistically-significant improvement in both local control and survival was observed in the cases treated in HPO. However, in other sites such as bladder, the results in HPO were the same as those obtained for irradiation in air. It is possible that advantages may be derived by modification of the X-ray fractionation schedule (i.e. the use of a few large dose fractions). On the basis of this, trials of the treatment of bronchial and bladder carcinomas have been carried out after the use of conventional fractionation had not given good results. It should be pointed out, however, that good results have been obtained in stage III Ca. cervix using conventional fractionation. In regard to normal tissue tolerance, more intense reactions and increased complication rates have been found in some tissues, i.e. larynx, intestine, etc.) following treatment in HPO. However, in cervix ca. treatments some conflicting results have been found.

Although it is recognised that treatment in HPO can modify the effect of radiation on carcinomas, prospects for its general use are severely limited because of the organisational and other practical difficulties involved. One may speculate as to how the experience with HPO may be useful in the clinical evaluation of chemical radio-sensitizers, particularly misonidazole. Initially it was felt advisable to use misonidazole, firstly in those sites where the use of HPO appeared to be promising, i.e. head and neck cancer, stage III ca. cervix using appropriate radiation schedules. However, it must be borne in mind that although there are similarities in the rationales for the use of HPO and electron-affinic sensitizers, there are also important differences. These can suggest the investigation of misonidazole in other disease sites in treatments employing various different radiation schedules.

CONCLUSIONS FROM CLINICAL STUDIES WITH MISONIDAZOLE

a) Phase I

Three consecutive phases have been developed for studies with radiosensitizers, radioprotective agents and antiproliferative drugs (4). As with oxygen, the radiosensitizing effect of electron-

affinic drugs depends upon the concentration in the blood and
hence in the neoplastic tissue.   Moreover, the effect may be
larger when large dose-fractions are used compared with the small
fraction regimes usually employed in clinical radiotherapy.

The most serious limitation in the use of misonidazole is
peripheral neurotoxicity.   The most relevant factor affecting this
toxicity is the total administered dose.   Phase I studies by
Dische (5) and confirmed by others (6), indicated that the total dosage
of misonidazole should not exceed $12g/m^2$ administered over a
minimum period of 18 days.   Usually with such dosage, neurotoxic
manifestations are of low intensity and are reversible.

b)   Phase II

The data from the phase I studies gave rise to various
proposals for fractionation of both misonidazole and the associated
radiation treatments.   These are:

i) Irradiation with conventional fractionation using 2Gy per
    fraction, 5 fractions per week, 20-30 fractions in 4-6 weeks
    and $0.4-0.6$ g/m^2 of misonidazole before each treatment.

ii) Conventional fractionation with the drug administered only one
    day per week at high doses ($2g/m^2$ for 6 weeks).

iii) Hypofractionation with high radiation doses, i.e. 6Gy twice-
    weekly for three weeks and $2g/m^2$ of misonidazole before each
    radiation fraction.   In some non-conventional fractionation
    schedules, in order to exploit the long metabolic half-life
    of the drug (about 12 hours) and reduce the number of
    administrations, daily multiple fraction schedules (DMF) have
    been used with 2, or more often, 3 radiation treatments in
    the same day at 4-hourly intervals with variable size of dose
    per fraction.

iv) 2Gy x 3 daily for 5 days with $1.2g/m^2$ of misonidazole given
    daily 2-3 hours before the first radiation treatment with
    repetition of the course after an interval of 2-3 weeks.

v) 1.6Gy x 3 daily for 10 days with the same drug dosage.   After
    2-3 weeks, a 20-30Gy boost is given.

vi) 1Gy x 3 daily, three weeks with $0.8g/m^2$ of misonidazole daily
    3 hours before the first radiation fraction.   20-25Gy boost
    after a 2-3 weeks' interval.

Such a wide range of possibilities concerning drug and
radiation dosages, fraction schedule and overall treatment time
clearly pose problems in identifying the best method of using
misonidazole.

Schedule (i)   From the low doses of drug per fraction, one
would expect only a small sensitizing effect.   However, the use
of this fractionation schedule may greatly reduce the extent of
tumour hypoxia because of re-oxygenation between fractions.

Schedule (ii)   Misonidazole administered on the first day of the
week after the course has been interrupted for 48 hours may be
effective on the hypoxic cell component which will be further
reduced by re-oxygenation during subsequent treatment.

Schedule (iii)   From the purely radiosensitization viewpoint, this
may appear to be the most rational schedule.   However, doubts may
arise in regard to the damage to the vascular endothelia that such
large dose-fractions may cause and possibly inhibit the diffusi-
bility of the drug.   Further, there are doubts concerning
tolerance thresholds of particularly sensitive anatomical structures
(larynx, heart, intestine, bladder, mucosa, etc.).   One must also
consider the question of repopulation during the longer intervals
between individual doses.

     The schedules employing daily multiple-fractions are based
upon possible different recovery times for sub-lethal damage in
neoplastic tissue compared with healthy tissue with the subsequent
increase in overall therapeutic index.   Misonidazole at 0.8-1.2g/
m^2 could increase the benefit.

Schedule (iv)   Single doses of 2g 3 times a day generally imply
very intense reactions which may become critical for some sensitive
structures (larynx, mouth).   Increased frequency of radiation
necrosis has sometimes been observed in head and neck carcinomas
which is almost the only site where this schedule has been studied.

Schedule (v)   This represents a proposal of the EORTC aimed partly
at reducing normal tissue damage in the treatment of carcinomas
of the head and neck.

Schedule (vi)   This schedule is based on the radiobiological
research of Revesz and Littbrand (7).   The influence of daily
multiple fractions with sensitizers may be to improve therapeutic
ratio by a possible reduction in the maximum OER combined with a
reduction in the extent of repair of sub-lethal damage.

     Clinical studies of the treatment of mouth and bladder
carcinomas (8) with daily multiple fractions of 1Gy x 3 and total
dosage of 84Gy in 8 weeks showed increased tumour response compared with conventional fractionation but, in general, failed to
show improvement in survival.

     This schedule has been used by us (9) (without sensitizers)
in the treatment of infiltrating bladder tumours but with smaller

total doses of 65-70Gy.   It is well tolerated and showed some
advantage with regard to conventional treatment also for survival.

Now we review some schedules proposed by various groups concerning different neoplastic sites and which we believe are worth
examining more thoroughly.

1) Highly malignant glioma grade III-IV (Table 1)

In the radiotherapy-only schedules, there are three programmes
utilising hypofractionation associated with misonidazole and one
using daily multiple fractionation.

Table 1. Phase II Studies of Misonidazole and Radiotherapy in the
          Treatment of Malignant Glioma (Gr.III-IV)

Author or Group	Radiotherapy Schedule	Misonidazole Dose Schedule
URTASUN R.	4.3Gy/day x9F in 3 weeks = 38.7Gy	1-1.5g/m^2 x 9
BLEEHEN N.	2.94Gy/Mon. and Wed., 5Gy on Fri. x 4 weeks	3g/m^2 before the 500 rad dose Q week x 4
RTOG Prot.M.78/01	4Gy on Mon. 1.5Gy Tues-Thur-Fri x 6 weeks + Boost dose 1.8Gy x 5 = 60Gy T.D.	2.5g/m^2 Q week x 6
EORTC	2Gy x 3/day x5 in 1 week After 2-3 weeks interval 2Gy x3/day x5 day = 60Gy T.D.	1g/m^2 x 10 (ref. 10)
BTSG	1.7-2Gy/day x5F x 6-7 weeks = 60Gy T.D. + BCNU, 80mg/m^2 x 3 days of 8 weeks	1.5g/m^2 on Mon. and Thur. x 6 weeks
NCOG	Whole brain 1.8-2Gy/day x 5F x5-6 weeks Tumour boost 1.8-2Gy/day = 60Gy T.D.	1.75g/m^2 Tues., Thur. (ref. 11)

2) Advanced head and neck tumours (Table 2)

In addition to one protocol using hypofractionation, there
are three using a uniform daily multifraction with three treatments
every 4 hours, and one administration of misonidazole given 2-3
hours before the first daily X-ray treatment.

Table 2. Phase II studies of misonidazole and radiotherapy in the
treatment of advanced head and back cancers

Author or Group	Radiotherapy Schedule	Misonidazole Dose Schedule
MRC	4Gy/day x 10/F on alt. day x 3 weeks = 40Gy T.D.	1.2g/m^2 x 10
ARCANGELI G. et al.	2+1,5+1,5Gy/day x 5 Repeat after 1 week	1.2g/m^2 x 10 (ref. 12)
RTOG Prot. n. 78/02	2.5Gy 4h. after miso.) 2.1Gy 8h. after miso.) 1.8Gy/day x3F/week x 5 week = 50Gy T.D. Then 1.8Gy/day x5F x 2-3 week = 6.6-7.2Gy T.D.	2-2.5g/m^2 Q week x6
EORTC .	1.6Gy x3/day x 5 x 2 weeks = 48Gy + booster dose 15-25Gy	0.8-1.2g/m^2 x 10 (ref. 13)

3) Lung tumours (Table 3)

      The table includes three schedules for treatment of differ-
entiated, non-oat cell, inoperable carcinomas of the bronchus in
which hypofractionation is the preferred scheme. In addition,
our own proposal is included which utilises daily multiple fractionation at low values of single dose. We have observed a good
tolerance and a high percentage of immediate objective responses.
However, there is a rather high incidence of fibrosis. As yet,
we cannot evaluate how closely the fibrosis is linked to the
particular fractionation and the misonidazole and how much it is
associated with better survival of the responders. As of this
time, the treatment has only been used in the differentiated types
and we have not yet established a programme of treatment integrated
with chemotherapy.

Table 3. Phase II studies of misonidazole and radiotherapy in the
treatment of inoperable non-oat-cell lung cancers

Author or Group	Radiotherapy Schedule	Misonidazole Dose Schedule
DISCHE S.	6Gy x6 BIW / 3 weeks = 36Gy T.D.	2g/m^2 x 6
RTOG	6Gy x 6 BIW / 3 weeks	1.75-2g/m^2 x 6
D.Ra.O.M.	1Gy x3/day x 5/week x 3 weeks (ext. fields) + tumour boost 15-20Gy 1.5-2 weeks	0.8g/m^2 x 15
EORTC	4Gy/day x 5/week After 2-3 weeks interval 4Gy/day x 5/week = 40Gy T.D.	0.8-1.2g/m^2 x 10 (ref. 14)

4)   Carcinoma of the cervix - stage III (Table 4)

Two protocols utilise low doses of misonidazole and conventional radiotherapy with 20-30 fractions followed by intra-cavity irradiation.   Another protocol involves hypofractionation. Our own proposal involves daily multiple fractionation at reduced single doses together with brachytherapy.   Three of the schedules involve misonidazole administration during intra-cavity therapy carried out with a low-intensity technique.   Our schedule is well-tolerated and the immediate objective response, usually assessed 3 weeks after the end of treatment, has proved to be notable in almost all patients so far treated.

Table 4.   Phase II studies of misonidazole and radiotherapy in the treatment of Stage III cervix carcinoma

Author or Group	Radiotherapy Schedule	Misonidazole Dose Schedule
MRC	2.1Gy/day x5F x 4 weeks = 42Gy T.D. + Intracavitary treatment 20Gy point A	$0.5g/m^2$ x 20 $0.5g/m^2$ x 4 (ref. 15)
D.Ra.O.M.	1Gy x3/day x 5/week x 3.5 weeks 20Gy intracavitary brachitherapy	$0.7g/m^2$ x 17
RTOG	4Gy BIW x 5 = 40Gy T.D. + intracavitary boost	$1.25g/m^2$ x 10 $1.25g/m^2$ x 2
EORTC	1.7Gy/day x 5F x 6 weeks = 51Gy T.D. + Endocurietherapy	$0.9g/m^2$ on 1st, 3rd, 5th weeks (ref. 16)

5)   Locally-advanced bladder carcinoma (Table 5)

The proposals given in Table 5 include conventional fraction-ation with rather reduced misonidazole doses, hypofractionation (4Gy fractions) with high misonidazole doses once weekly, and a daily multiple fractionation schedule.   This last schedule, already adopted by us without the use of sensitizers, has given more encouraging results than those obtained with a conventional X-radiation schedule both in regard to local control and survival.

The final schedule given in the Table has been used in pre-operative and radical treatment of squamous cell carcinoma of the bladder associated with Bilharzia.

Table 5. Phase II studies of misonidazole and radiotherapy in the
          treatment of locally advanced bladder carcinoma

Author or Group	Radiotherapy Schedule	Misonidazole Dose Schedule
DISCHE S.	2.6Gy/day x 5F x 4weeks = 52Gy T.D.	$0.6g/m^2$ x 20
RTOG Prot. N. 78/21	4Gy on Mon. x8 weeks 2Gy on Wed-Fri. x 6 = 48 Gy T.D. + bladder boost 20Gy/2 weeks	$1.5g/m^2$ x 8
D.Ra.O.M.	1Gy x 3/day x 5/week x 3 weeks (ext. fields) After 3 weeks rest period bladder boost of 20-25Gy /2-2.5 weeks	$0.8g/m^2$ x 15
AHWAD et al.	Preop.: 4Gy x 5F in a week or 6Gy x 2 Radical: 1) 2Gy x 10F in 2 weeks After a week interval 2Gy x 10F/2 weeks 2) 0.6Gy x 17F, 1F each hour = 10Gy in 2 days After 1 week same doses and schedule	$1.2-1.5g/m^2$ x 5 or 2 $0.5g/m^2$ x 20 $1.5g/m^2$ each day

6) Soft tissue sarcomas (Table 6)

    In addition to the hypofractionation schedules being
investigated for the treatment of these radiation-resistant tumours,
we present our own proposals for two daily fractions of 2g for 5
days a week up to a total dose of about 20Gy.   Metronidazole 4g/
m^2 is given every second day.

Table 6. Phase II studies of misonidazole or metronidazole and ra-
          diotherapy in the treatment of soft tissue sarcomas

Author or Group	Radiotherapy Schedule	Misonidazole or Metronidazole Dose Schedule	
RTOG 78/15	7Gy Q week x 6 weeks = 42Gy T.D. 6Gy x 6 BIW/3 weeks = 36Gy T.D.	$2.5g/m^2$ x 6 $1.75g/m^2$ x 6	(Miso.) (")
D.Ra.O.M.	2Gy x 2/day x 5/week x 3.5 weeks = 68-72 Gy T.D.	$4g/m^2$ each other day	(Metro.)

DISCUSSION

At present, a definitive view is not available concerning the optimal conditions for using misonidazole and radiotherapy. However, on the basis of radiobiological and other experimental data, as well as clinical experience with hyperbaric oxygen, the prevalent trends seem to favour hypofractionation with miso-nidazole administered either before each X-ray treatment (2-3 times per week) or once-weekly when the radiation fraction is increased to 4-5Gy for that day only.   However, it should be noted that experience with some published randomized clinical trials (not involving sensitizers) has shown worse results compared with those obtained with conventional five-fractions-a-week treatments (see Sixth Progress Report of the British Institute of Radiology Fractionation Study of 3F/week versus 5F/week in Radiotherapy of Laringopharynx) (17) and other reports (18,19).   If it is generally true that hypofractionation gives inferior results then the addition of sensitizers would have to compensate for this disadvantage.before any overall therapeutic gain could be obtained (18).   Reactions are not well known, except for CNS where it may be presumed that they are reduced because of the use of medical support therapy with corticosteroids and anti-convulsant drugs.

The use of misonidazole at small doses of 0.4-0.6 g/m^2 with each fraction in   conventional treatments of 20-30F in 4-6 weeks has been discussed by Dische (5).   There are doubts that with these schedules, the individual dose-per-fraction of misonidazole is insufficient to produce significant radiosensitization.   However, other factors may be relevant.   The metabolic half-life of the drug is 5-10 times longer than in rodents.   There is therefore a possibility of better diffusion into human tumours compared with that in rodent tumours.   Further, the proportion of hypoxic cells in human tumours may be smaller than in experimental tumours and may be reduced even more by re-oxygenation processes occurring during a conventional fractionation treatment.   There is also the possible involvement of the direct cytotoxic effect of misonidazole on hypoxic cells which is independent of the radiosensitizing effect.   The cytotoxic action is linked mainly to the duration of contact of the drug with the hypoxic cells in the tumour.

The tolerance of healthy tissues included in the radiation field in conventional treatments does not seem to be significantly affected by the use of radiosensitizers.

Advantages of sensitizers with daily multiple fractionation may be summarised by the use of single daily doses of 0.8-1.2g/m^2 of misonidazole given before the first of 3 daily fractions at 4-hourly intervals with either continuous treatment or a 2-3 weeks split course.   Due to the long half-life of the drug in man,

three sessions of radiotherapy can be given in the same day following one administration of misonidazole 3 hours before the first
radiation fraction with drug still present during the third treatment.   However, the level is somewhat reduced by this time.   Thus
the total number of oral administrations is reduced, which allows
the drug-dose per fraction to be increased.   Further, the overall
treatment time is reduced (20).   Suggested daily doses are 2Gy x 3
for treatment of glioma; cervica-facial tumours and 1Gy x 3, used
with good tolerance and immediate advantage for treatment of
tumours in the pelvic region (bladder, cervix, rectum) and for
lung tumours.

SOME CONCLUDING REMARKS

Even though misonidazole is currently the most active radiosensitizing drug for hypoxic cells, its properties are not optimal
for use in radiotherapy with fractionated irradiation.   As yet, no
real advantages have been proven in prospective randomised trials
but are suggested by results of some studies in some disease sites,
e.g. head and neck and cervix.   The present phase of clinical
research with misonidazole involves identifying optimal drug-dosage
schedules and the most beneficial fractionation regimes.   Hopefully,
this will lead to increases in the radiosensitizing effect on the
hypoxic cell component in tumours without increasing damage to
healthy tissues thus allowing a real therapeutic advantage to be
obtained.   Once the studies are completed the assessment of tumour
results and tolerance will provide useful information for the design
of further phase III trials.

It is likely that the optimal schedules for misonidazole will
not be the same for all tumour sites.   Misonidazole toxicity does
not depend on the tumour site but tolerance of radn. doses depends on
the site because of the specific reactivities of healthy tissues or
organs included in the treatment volume.

The use of large, single X-ray dose fractions twice-weekly or
with daily multiple fractions does not seem advisable at present,
for locations different from CNS in view of the extension of the
tumour volume. At the current stage of clinical research with
sensitizers, one deals more frequently with advanced tumours which
require the irradiation of both the primary lesion and the regional
lymph nodes.   Some of the above observations apply to treatment
of Ca. bronchus as far as acute reactions, fibrosis and possible
damage to the spinal cord are concerned.

With transcutaneal treatment of cervix carcinoma at a locally
advanced stage (Stage III), the prevailing trend is in favour of
conventional fractionation, particularly in view of the remarkable
intestinal sensitivity in association with intracavity curietherapy.   A similar trend can be observed also, for other pelvic

carcinomas (bladder and rectum).   In this regard, we underline the favourable preliminary results with daily multiple fractionation with reduced doses of 1Gy x 3 concerning tolerance and immediate reactions.

Due to the moderate radiosensitizing efficacy of misonidazole at tolerated doses, we do not suggest replacing conventional fractionation by hypofractionation which generally has more disadvantages than the former procedure. We point out that radio-biological research (21,22) indicates the advisability of exploit-ing the combined effect of misonidazole and re-oxygenation during conventional fractionation or even better, of using misonidazole with hyperfractionation, especially in a reduced total treatment time (23).

This work was supported by Grant N.8001 63496 of the finalized project "Control of the tumour growth".

REFERENCES

1. G. E. Adams, J. Denekamp and J. F. Fowler, Biological basis of sensitization by hypoxic cell radiosensitizers, Chemotherapy Vol.7, K. Hellmann and T. A. Connors, eds., Plenum Press, New York and London (1977).
2. J. R. Glassburn, L. W. Brady and H.P. Plenk, Hyperbaric oxygen in radiation therapy, Cancer 39:751 (1977).
3. S. Dische, Hyperbaric oxygen: the MRC trials and their clinical significance, Brit. J. Radiol., 51:888 (1978).
4. T. L. Phillips, Design of clinical trials for hypoxic cell sensitizers and radioprotectors in Conference on combined modality cancer treatment: radiation sensitizers and protectors, Key Biscayne, Florida, Oct.3-9, Abstracts, p.5 (1979).
5. S. Dische, Hypoxic cell sensitizers in radiotherapy, Int. J. Radiat. Oncol. Biol. Phys., 4:157 (1978).
6. T. H. Wasserman, J. A. Stetz and T. L. Phillips, Clinical trials of misonidazole in the United States, Cancer Clin. Trials, 3 (1980) in press.
7. L. Revesz and B. Littbrand, Variation of the oxygen enhancement ratio at different X-ray level and its possible significance in "Advances in radiation research biology and medicine" *
8. B. Littbrand and F. Edsmyr, Preliminary results of bladder carcinoma irradiated with low individual doses and a high total dose, Int. J. Radiat. Oncol. Biol. Phys. 1:1059 (1976).
9. C. Rimondi and L. Busutti, Trattamento radiante di pazienti affetti da carcinoma vescicale (T3 NX MO) con tre sedute gionaliere in "Radiobiologia dei Tumori" EMSI (1978).
10. EORTC (Cooperative group of radiotherapy) Pilot study of the feasibility of a combination of daily multifractionation

radiotherapy and misonidazole in the treatment of high grade
malignant gliomas.   Personal communication (1979).

11. NCOG: Protocol No. 6G91.

12. G. Arcangeli, F. Mauro, D. Morelli and C. Nervi, Multiple daily
     fractionation in radiotherapy: biological rationale and pre-
     liminary clinical experiences. Eur. J. Cancer, 15:1077
     (1979).

13. EORTC (Cooperative group of radiotherapy) Protocol 22801, Pilot
     study on the combination of daily multifraction radiotherapy
     and misonidazole in the treatment of advanced head and neck
     cancer. Personal communication (1979).

14. EORTC (Cooperative group of radiotherapy) Randomized clinical
     trial on the influence of misonidazole in association with
     ·split course radiotherapy for epidermoid carcinoma of the
     bronchus. Personal communication (1979).

15. MRC (Cancer therapy committee) A study of misonidazole in con-
     junction with radiotherapy for the treatment of stage III
     carcinoma of the uterine cervix. Personal communication
     (1979).

16. EORTC: Protocol Ca. uterine cervix, stage III exclud. ETLA
     stage IV in association with misonidazole. Personal
     communication (1979).

17. G. Wiernik et al., Sixth interim progress report of the British
     Institute of Radiology fractionation study of 3F/week
     versus 5F/week in radiotherapy of the laryngo-pharynt, Brit.
     J. Radiol., 51:241 (1978).

18. J. D. Cox, R. W. Byhardt, R. Komaki and M. Greenberg, Reduced
     fractionation and the potential of hypoxic cell sensitizers
     in irradiation of malignant epithelial tumours, Int. J.
     Radiat. Oncol. Biol. Phys. 6:37 (1980).

19. E. R. Watson, K. E. Halnan, S. Dische, M. I. Saunders and I.S.
     Cade, Hyperbaric oxygen and radiotherapy: a MRC trial in
     carcinoma of the cervix, Brit. J. Radiol. 51:879 (1978).

20. C. Rimondi, Metronidazole: a radiosensitizer of the hypoxic
     cells, in: "Bladder Tumors and Other Topics in Urological
     Oncology", M. Pavone Macaluso, P.H. Smith and F. Edsmyr,
     eds., Plenum Press, New York and London (1980).

21. J. Denekamp, N. J. McNally, J. F. Fowler and M. C. Joiner,
     Misonidazole in fractionated radiotherapy: are many small
     fractions best? Brit. J. Radiol. 53 (1980) in press.

22. J. F. Fowler, New horizons in radiation oncology, Brit. J.
     Radiol. 52:523 (1979).

23. J. F. Fowler, In vivo radiosensitization: principles and
     methods of study, in: "Radiosensitizers in Hypoxic Cells",
     A. Breccia, C. Rimondi and G. E. Adams, Elsevier North
     Holland (1979).

* J.F. Duplan and A. Chapiro, eds., Gordon & Breach, London, 1215
     (1973).

THE DESIGN OF CLINICAL TRIALS AND CLINICAL TOXICOLOGY OF THE
NITROIMIDAZOLE MISONIDAZOLE IN PHASE I TESTING IN THE RADIATION
THERAPY ONCOLOGY GROUP*

Theodore L. Phillips and Todd H. Wasserman

Department of Radiation Oncology

University of California San Francisco, and
Department of Radiation Oncology
Washington University School of Medicine
St. Louis, Missouri, USA

*Supported by the Radiation Therapy Oncology Group CA 21439

INTRODUCTION

The Radiation Therapy Oncology Group (RTOG) is the only
organized cooperative group within the United States dedicated to
the investigation of therapeutic radiology in the treatment of
malignant disease.   More than 25 institutions have joined together
with support from the National Cancer Institute for a series of
cooperative clinical trials in a number of disease sites and a
wide range of new modalities.   The goal of the RTOG is to improve
the results of radiotherapy in the cure of cancer and in the
palliation of metastatic disease.

The use of hypoxic cell sensitizers and in particular the
nitroimidazoles, is one of the most important activities at this
time within the RTOG (2).   It would appear that radiotherapy is
reaching a plateau in terms of the gains that may be reached through
improvement in physical dose distribution while exploitation of
biological differences between tumour and normal tissue have just
begun.   The most important activities of the RTOG now focus on the
introduction of new modalities into clinical radiotherapy.   These
modalities include hypoxic cell radiosensitizers, radioprotectors,
hyperthermia, large field irradiation, high LET radiation and
isotopic immunotherapy.

ORGANIZATION OF MODALITY STUDIES WITHIN THE RTOG

Each of the new modalities involves a combination of expertise
in biology, physics and clinical radiotherapy.   In order to best

197

exploit the potential advantages of new modalities, the RTOG has organized a series of modality subcommittees, the Chairmen of which form the modality committee. These subcommittees are charged with introducing their new methods into clinical trials at all levels and exploring the potential for the modalities to improve clinical radiotherapy results.

Each modality subcommittee is charged with developing Phase I, Phase II and Phase III studies in its area of expertise. The parent modality committee is charged with coordinating these studies, avoiding overlap in the need for patient resources and giving peer review to protocols proposed by each modality.

THE ORGANIZATION AND TYPES OF SENSITIZER TRIALS

The definition of various stages of clinical trials in the area of hypoxic cell sensitizers is somewhat different than in terms of classical chemotherapy. Although the Phase I studies may be rather similar, those at the Phase II and III level are not.

Phase I investigations of hypoxic cell sensitizers involve the elucidation of the basic toxicity to be expected from a new agent, derivation of the maximum tolerated dose and preliminary observations on the effectiveness of the compound. A number of differences exist in hypoxic cell sensitizer trials in that patients should be receiving palliative radiotherapy for advanced local disease or metastases, should have an adequate functional status and will be receiving the sensitizer on a scheme compatible with some acceptable form of radiation fractionation. It is this latter requirement that separates hypoxic cell sensitizer trials from cytotoxic chemotherapy trials in that multiple drug administrations are required and ideally the drug should be administered daily. From the Phase I trial comes information as to the effect of overall time and number of dose administrations on the total tolerated dose and the maximum tolerated dose for each of the possible schedules of administration. Preliminary observations may be made on the efficacy of the compound in enhancing radiation response.

Phase II studies with hypoxic cell sensitizers focus the investigation on a specific cancer site and histology and a specific combination of radiation and drug fractionation/administration schemes. This is an important part of the study in that it may determine that a given drug administration scheme is too toxic or that the given radiation scheme with which it is to be combined turns out to be too toxic or less than optically effective. If 30-40 patients are entered into the Phase II evaluation it is possible to statistically compare the results with former trials and historical controls and determine that the result is at least as good as in previous experience, thus allowing a Phase III investigation.

The experience in the RTOG has been that Phase II trials are valuable in adjusting drug doses, adjusting radiation doses, and rejecting schemes that will not be acceptable to the group or which will yield unacceptable toxicity. Some specific examples may be cited from the recent experience of the RTOG in Phase II sensitizer trials.

After introduction of misonidazole into Phase II testing, it was found that the established maximum tolerated doses from the Phase I trial, i.e. 12 g/m^2 in 3 weeks and 15 g/m^2 in 6 weeks, were not acceptable in trials other than those involving tumours of the central nervous system (6). It then became evident that patients ingesting dexamethasone and phenytoin sodium, the usual situation in the presence of cranial primaries or metastases, had a much lower incidence of peripheral nervous system damage and CNS toxicity than patients receiving an identical misonidazole scheme without those other drugs (5). Examples of this are seen in Table I. Thus, it became necessary to modify the doses in the remainder of the Phase II trials with new limits of 10 g/m^2 in 3 weeks and 12 g/m^2 in 6 weeks established. Following this, major toxicities disappeared and the incidence of Grade I and II toxicities reduced from 25 to 20%.

Other examples of the usefulness of Phase II studies include the decision to reduce the overall time for treatment of melanoma and sarcoma from 6 to 3 weeks because of poor response in the prolonged schema protocol with treatment once per week. Response has improved with twice weekly 600 rad fractions for 3 weeks.

Table 1. Relationship of misonidazole toxicity to dexamethasone and phenytoin ingestion.

INST	DOSE SCHEDULE	± PHENYTOIN SODIUM	± DEXAMETHA- SONE	INCIDENCE P.N.	INCIDENCE CNS
UCSF	2 g/m^2 BIW x 3 wks	+	+	0/15	0/15
UCSF	same	−	−	4/5	1/5
UCSF	1.25 g/m^2 BIW x 6 wks	+	+	0/4	0/4
UCSF	same	−	−	6/7	0/7

Toxicity was unacceptably high from radiation damage to the small bowel in the bladder protocol, which included 400 rads weekly for 8 weeks with additional small fractions.   Acceptance of 400 rads twice weekly was poor in carcinoma of the cervix and this protocol was modified to utilize standard daily fractionation.   It became evident during Phase II trial in carcinoma of the oesophagus that an intravenous medication was required and this study will soon be switched to the new compound desmethylmisonidazole which will be available as an intravenous preparation.

Phase III trials in sensitizers are basically built upon the results of Phase II trials.   Those Phase II studies which have been successful and have had acceptable toxicity from drug and radiation can then be used as one arm of a randomized trial.   The experimental arm may be compared with conventional radiotherapy, to the same altered fractionation scheme without misonidazole, or to controls involving both altered fractionation and conventional radiotherapy without misonidazole.   Examples of all three types of controls exist within the RTOG Phase III studies now activated (6).   These include a randomized trial in brain metastases with 300 rads x 10 and 500 rads x 6 with and without misonidazole.   Other studies in carcinoma of the lung include conventional fractionation with and without sensitizer for moderately advanced disease and 600 rads x 6 with and without sensitizer for very advanced disease.   In glioblastoma multiforme, patients are given 400 rads once weekly with misonidazole followed by 3 conventional fractions for a total of 6-7 weeks.   For carcinoma of the head and neck, patients are given 2 fractions each Monday with misonidazole and 3 additional fractions without sensitizer for a total of 6-7 weeks.   In carcinoma of the cervix, patients are given conventional radiotherapy with and without misonidazole including drug during the brachytherapy. Finally, in hepatic metastases, patients are given 300 rads x 7 with and without sensitizer.

DATA COLLECTION, REPORTING AND REVIEW

When one conducts Phase I, II and III studies within a cooperative clinical trials group, it is essential to collect the information in a uniform manner.   The RTOG does this through the use of a sensitizer flow sheet which is submitted to headquarters throughout the patient's treatment course and which records each treatment given.   Information collected includes details of the radiotherapy, the sensitizer dose and cumulative dose as well as blood levels. Other administered medication is recorded as well as the performance status of the patient.   Response of the primary, lymph nodes, and metastases are recorded, and toxicity is evaluated in the central nervous system, peripheral nervous system, ears, gastrointestinal tract, and other critical organs including kidney, liver, bone marrow and skin.   Simple serum chemistries are followed routinely as is the haematologic profile.

The information collected on flow sheets is desseminated to each study manager and abstracted for inclusion in the headquarters computer.   In particular, the computer monitors the drug levels, the toxicity, and the tumour response and gives a frequent printout to the study managers and toxicity monitors on a patient-by-patient basis.

TOXICITY EVALUATION

In order to record the toxicity of a new sensitizer, it is essential to have adequate toxicity grading systems.   This toxicity grading must not be confined to only those systems which may be thought to cause toxicity but all important body systems. The toxicity grading system of the RTOG for sensitizers evaluates not only the GI and nervous systems but also the haematologic, renal, hepatic, pulmonary, cardiac and other systems.   This is essential to discover other unexpected toxicities.

This more recently derived system divides peripheral nervous systems into a number of sub-systems including reflexes, strength, sensory system and GI motility and divides the central nervous system effects between mental status, mood, motor paresis, cerebellar function and seizures.

The earlier toxicity grading system, which is much simpler, was utilized during the Phase I evaluation of misonidazole in the United States (1,3.4).   This system is shown in Tables 2a to 3d for nausea and vomiting, the peripheral nervous system, the central nervous system and for ototoxicity.

Table 2a.   Nausea and vomiting
toxicity scale

Grade

0 = No nausea or vomiting

1 = Nausea, no vomiting

2 = Nausea and occasional vomiting

3 = Nausea and frequent vomiting

4 = Continuous vomiting

Table 2b.   Peripheral nervous system toxicity scale.

Grade

0 = None measurable.

1 = 50% reduction in vibratory sense to 128 cps tuning fork or
      perception of pin-prick in lower extremity. Mild pares-
      thesias.

2 = 80% reduction in vibratory sense to 128 cps tuning fork or
      perception of pin-prick in both upper and lower extremities.
      Moderate paresthesias. Muscle cramps.

3 = Disabling sensory loss or pain. Peripheral nerve weakness
      or foot drop. Severe paresthesias. Severe weakness.

4 = Patient unable to walk or sleep because of paresthesias or
      pain.   Patient confined to bed or wheel-chair because of
      peripheral neurologic deficit.

Table 2c.   Central nervous system toxicity scale.

Grade

0 = None measurable.

1 = Mild CNS toxicity, confusion.

2 = Moderate CNS toxicity, lethargy, marked confusion.

3 = Seizures or complete coma due to CNS injury by misonidazole.

4 = CNS-type death thought due to misonidazole.

Table 2d.   Ototoxicity scale.

Grade

0 = None measurable.

1 = Difficulty only with faint speech.

2 = Frequent difficulty with faint speech.

3 = Frequent difficulty with loud speech.

4 = Essentially deaf.

Table 3.   Schema of patient entry by dose level and number of doses.

DOSE SCHEDULE	DOSE (gm/m^2)	TOTAL DOSE (gm/m^2)	PATIENT COURSES	PATIENT COURSES COMPLETED
Weekly x 3 weeks	1.0	3	3	3
(3 doses)	2.0	6	4	4
	3.0	9	4	2
	4.0	12	3	2
	5.0	15	4	2
Weekly x 6 weeks	1.0	6	3	1
(6 doses)	2.0	12	9	5
	2.5	15	5	3
	3.0	18	5	0
Twice/week	2.0	12	12	10
x 3 weeks	2.5	15	6	4
(6 doses)				
Twice/week	1.25	15	14	10
x 6 weeks	1.5	18	6	2
(12 doses)	1.75	21	1	1
Thrice/week x 2 weeks (6 doses)	1.5	9	2	2
Thrice/week	1.5	10.5	3	3
x $2^1/_3$ weeks	1.75	12.25	4	3
(7 doses)				
Once/day x 5 days (5 doses)	1.5	7.5	6	6
Once/day	1.5	10.5	6	3
x 7 days	1.75	12.25	4	2
(7 doses)				
			104	68

OBSERVED TOXICITY IN RTOG PHASE I STUDIES

     The initial Phase I study of misonidazole in the United States involved a total of 102 patients with 104 patient courses of drug (3). Two patients had second courses of drug remote from the first course. In Table 3 is shown the scheme of administration of drug in terms of individual doses, dose schedule and total dose for the entire initial Phase I evaluation. This study involved patients with a wide range of histologic types and primary sites and many patients with distant metastases. The various histologic diagnoses are shown in Table 4.

     As the total doses were escalated, toxicity in terms of nausea and vomiting, peripheral neuropathy with sensory and motor changes, central nervous system effects with lethargy and confusion and oto-toxicity with transient deafness were observed. In all cases the symptoms were reversible although some of the most severe peripheral neuropathies took 6-12 months to resolve completely. The CNS and ototoxicity effects were rather short-lived, reversing in almost all patients within 2 weeks. The incidence of the various toxicities as a function of individual dose for nausea and vomiting and total dose (in g/m^2) for the other toxicities are shown in Tables 5 to 8.

     Subsequent to the completion of the Phase I study, a second study which entered a total of 43 patients, was begun to compare the bioavailability of misonidazole in the original tablet form to the newly adopted capsule form (7). Administration of tablets was difficult in some patients who required liquid suspension of the drug and for careful adjustment of the exact dosage. For this

Table 4. Misonidazole Phase I Study.

Histologic Diagnosis	No. of Patients
Squamous cell carcinoma	27
Adenocarcinoma	25
Sarcoma	3
Melanoma	6
Glioma	17
Other and unclassified	24
Total	102

Table 5.   Nausea and vomiting incidence and grade.

DOSE (gm/m^2)	TOTAL INCIDENCE	GRADE 1	GRADE 2	GRADE 3	GRADE 4
1.0	1/6	1	-	-	-
1.25	4/14	2	1	-	1
1.5	10/21	4	6	-	-
1.75	1/9	-	1	-	-
2.0	11/25	7	3	1	-
2.5	8/11	5	3	-	-
3.0	6/9	2	1	1	2
4.0	3/3	1	1	-	1
5.0	4/4	1	2	1	-
	48/102	23	18	3	4

Table 6.   Peripheral neuropathy incidence and grade.

TOTAL DOSE (gm/m^2)	TOTAL INCIDENCE	GRADE 1	GRADE 2	GRADE 3	GRADE 4
0 - 3	1/6	-	1	-	-
3+ - 6	1/11	1	-	-	-
6+ - 9	7/17	-	5	2	-
9+ - 12	14/30	4	7	3	-
12+ - 15	23/31	2	15	5	1
15+ - 18	1/2	-	-	1	-
18+ - 21	2/2	1	1	-	-
	49/99 (49%)	8	29	11	1

Table 7.   Central nervous system toxicity incidence and grade.

TOTAL DOSE (gm/m^2)	TOTAL INCIDENCE	GRADE 1	GRADE 2	GRADE 3	GRADE 4
0 - 3	0/6	-	-	-	-
3+ - 6	0/11	-	-	-	-
6+ - 9	1/17	-	1	-	-
9+ - 12	4/30	3	-	1	-
12+ - 15	3/31	1	2	-	-
15+ - 18	1/2	-	1	-	-
18+ - 21	0/2	-	-	-	-
	9/99 (9%)	4	4	1	0

Table 8.   Ototoxicity incidence and grade.

TOTAL DOSE (gm/m^2)	TOTAL INCIDENCE	GRADE 1	GRADE 2	GRADE 3	GRADE 4
0 - 3	0/6	-	-	-	-
3+ - 6	0/11	-	-	-	-
6+ - 9	1/17	1	-	-	-
9+ - 12	2/30	-	-	2	-
12+ - 15	6/31	-	5	1	-
15+ - 18	0/2	-	-	-	-
18+ - 21	0/2	-	-	-	-
	9/99 (9%)	1	5	3	-

Table 9.　Bioavailability of Misonidazole.

	DOSE SCHEDULE	T.D. g/m^2	OTO.	P.N.	GI
CHILDREN N=9					
	Intermittent				
(N=2)	1.5 g/m² 3/wk x 6 doses	12	I 1/2	I 1/2	I 2/2
(N=1)	1.5 g/m² 1/wk x 4 doses 2/wk x 4 doses	12	I 1/1		
	Daily				
(N=1)	1 g/m² qd x 10	10		II 1/1	III 1/1
(N=1)	1.75 g/m² 1/wk x 1 .5 g/m² d. x 25 doses	14.25		II 1/1	
	TOTAL INCIDENCE		2/9	3/9	3/9
ADULTS N=32					
	Intermittent				
(N=1)	2.5 g/m² 1/wk x 6 doses	15		II 1/1	II 1/1
(N=1)	2 g/m² 3/wk x 5 doses	10			I 1/1
(N=1)	1.25 g/m² 2/wk x 6 doses	12.5		I 1/1	
(N=1)	1 g/m² 2/wk x 11 doses	11		III 1/1	
	Daily				
(N=2)	1.5 g/m² qd x 7 doses	10.5		I 1/2	
(N=1)	0.5 g/m² qd x 15 doses	7.5			I 1/1
(N=3)	0.5 g/m² qd x 25 doses	12.5		I 2/3	I 1/3
(N=12)	0.5 g/m² qd x 30 doses	15		I 2/12	
	TOTAL INCIDENCE			8/32	4/32

[+]Roman numeral indicates grade.

reason the format was changed to capsules rather than tablets and it was desired to determine that the pharmacology of capsules was similar to tablets.   This study was also expanded to include 9 children as well as 32 adults since the initial Phase I study had not involved children.

In Table 9 is shown the toxicity data for patients treated in this bioavailability study.   The pharmacologic results will be presented elsewhere in this conference but it suffices to say there was no significant difference between capsules and tablets or between adults and children.   From the toxicity evaluation it can be seen that 2 of 9 children experienced Grade I ototoxicity and 3 of 9 Grade I or II peripheral neurotoxicity with 3 of 9 showing Grade I-III GI Toxicity.   The peripheral neuropathy is somewhat higher than expected from total doses of 10 and 12 g/m^2 and may represent a slight increase in sensitivity of children.

Among the adults, the overall peripheral neuropathy incidence was 8 of 32 and there was no central or ototoxicity.   This incidence is similar to that seen in the more recent Phase II trials and lower than that in the original Phase I trial which was close to 50%.   GI toxicity occurred in 4 of 32 adults receiving between 0.5 and 2.5 g/m^2 per dose.

SUMMARY

The division of trials into Phase I, Phase II and Phase III within the RTOG and the careful supervision by the modality sub-committee for sensitizers has led to a rapid introduction of misoni-dazole into clinical trials.   The initial impressions from the Phase I study as to maximum tolerated dose were refined in the Phase II studies and in some situations the total dose was reduced because of the recognition of increased tolerance in certain patients with central nervous system disease taking additional medication.   The extensive toxicity grading system of the RTOG has proven valuable in elucidating the various toxicities of nitro-imidazole sensitizers and the results of the Phase II studies are now in randomized trials in comparison with conventional radiotherapy to determine the true efficacy of hypoxic cell sensitizers of the misonidazole class.

REFERENCES

1.   T. L. Phillips, T. H. Wasserman, R. J. Johnson
       The hypoxic cell sensitizer program in the United States,
       Br. J. Cancer 37:suppl. III:276 (1978).
2.   T. L. Phillips, and T. H. Wasserman, Hypoxic cell sensitizer
       studies in the U.S., in: "Treatment of Radioresistant
       Cancers", Elsevier, North Holland Press, pp. 29-40 (1979).

3. T. L. Phillips, T. H. Wasserman, R. J. Johnson,
    Final report on the United States Phase I clinical trial
    of the hypoxic cell radiosensitizer misonidazole.
    Submitted to <u>Cancer</u> (1980).
4. T. H. Wasserman, T. L. Phillips, R. J. Johnson,
    Initial U.S. clinical and pharmacologic evaluation of
    misonidazole, an hypoxic cell radiosensitizer, <u>Int. J.</u>
    <u>Radiat. Oncol. Biol. Phys.</u> 5:775 (1979).
5. T. H. Wasserman, R. Urtasun, and J. Schwade, The neurotoxicity
    of misonidazole. Potential modifying role of phenytoin
    sodium and dexamethasone, <u>Brit. J. Radiol.</u> 53:173 (1980).
6. T. H. Wasserman, J. Stetz, and T. L. Phillips, Clinical trials
    of misonidazole in the United States, <u>Cancer Clinical</u>
    <u>Trials</u>, in press, (1980).
7. G. VanRaalte, T. L. Phillips, and T. H. Wasserman, (Abstract),
    <u>Int.J. Radiat. Oncol. Biol. Phys.</u>, in press, (1980).

MISONIDAZOLE CLINICAL TRIALS IN THE UNITED STATES RADIATION THERAPY

ONCOLOGY GROUP (RTOG)

Todd H. Wasserman,[1] JoAnn Stetz,[2] Theodore L. Phillips[3]

[1] Division of Radiation Oncology, Mallinckrodt Institute
of Radiology, Washington University School of Medicine
St. Louis, Missouri 63108
[2] Radiation Therapy Oncology Group, 925 Chestnut Street
Philadelphia, Pennsylvania 19107
[3] Department of Radiation Oncology, University of
California at San Francisco, San Francisco
California 94143.

ABSTRACT

This paper presents a review of the progressive clinical trials
of the hypoxic cell radiosensitizer, misonidazole, in the United
States.   Presentation is made of all the schemas of the recently
completed and currently active Radiation Therapy Oncology Group (RTOG)
Phase II and Phase III studies.   Detailed information is presented
on the clinical toxicity of the Phase II trials, specifically
regarding neurotoxicity.   With limitations in drug total dose, a
variety of dose schedules have proven to be tolerable, with a
moderate incidence of nausea and vomiting and mild peripheral
neuropathy, and a low incidence of more severe peripheral neuropathy
or central neuropathy.   No other organ toxicity has been seen,
specifically no liver, renal or bone marrow toxicities.   The clinical
pharmacologic monitoring of misonidazole blood levels has been
satisfactory with good correlation between the group-wide (Phase II)
UV values and the HPLC values from the Phase I study.   The patient
accrual of the trials has been rapidly increasing and an early
analysis suggests efficacy which is better when compared to previous
radiation experience.   A series of eight Phase III trials are
currently underway or proposed in the RTOG and the results of these
are pending.   An additional Phase III malignant glioma trial in
the Brain Tumor Study Group is described.

211

INTRODUCTION

The National Cancer Institute, Division of Cancer Treatment
(NCI-DCT), in conjunction with the Radiation Therapy Oncology Group
(RTOG), has embarked upon a program to develop and apply hypoxic cell
radiosensitizers to the treatment of advanced cancer (1,2,3).

The preclinical background for the presence of hypoxic cells in
solid tumors in animal models and man, for their known resistance to
the effects of ionizing radiation, and for the attempts to overcome
this resistance by the use of either hyperbaric oxygen, high linear
energy transfer radiation, and/or hypoxic cell radiosensitizers is
not the subject of this paper and has been discussed elsewhere (1,4).
That the nitroimidazoles appear to be the best class of compounds
tested to date as hypoxic cell radiosensitizers and that misonidazole
has been the primary compound in this class tested to date has also
been discussed elsewhere (3,4,5).

METHODS

As a first clinical step in this program, misonidazole was
obtained by the NCI-DCT and an application for initial clinical trial
was filed with the US Food and Drug Administration (FDA) and
approved for activation in July, 1977 via the RTOG. The objectives
of the Phase I trial were to determine the maximum tolerated dose of
misonidazole administered orally on a once per week dose schedule
for up to six weeks and then multiple doses per week schedules for
up to six weeks, to determine the qualitative toxicities of the
drug and to determine the pharmacologic properties of the drug with
regard to peak serum levels, half lives, excretion, metabolism, and
tumor tissue levels. The initial aspect of the study was previously
published (2). A detailed publication on the pharmacology of
misonidazole was published by Wasserman et al (5). The initial
Phase I clinical trial which opened at the University of California,
at San Francisco and Roswell Park Memorial Institute in Buffalo, New
York, accrued 104 patients on multiple dose schedules during its
time course of July 1977 through December 1978 (6).

The RTOG using the information from the Phase I study opened a
number of pilot Phase II studies starting in April 1978. As of
August 1980, five studies have been completed, three studies were
closed before completion, and seven active Phase II clinical trials
are ongoing. Six Phase III trials are currently open and two others
are in preparation.

The Phase II studies were designed to be cancer-site and stage-
specific, to use a fixed dose schedule of radiation, to use a fixed
dose schedule of misonidazole, and to enter between 30 to 40
patients. The end points of the study were to establish the
tolerance of any modifications in the dose schedule of radiation

that were necessary in order to use the misonidazole, to establish the tolerance of the misonidazole in a larger number of patients of a given cancer site and stage, to increase the clinical familiarity of multiple investigatives with misonidazole, to establish the reproducibility of the ultra-violet pharmacologic assay and to look for some information on the frequency of tumor clearance compared to the historical clinical experience of radiation alone in the specific cancer site and stage.   These studies were designed to be preparatory for randomized Phase III studies.   These Phase II studies in general either use conventional fractionation of radiation therapy with two fractions in 18 hours with misonidazole being given once or twice per week; or intermittent fractionation of radiation therapy and intermittent misonidazole with the misonidazole being given before every fraction of radiation; or a large weekly dose of radiation plus misonidazole and conventional fractionation without misonidazole for the rest of the week.

RESULTS

     The Phase I clinical trial established a safe initial starting drug dose on several dose schedules namely weekly for three weeks, weekly for six weeks, twice a week for three weeks, twice a week for six weeks, thrice a week for two weeks, daily for five days, and daily for seven days (6).   The study also established high-pressure liquid chromatography (HPLC) and ultra-violet (UV) pharmacologic data which established the qualitative and quantitative aspects of the dose limiting peripheral neurotoxicity and clearly showed that the major risk factor was total misonidazole dose in g/m^2.   The study established the lack of other major organ toxicities, such as renal, bone marrow, or hepatic.   The majority of the neurotoxicities occurred with total doses greater than 12 g/m^2.   Also the majority of the neurotoxicities were of grade I or II type with only severe peripheral neurotoxicities (PN) seen in 12% of the cases, overall. Table 1 gives the criteria for grading the neurotoxicity.   The incidence of central neurotoxicity (CN) was 9 out of 99 with 8 of the 9 toxicities grades I or II and only one grade III toxicity.   The incidence of ototoxicity was also 9 out of 99 (9%), and this was a new toxicity identified in the Phase I study.   One finding in reviewing those patients who did or did not develop neurotoxicity was a relationship of misonidazole toxicity to the administration of dexamethasone and dilantin.   Those patients who received either dexamethasone or dilantin had a lower incidence of neurotoxicity than those patients who did not at a similar dose schedule (7).

     The first Phase II study opened in April 1978 and 15 studies have been opened as of August 1980, with five studies completing accrual.   A total of 467 patients have been entered with 372 patients evaluable.

Table 1.   Misonidazole neurotoxicity grading

GRADE	PERIPHERAL	CENTRAL
I	OBJECTIVE SENSORY CHANGES OR MILD PARESTHESIAS OR DECREASED REFLEXES	MILD LETHARGY OR CONFUSION
II	MODERATE PARESTHESIAS OR PAIN OR DETECTABLE WEAKNESS OR ABSENT REFLEXES	MODERATE LETHARGY OR CONFUSION OR SEIZURE
III	SEVERE PARESTHESIAS OR PAIN OR SEVERE WEAKNESS	SEVERE LETHARGY OR CONFUSION UNCONTROLLED SEIZURES
IV	PARALYSIS	COMA

Table 2 gives complete information of the five closed studies, including the RTOG protocol number, the cancer site and stage, the inclusive dates of protocol entry, the number of patients entered, the number of patients evaluable, the radiation dose schedule, the misonidazole dose schedule, and any appropriate reference.

Table 2.   Completed RTOG Phase II misonidazole studies

RTOG No.	CANCER TYPE AND STAGE	DATE OPENED – CLOSED	No. Pts. ENTERED	No. Pts. EVALUABLE	RADIATION SCHEDULE	MISONIDAZOLE DOSE SCHEDULE	REF
78-01	MALIGNANT GLIOMAS – GRADE III, IV	4/78 11/79	59	54	WHOLE BRAIN – 400 RADS – MON 150 RADS – TU, TH, FRI X 6 WKS +180 RAD X 5 BOOST TOTAL DOSE = 6000 RADS	2.5 GM/M² Q WK X 6 = 15 GM/M²	8,9
78-02	HEAD & NECK CANCERS–T3, T4	4/78 6/79	50	45	250 RADS (4 HRS AFTER MISO) 210 RADS (8 HRS AFTER MISO) } Q WK X 5 WKS 180 RADS Q D X3 PER WK X5 WKS THEN 180 RADS Q D X 5/WK X2 – 3 WKS TOTAL DOSE = 6600-7200 RADS	2.5 GM/M² Q WK X 6 = 15 GM/M² MODIFIED TO 2.0 GM/M² Q WK X 6 = 12 GM/M²	10
78-12	BRAIN METASTASES (PTS WITH OTHER METASTASES ALSO)	7/78 5/79	40	34	600 RADS BIW X 3 WKS = 3600 RADS	2.0 GM/M² BIW X 3 WKS = 12 GM/M²	11
78-30	LIVER METASTASES	1/79 11/79	50	44	300 RADS DAILY X 7 D=2100 RADS	1.5 GM/M² D X 7 = 10.5 GM/M²	12
78-14	LUNG CANCER (STAGE III)	8/78 1/80	52 / 251	49 / 226	600 RADS BIW X 3 WKS=3600 RADS	2.0 (REDUCED TO 1.75) GM/M² BIW X 3 WKS = 12 (10.5) GM/M²	13

In gliomas, a Phase II trial (#78-01) of misonidazole with radiation but without the use of concomitant chemotherapy has been completed (8,9)(Table 2). The study looked at malignant gliomas, grade III and IV, receiving whole brain radiation in conjunction with misonidazole. The dose of radiation was increased on the day that the misonidazole was given, and both the large dose of radiation and misonidazole were given weekly. The incidence of peripheral neuropathy (PN) in this study was 7/54 = 13% and is lower than that seen in the overall Phase II experience. This is presumed to be secondary to the fact that most of these patients were receiving concomitant, dexamethasone and/or dilantin. The incidence of central neurotoxicity was 8 grade 1 (15%) and many of these may be related to the primary glioma and not to misonidazole. The overall median survival was 52 weeks despite the lack of initial chemotherapy. The conclusion of this study was that the survival was equivalent to previous experience with radiation therapy only and that a randomized study should be undertaken in this disease which has been started (#79-18)(Table 9). It was felt that the toxicity of the radiation and misonidazole was minimal and that the regimen was acceptable.

A Phase II study in head and neck cancers (#78-02), has been completed, using misonidazole and a unique schedule of radiation therapy in advanced primaries (T3 and T4). The radiation schedule involved two fractions of irradiation given in one day in conjunction with misonidazole and repeated weekly for five weeks; with conventional fractionation given during the course of the rest of the week. This study which has been reported by Frazekas (10), has shown a good tumor clearance rate at the end of therapy with moderate toxicity. The misonidazole dose schedule was modified from 2.5 g/m^2 weekly x 6 weeks to 2 g/m^2 weekly x 6 weeks, lowering the total dose from 15 g/m^2 to 12 g/m^2. This patient population is susceptible to developing dehydration secondary to radiation reaction, or primary tumor reaction and this has led to some higher than expected serum levels of misonidazole with prolonged half-lives. The incidence of neuropathy decreased with the dose reduction, and with the study also modified to assure adequate hydration. Prior to the dose reduction there were three cases of misonidazole encephalopathy, two of which were associated with the ultimate death of the patient with misonidazole felt to be a contributing factor. Only one case of mild encephalopathy out of twenty patients has been reported since the dose reduction. The overall incidence of PN was 16/45 = 36% with grade 1 = 7; grade 2 = 7; grade 3 = 2. No increased mucosal toxicity was seen. It was recommended that this study proceed into a Phase III randomized study which has been started (#79-15) (Table 9).

A Phase II trial in patients with brain metastases (#78-12)(who also had involvement of other metastatic sites) has been completed (11)(Table 2). This study used a bi-weekly fractionation of radiation therapy in conjunction with bi-weekly misonidazole. Again

Table 3.   Ongoing Phase II misonidazole studies

RTOG NO.	CANCER TYPE AND STAGE	DATE OPENED	RADIATION SCHEDULE	MISONIDAZOLE DOSE SCHEDULE
78-13	WIDESPREAD METS.	7/78	600 RAD - HEMIBODY	5 (REDUCED TO 4) GM/M^2 ONE DOSE
78-15	ADVANCED OR RECURRENT SARCOMAS OR MELANOMAS	7/78 (MODIFIED 7/79)	700 RAD Q WK X 6 WKS = 4200 RAD (600 RAD BIW X 3 WKS = 3600 RAD)	2.5 GM/M^2 Q WK X 6 = 15 GM/M^2 (1.75 GM/M^2 BIW X 3 WKS = 10.5 GM/M)
78-23	PEDIATRIC CNS TUMORS RECURRENT	12/78	300 RAD X 10/2 WKS = 3000 RAD	1.5 GM/M^2 TIW X 2 WKS = 9.0 GM/M^2
78-32	ESOPHAGUS - LOCALLY ADVANCED	1/79	400 RAD/12 FXS/4-1/2 WKS = 4800 RAD	1.0 GM/M^2 X 12 = 12 GM/M^2
79-03	GLIOMAS - NEUTRONS	7/79	300 (NEUTRONS) X 4 + BOOST OF 300 (NEUTRONS) X 2	2.5 GM/M^2 X 6 = 15 GM/M^2
79-04	HEAD & NECK - STAGE III, IV	6/79	400 RAD X 12 FX/2-1/2 WKS = 4800 RAD SAME + MISONIDAZOLE	1.5 GM/M^2 TIW X 7 = 10.5 GM/M^2
79-05	PELVIC - ADVANCED LOCAL CANCER	10/79	1000 RAD/1 FX/Q MO. X 3 = 3000 RAD	4.0 GM/M^2 Q MO X 3 = 12.0 GM/M^2

the incidence of neurotoxicity was lower in this group than
anticipated, probably due to protection by dexamethasone and/or
dilantin with twenty-nine of thirty-four evaluable patients taking
either medication.   The incidence of peripheral neuropathy was
2/33 = 6% (all grade 1) and that of central neuropathy 1/33 = 3%.
Most patients had good improvement of neurological function and
there were some patients with serial CT scans who had good reduction
of mass on CT scan.   It was felt that this regimen was equally
tolerable to previous best regimen in the RTOG of 3000 rad in 10
fractions in two weeks.   A comparative Phase III study has been
started (#79-16)(Table 9).

Another Phase II study has been completed in patients who have
hepatic metastases (#78-30)(12)(Table 2).   This study looked at
daily fractions of radiation and of misonidazole for a total of
seven days, radiation dose totalling 2100 rads, misonidazole dose
totalling 10.5 g/m^2.   The study has been well tolerated with

acceptable incidence of neurotoxicity (8/44 = 18%).   There has been
no cases of radiation hepatitis or nephritis.   This therapy yielded
a high response rate of 40-60% for pain relief, increased Karnofsky
score, decreased liver size, and decreased liver function tests.   A
Phase III randomized trial has been started in liver metastases
(#80-03)(Table 9).

A Phase II trial of intermittent twice a week radiation therapy
for advanced, stage III, non-oat cell lung cancers has been completed
(#78-14)(13)(Table 2).   This study had an incidence of peripheral
neuropathy of 43% (21/49) (grade 1 = 9, grade 2 = 10, grade 3 = 2)
and an incidence of central neuropathy of 12% (6/49).   Complete and
partial responses of 17% and 54% respectively were observed on serial
chest x-rays.   The median survival is 7 months (60% dead to date)
with 32% alive at 1 year.   This regimen also proved to be quite
tolerable and has been put into a Phase III randomized study in
locally advanced lung cancer (#79-25)(Table 9).

A number of other Phase II studies in other cancer types and
stages are currently ongoing in the RTOG (Table 3).   Several studies
have closed before completion of patient accrual and they are shown
in Table 4 with the reasons for incompletion given.

Table 5 shows the relationship of misonidazole mean four-to-six
hour serum levels to the dose of misonidazole in g/m^2.   A
comparison is made between the determinations of the Phase I study
and Phase II studies.   The determinations in the Phase I study were
primarily using HPLC while those in Phase II studies were primarily
UV spectrophotometry and involved multiple institutions.   As can be
seen there is generally good agreement between the values of the

Table 4.   Closed RTOG Phase II Misonidazole studies

RTOG NO.	CANCER TYPE & STAGE	DATE OPENED/CLOSED	NO. PTS. ENTERED	NO. PTS. EVALUABLE	RADIATION SCHEDULE	MISO SCHEDULE	COMMENTS
78-21	BLADDER-LOCALLY ADVANCED	10/78-2/80	11	9	400 RAD Q MON X 8 WKS 200 RAD Q WED, FRI X 8 WKS = 4800 RAD BLADDER BOOST = 2000 RAD/2 WKS	1.5 GM/M²Q WK X 8 WKS = 12 GM/M²	GOOD LOCAL TUMOR CONTROL-7 CR's LITTLE MISO TOXICITY-4 GR I NEURO STUDY CLOSED DUE TO 3 SMALL BOWEL OBSTRUCTIONS
78-24	HEAD & NECK - STAGE III, IV	12/78-8/79	11	10	400 RAD 2 X/WK THEN 3 X/WK = 4800-5600 RAD	1.25 GM/M² (REDUCED TO 1.0 GM/M²) BIW-TIW X 5 WKS = 12-15 GM/M²	STUDY CLOSED DUE TO COMPLETING STUDY
79-06	CERVIX-IIIB, IVA	7/79-7/80	10	7	400 RAD BIW X 5 WKS= 4000 RAD + INTRACAVITARY BOOST	1.25 (REDUCED TO 1.2) GM/M² BIW X 5 WKS=12.0-12.5 GM/M² (1.25 GM/M² X 2 DURING BOOST = 15 GM/M²	5/7 GRADE I NEUROTOXIC. 1/7 GRADE II POOR ACCRUAL DUE TO HIGH DOSE FXS.

Table 5.   Misonidazole Phase I and II studies

RELATIONSHIP OF DOSE TO MEAN 4-6 HOUUR SERUM LEVEL

DOSES GM/M²	NO. OF DOSES (DETERMINATIONS)		MEAN 4-6 HR. SERUM LEVEL µg/ml		+/- STANDARD DEVIATION		OBSERVED RANGE	
	PHASE I	PHASE II	PHASE I	PHASE II	PHASE I	PHASE II	PHASE I	PHASE II
1.0	17	10*	30	49	9	13	21-57	25-72
1.25	116	65	46	44	6	17	31-61	6-74
1.5	78	225	60	57	18	23	16-95	3-179
1.75	18	50	70	64	18	17	39-107	3-102
2.0	99	306	76	68	14	22	51-120	2-141
2.5	43	324	98	83	23	29	35-148	4-165
3.0	25	-	116	-	26	-	39-155	-
4.0	8	7	175	146	56	44	83-238	68-204
5.0	7	7	183	170	60	47	91-245	85-210
	411	994						

* 1 PATIENT

PHASE I VALUES   HPLC (0582 + 9963)
PHASE II VALUES   UV

Table 6.   Misonidazole RTOG Phase II Studies

PERIPHERAL NEUROPATHY

TOTAL DOSE GM/M²	TOTAL INCIDENCE		GRADE			
	NO.	%	I	II	III	IV
0 - < 5	0/32	0	-	-	-	-
5 - < 7	3/16	19	2	1	-	-
7 - <10	17/83	20	7	8	2	-
10 - <12	42/127	33	21	18	3	-
12 - <15	33/86	38	14	16	3	-
15 - <18	6/28	21	2	2	2	-
	101/372	27	46(12%)	45(12%)	10(3%)	

Phase I and II studies with both sets of data showing increased blood
level expected for increased oral dose given. Any variance between
the Phase I and Phase II studies are probably due to several compoun-
ding factors. First, the determination of m^2 can vary from
institution to institution. Second, the rounding of the doses to
the nearest g/m^2 varied somewhat during the course of the studies
depending upon the pharmacologic preparation available. Initially
there was only a 500 mg enteric coated tablet and then subsequently
there were 500 and 100 mg capsules. There is no apparent pharmacological difference between the tablet or the capsule (14) but the
capsules allowed for a closer dose approximation. The third reason
for any variance is due to the multiple institutions which provided
the assay data and explains the larger observed ranges in the Phase II
studies. However, we feel it can be generally concluded that the
pharmacologic assay is reproducible and reliable, because the
variance is small.

The acute toxicities of misonidazole can be divided into two
categories, gastrointestinal toxicity and neurotoxicity. The
gastrointestinal toxicity consists primarily of nausea and vomiting.
The incidence of this toxicity overall is 58% in 226 evaluable
patients. Most of the toxicities are of a grade I or II type with
nausea and occasional vomiting. There is clearly a relationship of
the incidence to the anatomic area being treated with radiation, and
it is difficult to separate radiation induced nausea and vomiting
from drug induced nausea and vomiting. There was a higher incidence
of nausea and vomiting in the hemi-body study, sarcoma study and
liver mets study and a lower incidence in the brain metastases
study and head and neck study.

The second major toxicity is that of neurotoxicity. The
primary manifestation is that of peripheral neurotoxicity consisting
primarily of objective sensory changes, mild paresthesias and
occasional sensory pain or severe paresthesias. There is some, but
not a major component of motor neuropathy. The overall incidence
of peripheral neuropathy in the 372 evaluable patients was 27%.
This is a lower overall incidence than the 49% seen in the Phase I
study (6) and is due to the more limited total doses of the Phase II
studies. Table 6 gives the incidences of toxicity in patients
that were evaluable for total dose of misonidazole given. The
incidence of neurotoxicity increases with increasing total dose. The
incidence of peripheral neuropathy is related to total dose within
the narrower total dose range of the Phase II studies by a linear
relationship with a correlation coefficient of 0.777. The slope,
however, of this linear relationship is much shallower than the slope
of the same relationship in the Phase I study as given in Figure 1.
(The data in Figure 1 is based on only 324 patients.) We assume
that the reasons for this are several fold. There was probably a
tendency to over-call the perioheral neurotoxicity in the Phase I
study because of very careful follow-up of these patients for minor

Table 7. Misonidazole RTOG Phase II studies

CNS TOXICITY

TOTAL DOSE GM/M²	TOTAL INCIDENCE NO.	%	GRADE I	II	III	IV
0 - < 5	2/32	6	-	1	1	-
5 - < 7	1/16	6	1	-	-	-
7 - < 10	10/83	12	6	2	2	-
10 - < 12	7/127	6	4	-	1	2
12 - < 15	10/86	12	7	2	-	1
15 - < 18	2/28	7	2	-	-	-
	32/372	9	20(5%)	5(1%)	4(1%)	3(1%)

changes in neurologic function. Second, the patients in the Phase I study were generally more advanced than those in the Phase II studies and had other nutritional, cancer-related, and age-related reasons for developing neuropathies. It has been generally assumed throughout all the studies that any changes in the neurologic exam which have occurred after the administration of misonidazole have been causally related, even though they may only be temporally related. The majority of neurotoxicities are of a grade I and II nature, with only an overall 3% incidence of severe neurotoxicity (grade III or IV). Most of the neuropathies occurred after the patient approached 10 g/m² usually within several weeks of that dose; some of the neuropathies occurred within the first two weeks after completing the total drug dose schedule. None of the neuropathies significantly progressed when the drug was stopped; instead, the neuropathy improved with time, lasting up to several weeks and occasionally months. Patients who have had prior vincristine neuropathy developed rapid severe misonidazole neuropathies suggesting an added toxic effect and these patients should be excluded from the clinical study with misonidazole (5). Other conditions which are associated with neuropathies, such as diabetes, alcoholism, cancer, poor nutritional state, do not seem to predispose to an increase of misonidazole toxicities. The grade I and II peripheral neuropathies as defined above, are not inconsistent with peripheral neuropathies expected clinically in association with other anti-cancer drugs, such as vincristine, hexamethylmelamine, cis-platinum.

The second type of neurotoxicity is that of the central neurotoxicity consisting primarily of confusion, lethargy, and decrease in mental function. The overall incidence of this toxicity in 372 evaluable patients was 8%. Table 7 presents the incidence by total

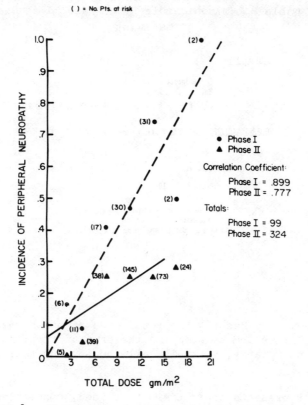

Figure 1. Neuropathy vs misonidazole total dose

misonidazole dose.   Also it shows the grade of the toxicity and again
the majority of the toxicities are of a grade I or II type.   Again
the incidence of severe central nervous toxicity is in the order of
3%.   As a result of some initial severe toxicities, some of the
Phase II studies had modifications in misonidazole dose and other
factors (Tables 2 and 3).   Modifications in the protocols have
included careful monitoring of hydration, total body weight, and
lowering of the age of patients eligible for the studies to that of
75.   Indeed such modifications have lowered the overall incidence of
neurotoxicity somewhat and virtually eliminated all the serious
neurotoxicities (grade III and IV).   Central neurotoxicity was
uncommonly seen (9 cases) in the absence of peripheral neurotoxicity
and when it did occur it was always a grade I, and potentially not

Table 8.   Misonidazole RTOG Phase II studies
OTHER TOXICITIES

OTOTOXICITY

TOTAL INCIDENCE
No.   %
23/372   6   (14 GRADE 1, 9 GRADE 2)

OTHER TOXICITIES   -   372 EVALUABLE PATIENTS

FEVER   7

SKIN RASH   9

ALLERGY   10

SOME TOXICITIES TEMPORALLY RELATED BUT
QUESTIONABLE CAUSALLY RELATED.
NO LIVER, BONE MARROW OR RENAL TOXICITIES.

drug related.   By keeping the total dose of misonidazole within
prescribed limits and by stopping the drug at the first sign of any
peripheral neuropathy, virtually all the serious toxicities have been
eliminated.

Table 8 presents other toxicities seen, consisting of occasional
ototoxicity, fever, skin rash and allergic symptoms.   As can be
expected some toxicities are temporally related but questionably
causally related.   The Phase II studies confirmed the lack of any
liver, bone marrow, or renal toxicities or toxicities of other organ
systems.

DISCUSSION

The Phase II studies confirmed the dose limiting neurotoxicity
and established an acceptable incidence of mild peripheral neuropathy
with total dose limitations of between 10.5 and 12 g/m^2.   The
acceptable dose schedules are :

- 3-4 g/m^2 single dose
- 1.25-1.5 g/m^2 daily x 5-7 days (6.25-10.5 g/m^2)
- 10.5 g/m^2 divided doses over 3 weeks
- 12.0 g/m^2 divided doses over 6 weeks.

There was a tendency to find toxicity in patients who were
elderly and became dehydrated secondary to their primary cancer, such
as head-neck cancer, and to the radiation therapy fields.   As in the
Phase I study most of the serious toxicities, central and peripheral,

Table 9. Ongoing RTOG Phase III Misonidazole studies

RTOG NO.	CANCER TYPE AND STAGE	DATE OPENED	RANDOMIZATION ARMS
79-15	HEAD & NECK CANCERS - STAGE II, III, IV	9/79	1. XRT - 6600-7380 RADS/33-41 FXS AT 180-200 RADS/FX, 5 FXS/WK 2. XRT + MISO XRT - 2 FXS Q MON, 1 FX Q TUES, THURS, FRI 6600-7380 RADS/6-1/2-7 WKS MISO - 2.0 GM/M² Q WK X 6 = 12 GM/M²
79-16	BRAIN METASTASES	9/79	1. XRT - 300 RADS QD X 5 X 2 WKS = 3000 RADS 2. XRT - 500 RADS BIW X 3 WKS = 3000 RADS 3. XRT (AS IN 1.) + MISO. 1 GM/M² QD X 5 X 2 WKS = 10 GM/M² 4. XRT (AS IN 2.) + MISO. 2 GM/M² BIW X 3 WKS = 12 GM/M²
79-17	LUNG CANCER STAGE III-T₁-T₂, T₃, N₂)	4/80	1. XRT 200 RADS QD X 5 X 5 WKS = 5000 RADS + 500 - 1000 RADS BOOST 2. XRT + MISO. 400 MG/M² D X 5 FOR 6 WKS = 12 GM/M². XRT AS ABOVE.
79-18	MALIGNANT GLIOMAS - GRADE III, IV	11/79	1. XRT + BCNU XRT - 200 RADS QD X 5 X 6 WKS = 6000 RADS BCNU - 80 MG/M² QD X 3 Q 8 WKS. 2. XRT + BCNU + MISO XRT - 400 RADS Q MON, 150 RADS Q TUES, THURS, FRI X 6 WKS + 900 RADS BOOST = 6000 RADS BCNU - AS ABOVE MISO - 2.5 GM/M² Q WK X 6 = 15 GM/M²
79-25	LUNG CANCER - T₄ OR N₃	1/80	1. XRT - 600 RADS BIW X 3 WKS = 3600 RAD 2. XRT + MISO XRT - AS ABOVE MISO - 1.75 GM/M² BIW X 3 WKS = 10.5 GM/M²

were preceded by milder peripheral neurological signs of symptoms.
Current protocols require that any patient who develops a grade II
or greater peripheral neuropathy be discontinued from the administration of misonidazole.   This we feel will prevent any subsequent
incidence of more serious neurotoxicity.   There has been continued
monitoring of patients who are receiving dilantin or dexamethasone,
and this seems to be associated with a lower incidence of
neurotoxicity.   For instance, in the glioma study #78-01, the
incidence of peripheral neuropathy was 13% and the incidence of
central neuropathy was 15%.   This is lower than the overall incidence
given above.   The same was true in the brain-mets study #78-12,
where the incidence of peripheral neuropathy was 6% and the incidence
of central neuropathy was 3%.   Patients on both of these studies were
usually receiving dexamethasone and/or phenytoin sodium.

The results of the Phase II studies have established that the UV
pharmacologic assay is reliable, that the drug can be given with a
high degree of safety and a low degree of mild to moderate peripheral
neuropathies.   There has been some evidence to suggest that a higher
than expected tumor control has been seen with the addition of the
misonidazole to the radiation.   As a result of these pilot studies,
eight Phase III studies have now been started or proposed in the RTOG.
These are again disease-specific and designed to look at a fixed dose

schedule of radiation and misonidazole. They are generally,
randomized, stratified comparisons of radiation and misonidazole
against the best standard radiation.   There is some comparison of
radiation dose schedules contained in the brain metastases study.
The end points of the study are tumor clearance, toxicity short term
and long term, tumor-free interval and relapse rate.   Continued
pharmacologic monitoring is done for efficacy analysis.   The
details of these studies are presented in Table 9.   Patient
accrual to these studies is proceeding nicely with overall 382
patients entered, 207 patients receiving misonidazole.   The
toxicity analysis shows no apparent change in the toxicity spectrum
described above for the Phase II studies but more time is needed
before any efficacy information will be forthcoming.

A randomized, stratified clinical trial of misonidazole in the
treatment of malignant gliomas has been undertaken by the Brain
Tumor Study Group (BTSG).   The study which opened in May, 1978 and
is still ongoing with data coded and in analysis, accrues the
patients to one of four randomization arms (Table 10) one arm of which

Table 9 (continued) Ongoing RTOG Phase II misonidazole studies

RTOG NO.	CANCER TYPE AND STAGE	DATE OPENED	RANDOMIZATION ARMS
80-03	LIVER METS	5/80	1. XRT - 2100 RAD/7FX/1-1/2 WKS 2. XRT + MISO - 1.5 GM/M²/DX7 = 10.5 GM/M²
80-05	CERVIX - III B IV A	--	1. XRT - 4600 RAD PELVIS + 1000 RAD PARAMETRIAL BOOST + INTRA-CAVITARY OR EXTERNAL BOOST 2. XRT + MISO - 0.4 GM/M²QD X 30 = 12 GM/M²
80-xx	BLADDER B₂, C	--	1. XRT - 2000 RAD/5 FXS/1 WK PRE-OP 2. XRT + MISO 1 GM/M² QD X 5 = 5 GM/M² 3. XRT PRE-OP (500 RAD/ 1 FX) + XRT POST-OP (4500 RAD/5 WKS)

Table 10.   Misonidazole glioma protocol: BTSG

STRATIFY BY GRADE. RANDOMIZE TO FOUR TREATMENT ARMS.

1. CONVENTIONAL RADIOTHERAPY + BCNU
2.   "   "   + MISONIDAZOLE + BCNU
3.   - "   "   + STREPTOZOTOCIN
4. HYPERFRACTIONATED "   + BCNU

CONVENTIONAL XRT: 6000 RADS (1700 RETS)
                      30-35 FXS. OF 172-200 RADS IN 6-7 WKS.
BCNU: 80 MG/M² FOR 3 DAYS Q. 8 WKS.
MISONIDAZOLE: 1.5 GM/M² IN P.M. EACH M. & TH. DURING XRT. WITH NEXT
                  DAILY DOSE OF XRT. IN A.M.
STREPTOZOTOCIN: 1.25 GM/M² ONCE PER WK. FOR 8 WKS.
HYPERFRACTIONATED XRT.: 6600 RADS (1633 RETS) 2 FXS. OF 110 RAD EACH
                  DAY FOR 60 FXS. IN 6 WKS.

includes the use of misonidazole in conjunction with conventional radiotherapy and BCNU. The dose schedule of radiotherapy has been left unmodified in conjunction with the misonidazole but the timing of the doses have been modified slightly to give the dose of radiation after the misonidazole at approximately 4 hours and then another dose early the next morning at approximately 18 hours after the misonidazole. Misonidazole (1.5 g/m^2) is repeated twice a week for 6 weeks for a total dose of 18 g/m^2. Most of the patients having malignant gliomas are also on dilantin and/or dexamethasone. In a preliminary report of the trial (15), the toxicity is tolerable with a moderate nausea and vomiting and an incidence of minor reversible peripheral neuropathy of 19%, of 21 patients.

It is unlikely that misonidazole will be the ideal radio-sensitizer since it will not be possible to administer it in frequent dose schedules for periods up to 6 weeks, and at doses which are going to yield good blood levels, (more than 50 to 100 micrograms per ml), due to the total dose limiting neurotoxicity. The clinical efficacy of misonidazole with radiation is not yet known but the RTOG is encouraged to continue to pursue the clinical usefulness of this and other hypoxic cell radiosensitizers with the understanding of their limitations. Misonidazole is sufficiently tolerable to continue clinical research into its efficacy. It will act as a basis for looking at newer expected analogs. There is an ongoing project of the NCI-DCT to develop better analogs of misonidazole with lesser neurotoxicity. One of these analogs, desmethylmisonidazole (RO-05-9963) has been identified as the principle endogenous metabolite of misonidazole in man (5). It has the advantage of being more water soluble, and less lipid soluble, allowing for a parental preparation, better urine excretion, and perhaps less penetration into peripheral nerves and the central nervous system. It is anticipated that within 6 months, initial clinical trials with this compound will be instituted within the RTOG. Other analogs are being tested pre-clinically in toxicologic and pharmacologic systems looking for other therapeutically improved compounds (2,3).

The clinical trials of misonidazole in the United States, primarily through the RTOG, have resulted in progressively increasing patient accrual (over 775 patients) and clinical familiarity with misonidazole. The dose formulation and pharmacologic monitoring are both effective. The toxicities are primarily that of mild to moderate nausea and vomiting and mild to moderate peripheral neuro-pathy and are acceptable to the cancer clinician. The Phase II clinical studies are undergoing continued analysis for information on the efficacy of the misonidazole radiation combination. Preliminary evidence suggests better efficacy than that which would have been expected from radiation alone. The major effort to establish the efficacy of misonidazole rests with the currently on-going Phase III trials. It will be at least another year or two before preliminary answers can be sought from these studies.

ACKNOWLEDGMENT

We gratefully acknowledge Mary Kane Schmitt and Josie Garcia for their secretarial assistance.

REFERENCES

1. Committee on Radiation Oncology Studies Research Plan :
    Radiation Sensitizers, Cancer 37:2062 (1976).
2. T.L. Phillips, T.H. Wasserman, R.J. Johnson, C.J. Gomer,
    G.A. Lawrence, M.L. Levine, W. Sadee, J.S. Penta and
    D.J. Rubin, The Hypoxic cell sensitizer programme in the
    United States, Br. J. Cancer 37: Suppl.III, 276 (1978).
3. P. Rubin, R.B. Cowan and D.J. Rubin, The radiation oncology
    research program, B. Radiosensitizers/radioprotectors
    working group, Int.J.Radiation Oncology Biol.Phys. 5:651
    (1979).
4. J.D. Chapman, Current concepts in cancer: Hypoxic sensitizers-
    implications for radiation therapy, New.Eng.J.Med.
    301:1429 (1979).
5. T.H. Wasserman, T.L. Phillips, R.J. Johnson, C.J. Gomer,
    G.A. Lawrence, W. Sadee, R.A. Marques, V.A. Levin and
    G. VanRaalte, Initial United States clinical and
    pharmacologic evaluation of misonidazole (RO-07-0582) an
    hypoxic cell radio sensitizer, Int.J.Radiation Oncology Biol.
    Phys. 5:775 (1979).
6. T.L. Phillips, T.H. Wasserman, R.J. Johnson, V.A. Levin and
    G. VanRaalte, Final report on the United States Phase I
    clinical trial of the hypoxic cell radiosensitizer,
    Misonidazole, Cancer, In press (1980).
7. T.H. Wasserman, T.L. Phillips, G.V. VanRaalte, R.C. Urtasun,
    J. Partington, A. Kozio, J.G. Schwade, D. Ganji and
    J.M. Strong, The neurotoxicity of misonidazole: Potential
    modifying role of phenytoin sodium and dexamethasone,
    Br. J. Radiol. 53:172 (1980).
8. S.C. Carabell, L.A. Bruno, A.S. Weinstein, M.P. Richter,
    C.B. Weiler and R.L. Goodman, Misonidazole and radiotherapy
    in the treatment of malignant glioma : A Phase II trial,
    Int.J.Radiation Oncology Biol.Phys. 5:Suppl.2, 194 (1979).
9. S.C. Carabell, L.A. Bruno, A.S. Weinstein, M.P. Richter,
    C.H. Chang, C.B. Weiler and R.L. Goodman, Misonidazole and
    Radiotherapy in the treatment of malignant glioma: A
    Phase II trial of the Radiation Therapy Oncology Group,
    Int.J.Radiation Oncology Biol.Phys. In Press (1980).
10. J.T. Fazekas, The value of adjuvant misonidazole in the
    definitive irradiation of advanced head and neck squamous
    cancer: An RTOG pilot study (#78-02), Int.J.Radiation
    Oncology Biol.Phys. 5:Suppl.2, 186, (1979).

11. T.L. Phillips, J. Newall, S.E. Order, P. Rubin, W.M. Wara and
     T.H. Wasserman,   A Phase II Evaluation of misonidazole in
     patients with brain metastases. Abstract ASTR. (1980).
12. S. Leibel et al. Abstract ASTR. (1980).
13. J.R. Simpson, C.A. Perez, T.L. Phillips, J.P. Concannon,
     R.J. Carella,   Large fraction radiotherapy plus misonidazole
     in the treatment of advanced lung cancer: Report of Phase
     I/II trial. Abstract ASTR. (1980).
14. T.H. Wasserman, T.L. Phillips and G. VanRaalte,   Evaluation of
     the bioavailability of misonidazole in capsule, and tablet
     form,   Abstract,   ASTR, Int.J.Radiation Oncology Biol.Phys.
     In press, (1980).
15. M.D. Walker and T.A. Strike,   A phase II evaluation of
     misonidazole in the treatment of malignant glioma, Abstract,
     Proc. Amer.Soc.Clinical Oncology 20:433 (1979).

MISONIDAZOLE AND DESMETHYLMISONIDAZOLE IN CLINICAL RADIOTHERAPY

S. Dische

Marie Curie Research Wing for Oncology
Regional Radiotherapy Centre, Mount Vernon Hospital
Northwood, Middlesex HA6 2 RN, England

The first administration of misonidazole to a patient receiving radiotherapy was performed at Mount Vernon on the 1st November 1974. In the first phase of the work, when large single doses were given to 8 patients, we showed that good serum concentrations could be achieved in man with doses which were fairly well tolerated when given orally. The curve of plasma concentration showed a peak at 1 to 2 hours and then a period of slow-fall called the plateau period extending up to 4 or 5 hours. The concentration then fell away with a half-life of approximately 12 hours. Enhancement of radiation response in skin made artificially hypoxic was demonstrated in all 6 cases studied and concentrations up to 100% of the plasma concentration were found in biopsies of human tumours. An enhancement of tumour response was observed in 3 of 4 patients with multiple deposits of tumour where a comparison could be made of treatment with or without the drug (1,2,3).

In the second phase of the work commencing in July 1975 multiple doses of the drug were given. It was then found that the drug was neurotoxic, causing convulsions and peripheral neuropathy. In 1977 we showed evidence that neuropathy was directly related to the dose given and even more closely to the tissue exposure of the drug as shown by the curve of plasma concentration (4). On the basis of our experience we suggested that a total dose of 12 g per square metre of surface area should be set as a maximum when the dose is administered over a period of no less than 18 days (5). Some reduction of dose is necessary when the number of administrations and overall period is reduced and some increase is permitted if the dose is given only once a week, particularly if the duration of treatment is extended to 6 or more weeks. With monitoring so as to recognize the occasional patient who showed unusually high concentrations in the

229

plasma for the dose given, and also so as to reduce the dose for
those showing levels high in the normal range, the incidence of
peripheral neuropathy can be reduced to 20-25%.   Most of the cases
which occur under these conditions are mild;   however, an occasional
troublesome or very troublesome neuropathy will be encountered.
Following this practice, central neurotoxicity is uncommon, but a
number of cases of encephalopathy have been reported, particularly in
elderly, anaemic patients when total doses within the 12 g per square
metre of surface area have been given and normal plasma concentrations
demonstrated.   Usually there is a complete recovery but, in some,
severe changes have persisted and have contributed to death.   Careful
clinical observation is essential and drug administration discontinued
at the first suspicion of a neurotoxic effect (6).

      Our experience with misonidazole now extends to 240 patients.
The incidence of toxic effects is shown in Table I and the pharmacokinetic data in Table II.   These findings are similar to those
already recorded (6).

Table 1.   Mount Vernon - Misonidazole.   October 1974-July 1980.
            Toxic effects seen in 240 patients.

(1)	Nausea and vomiting	
(2)	Neurotoxicity	
	(a) convulsions	2
	(b) transient confusional state	2
	(c) peripheral neuropathy	59
(3)	Hypersensitivity rashes	3
(4)	Auditory	0

      There has been much consideration as to the best way to employ
the dose which may be given to a patient during a course of radiotherapy (7).   Ways which are being employed at the moment may be
grouped under four headings:-

(1) The giving of misonidazole with radiotherapy on a few occasions.
On theoretical grounds the addition of a sensitizer in such a fractionation should give the maximum enhancement of response when compared with patients given identical radiotherapy without the drug
(8).   We have performed a trial with this type of dose and fractionation in locally advanced carcinoma of the bronchus.   A total of 60
patients have been entered in this study, now in its fourth year.
We have not been able to demonstrate any improvement in result with
use of the drug.   However, our close observation of these patients

Table II.   Mount Vernon - Misonidazole.   October 1974-July 1980.

Calculated plateau concentrations in plasma when 1 g given per square metre of surface area.

	Cases	No. of estimates	mean μg/ml	S.D. μg/ml
Males	118	583	38.2	7.1
Females	102	448	41.2	9.0

Half lives - calculated from plateau and 24 hour concentrations.

	Cases	No. of estimates	mean (hr)	S.D. (hr)
Males	114	193	13.4	2.8
Females	92	139	12.3	3.2

suggests that gross tumour remained in nearly all cases.   We are unlikely to show benefit with an hypoxic cell sensitizer unless we approach more closely a cure situation - we must destroy all oxic cells before the hypoxic ones can matter.   Professor Sealy in Cape Town using a similar fractionation and a similar total dose in patients with locally advanced oral cavity tumours showed a margin of benefit in the early months following treatment (9).   However, this seemed to have been mostly lost by the time 18 months had passed, but we await his final report.

(2)   As a means of taking advantage of the enhancement to be expected with a high dose of radiosensitizer some have treated patients once weekly with a high dose of radiation.   Professor Bleehen gave the drug at a dose level of 3 g per square metre once a week and on that day gave a higher dose of radiation, 500 rad, with only 294 rad when treatment was given without sensitizer, on Mondays and Wednesdays. The overall duration of the course was 4 weeks.   In his trial no benefit has been shown with misonidazole in the treatment of these glioblastomas Grades III and IV (10).   In Vienna, Kogelnik and his colleagues have, in similar patients, used single large doses of misonidazole, but here they have given the drug at the beginning and at the end of the course of radiotherapy.   Those given the sensitizer seem to be faring better than those without, but we must wait completion of the study (11).

(3) An extension of the single dose of sensitizer each week has been used by the Radiation Therapy Oncology Group in the United States and by Bataini at the Fondation Curie in the treatment of head and neck tumours (12,13). Radiotherapy is given twice on the day when the sensitizer is given and also again early on the following day when appreciable concentrations are still available in the tumour. In this way a greater proportion of the radiotherapy is given with the sensitizer, despite the single administration each week.   There is evidence that when giving a single dose each week a total dose in excess of 12 g per square metre of surface area can be administered with safety.   Bataini has noted in the early results of a trial in advanced oral cancer a margin of benefit in those given the drug (13). Multiple treatments in one day with sensitizer can be given on several days of the week and so all, or a great part of a course of such therapy, can be given with sensitizer.   Explorations here in Italy and in other European centres have yielded promise in pilot studies and in the early stages of randomized trials.

(4) The sensitizer can be given with every treatment in a conventional course of radiotherapy.   This is the most frequently used form of administration, but unfortunately due to the dose limitation only modest sensitizing concentrations may be achieved in the tumour on each occasion.   We have performed trials in our own centre in carcinoma of the breast and bladder, including 30 and 42 cases respectively, and so far no advantage has been demonstrated with misonidazole.   However, in a limited series of patients, 10 in all, given misonidazole in the radiotherapy of carcinoma of cervix, all have shown a complete regression of tumour by the conclusion of treatment, a most promising prognostic sign, as shown in our previous experience with hyperbaric oxygen.

Variations of this form of administration include the giving of the drug with every treatment in the first two and the last two weeks of a 7-week course of radiotherapy, as used by Bataini in pharyngeal carcinomas where he has reported a margin of benefit in the early months following treatment.   In other trials the drug is given in the earlier weeks of treatment while in others only in the final weeks.

We must await the definitive results of these many studies which are being performed in all parts of the world.   There is no doubt some disappointment in that clear benefit has not already been shown in some of the studies.   One has the impression that benefit is being most often observed where most of a multi-fraction course is given with a reasonably high concentration of sensitizer present with most of the treatments.   Further, such benefit may only be shown in these tumours where after conventional fractionated radiotherapy the resistance of hypoxic tumour cells remains the dominant problem.   We have evidence from the hyperbaric oxygen trials that this situation may exist in squamous carcinoma in the head and neck and in the uterine cervix (14).

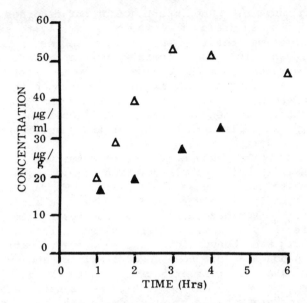

Fig. 1. Patient K3: Advanced carcinoma of breast. Simultaneous administration of both drugs. All values normalized to an administration of 1 g per sq/m of surface area. The plasma concentrations of MISO (Δ) and tumour concentrations (▲) are shown.

With Professor Adams and other colleagues we presented the relationship between concentration of radiosensitization as a guide to clinical application in 1977 (4). We know that in the majority of cases tumour concentrations lie between 60 and 100% of the plasma concentration at the time the sample is taken. In our experience plasma concentrations and tumour concentrations are closely linked and only occasionally will any lag be shown (Fig. 1.). We have found that there is a relationship between the amount of necrosis seen in a tumour sample and the concentration of misonidazole in an adjacent one (15). In our experience low concentrations are usually to be found in tumour samples showing a great deal of gross necrosis as revealed by histological study. However, we are unaware of the appearance of hypoxic though viable tumour cells under the microscope. The histological or cytological appearance of hypoxic cells are not likely to be different from those of oxic ones and we must interpret

our results with caution.   The importance of our findings as to the
concentration of drug in areas of necrosis is firstly to explain why
low values are sometimes obtained when tumour samples are examined for
concentration of sensitizer and, secondly, when correlation with
histological appearances is made to give a crude indication as to the
extent to which a sensitizing drug may diffuse through the oxic areas
of a tumour into the hypoxic ones.   We can argue that the higher the
concentration achieved in necrotic tissue the higher the level which
will occur in hypoxic cells with the tumour and sensitizer under study

Reviewing our work, a concentration of sensitizer in hypoxic
cells equal to half that in the plasma would seem to be a realistic
figure with which to predict possible benefit.   We can see in Fig.
2 the enhancement ratios likely to be achieved.   We are with the
present sensitizer, misonidazole, and the dose restriction imposed
upon it, achieving only a limited degree of sensitization of hypoxic
cells, particularly when conventional dose and fractionation regimes
are employed.   A doubling of those concentrations, and even better
a tripling, should be much more effective.   With the drug doses
presently being given we may only expect to see benefit where in
conventional radiotherapy hypoxic cells remain the dominant problem
for radiation failure.

The work to develop new radiosensitizing drugs to achieve such
levels has already been described in this course.   We have known of
the desmethyl derivative of misonidazole (Ro-05-9963) for some years.
It is the first metabolic breakdown product of misonidazole and has
long been detected in the blood and urine of our patients.   It has
a relatively low lipophilicity compared with misonidazole so it can
be expected to show those characteristics relevant to improving
sensitization - a shorter half-life in plasma - an effect related
to a more rapid renal clearance and a reduced rate of uptake into
nervous tissue.

In work commencing in January this year we were able to show
that the drug is surprisingly well absorbed (16).   Peak plasma concentrations are reached between 30 and 90 minutes after absorption
which are between 80 and 100% of the plateau concentrations which
have been obtained with misonidazole.   With the completion of a
satisfactory trial in normal volunteers, we were given permission to
proceed to a study in patients and have now accumulated experience in
over 30 patients.   A similar pattern of plasma levels has been
obtained as for the normal volunteers.   The half-life of the drug
appears to be about 50% of that with misonidazole.   The mean of the
area under the curve of plasma concentration is approximately 55%
of the mean of comparable misonidazole curves.   We now have observations upon the drug level in cerebro-spinal fluid in 8 patients where
it was possible to obtain one sample in each case at an interval
after administration of desmethylmisonidazole.   A comparison with
the CSF levels of misonidazole reported by Ash et al.(17) shows that

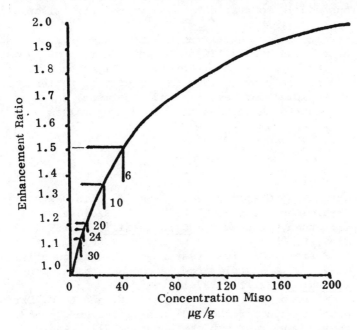

Fig. 2.   Division of 1.2 g/sq m into 6, 10, 20, 24 and 30 fractions.
Concentrations which may be achieved in hypoxic tumour
cells related to enhancement ratio.

the area under the curve of CSF concentration is approximately one-
third of that with misonidazole.   One can presume a similar reduction in exposure to the drug in the central nervous system and
possibly also in peripheral nerves (18).

Of particular importance is the concentration to be obtained in
human tumours and we have now the results in 13 patients.   A total
of 60 samples have been analysed for nitroimidazoles and in each case
a matching sample has been examined histologically.   Good concentrations were achieved and there is some suggestion that in comparison
with misonidazole slightly higher concentrations build up in areas
showing necrosis.   The optimum time for radiotherapy will be around
1½ hours after administration of desmethylmisonidazole compared with
3½ to 4 hours for misonidazole.   When we compare desmethylmisonidazole we have calculated that approximately equal sensitization will
be achieved when equal doses by weight are given (18).

Work is now underway giving multiple doses to patients and
everything depends upon the toxicity which will be found.   If the
predictions from animal models are to be realised, and it is extremely
important to the whole programme of drug development to determine

this, when we can hope that we can safely achieve radiosensitizing concentrations double to triple those achieved with misonidazole.

In the treatment of animal tumours no new measure has shown such clear benefit as has followed the introduction of hypoxic cell sensitizers. We hope that their promise will be achieved in humans for the method not only brings hope of benefit to patients in large centres fully equipped for research and treatment, but also to those attending all centres throughout the world, regardless of size and affluence.

1. S. Dische, A. J. Gray and G. D. Zanelli, Clinical testing of the radiosensitizer Ro 07-0582. II. Radiosensitization of normal and hypoxic skin, Clin. Radiol. 27:159 (1976).

2. A. J. Gray, S. Dische, G. E. Adams, I. R. Flockhart, and J. L. Foster, Clinical testing of the radiosensitizer Ro 07-0582. I. Dose tolerance, serum and tumour concentration, Clin. Radiol. 27:151 (1976).

3. R. H. Thomlinson, S. Dische, A. J. Gray, and L. M. Errington, Clinical testing of the radiosensitizer Ro 07-0582. III. Regression and regrowth of tumour, Clin. Radiol. 27:167 (1976).

4. S. Dische, M. I. Saunders, M. E. Lee, G. E. Adams, and I. R. Flockhart, Clinical testing of the radiosensitizer Ro 07-0582: Experience with multiple doses, Br. J. Cancer 35:567 (1977).

5. M. I. Saunders, S. Dische, P. Anderson, and I. R. Flockhart, The neurotoxicity of misonidazole and its relationship to dose, half-life and concentration in the serum, Br. J. Cancer 37(Suppl.III):268 (1978).

6. S. Dische, M. I. Saunders, I. R. Flockhart, M. E. Lee and P. Anderson, Misonidazole. A drug for trial in radiotherapy and oncology, Int. J. Radiat. Oncol. Biol. Phys. 5:851 (1979).

7. S. Dische, M. I. Saunders, and I. R. Flockhart, The optimum regime for the administration of misonidazole and the establishment of multi-centre clinical trials, Br. J. Cancer 37(Suppl.III):318 (1978).

8. J. Denekamp, F. J. Fowler and M. C. Joiner, Misonidazole in fractionated radiotherapy: little and often? Br. J. Radiol. (Awaiting publication).

9. R. Sealy and W. Levin, Clinical experience with misonidazole as a radiation sensitizer and as a radiation sensitizer in conjunction with hyperbaric oxygen or hyperthermia, Cancer Clin. Trials (1980)(Awaiting publication).

10. N. M. Bleehen, The Cambridge glioma trial misonidazole and radiation therapy with associated pharmacokinetic studies, Cancer Clin. Trials (1980)(Awaiting publication).

11. H. D. Kögelnik, Clinical experience with misonidazole. High dose fractions versus daily low doses, Cancer Clin. Trials 3:179 (1980).

12. T. H. Wasserman and T. L. Phillips, Clinical trials of misonidazole in the United States, Cancer Clin. Trials (1980) (Awaiting publication).

13. J. P. Bataini, Personal communication (1980).

14. S. Dische, Hyperbaric oxygen. The Medical Research Council trials and their clinical significance, Br. J. Radiol. 51:888 (1978).

15. T. A. Rich, S. Dische, M. I. Saunders, M. Stratford and A. Minchinton, The influence of necrosis on the concentration of misonidazole in human tumors, Int. J. Radiat. Oncol. Biol. Phys. (Awaiting publication).

16. S. Dische, M. I. Saunders, P. Anderson, M. E. Lee, J. F. Fowler, M. Stratford and A. Minchinton, A drug for improved radio-sensitization in radiotherapy, Br. J. Cancer (1980) (Awaiting publication).

17. D. V. Ash, M. R. Smith and R. D. Bugden, The distribution of misonidazole in human tumours and normal tissue, Br. J. Cancer 39:503 (1979).

18. S. Dische, M. I. Saunders, P. J. Riley, J. Hauck, M. H. Bennett, M. R. L. Stratford and A. I. Minchinton, The concentration of desmethylmisonidazole in human tumours and in cerebrospinal fluid, Br. J. Cancer (1980) (Submitted for publication).

PROSPECTS FOR NEW HYPOXIC CELL RADIOSENSITIZERS

J.G. Schwade[*], D.A. Pistenma[**] and T.L. Phillips[+]

[*] Radiation Oncology Branch, Clinical Oncology Program,
Division of Cancer Treatment, NCI
[**]Radiation Development Branch, Cancer Therapy
Evaluation Program, Division of Cancer Treatment, NCI
[+] Department of Radiation Therapy, University of
California, San Francisco

INTRODUCTION

The hypoxic cell radiosensitizers misonidazole and metronidazole are currently being evaluated in clinical trials in North
America and Europe.   The usefulness of both compounds is limited
by toxicity and pharmacology.   Alternative routes of administration, or pharmacokinetic modification may decrease these problems.
However, it is likely that development of new compounds with desirable physical and biological properties may be necessary in order
to effect clinically useful radiosensitization.   The status of
currently available drugs, the National Cancer Institute program
for development of new radiosensitizers (1), and the prospects for
some compounds resulting from that program will be reviewed.

CURRENT COMPOUNDS

Metronidazole is generally administered in 250 mg tablets.
Nausea and vomiting are common, and significant incidence of
peripheral neuropathy occurs above cumulative doses of 90 g.   I.V.
administration has not been found to be advantageous, possibly the
result of the dilute formulation (500 mg/100 ml), necessitating
prolonged infusion.   Orally, plasma half-life ($T_{\frac{1}{2}}$) averages about
12 hours.

Misonidazole, in 100 or 500 mg capsules for oral administration,
while displaying less gastrointestinal toxicity, is likely to cause
peripheral neuropathy above 12-15 g/m^2 in fractionated doses over

5-6 weeks.   On a molar basis, misonidazole would appear to be a
more efficient sensitizer, displaying a higher dose modifying
factor (DMF) at lower concentrations.   Administered orally, plasma
and serum half-life of misonidazole averages about 12-14 hours, with
peak levels in the blood at about 3-4 hours, and probably at least
4-6 hours in tumours (2,3).   Intravenous administration (500 mg/
19.5 ml over 5 min.) results in a biphasic pharmacokinetic curve
with a rapid (5.8 min) distribution, and slower (9.3 hour) elimination phase (4).   A significant incidence of peripheral neuropathy
results at approximately the same total dose, however.   This is
not unexpected since the toxicity of misonidazole correlates with
the area under the pharmacokinetic curve (AUC) ((4) and Schwade et
al., unpublished).   Since intravenous administration of misonidazole results in a shorter plasma $T_{\frac{1}{2}}$, due primarily to the elimination of slow absorption kinetics, the theoretical AUC will be equal
with either I.V. or P.O. administration.   However, since bioavailability with oral misonidazole is only about 80% (5), actual
AUC is higher with I.V. misonidazole than with equal doses given
orally.

At the NCI, intraperitoneal administration of misonidazole is
also being performed in certain patients with ovarian carcinoma and
peritoneal metastases.   High concentration can be achieved within
the peritoneal cavity and removed rapidly by peritoneal dialysis.

An I.V. form of misonidazole, therefore, offers no major
advantage over oral administration on pharmacologic grounds.
However, I.V. administration is preferable in certain situations,
such as intraoperative radiation therapy (where logistics demand
I.V. use), in certain disease sites (such as esophageal carcinoma
where swallowing pills may be difficult or impossible), or
situations where accurate pharmocologic measurements are necessary.

PHARMACOKINETIC MODIFICATION

Modification of the pharmacology of misonidazole, though, may
increase the drug's usefulness.   Inducers of hepatic microsomal
enzymes, such as phenobarbital and phenytoin sodium (Dilantin®)
shorten the plasma $T_{\frac{1}{2}}$ of misonidazole (4,5).   This has been
observed with both oral (2,6,7) and I.V. administration (7).   Here,
however, this change is seen entirely in the <u>elimination</u> $T_{\frac{1}{2}}$.   Thus,
with shortened $T_{\frac{1}{2}}$ secondary to enzyme induction and an enhanced
metabolism, the AUC is actually reduced, while peak levels reveal
little change (6,8).   It is unclear at this time whether the use
of enzyme inducing agents will decrease toxicity for identical peak
drug levels in patients.   The rapid loss of the plasma cell concentration gradient caused by shortening the plasma $T_{\frac{1}{2}}$ could
possibly minimize diffusion into hypoxic tumour cells.   In fact,
even with the normally long elimination $T_{\frac{1}{2}}$, there is evidence of
poor penetration of misonidazole (or none at all) into necrotic

regions of at least some tumours ((9) and Hurwitz et al., personal communication).

Phenytoin may decrease the incidence or severity of peripheral neuropathy by a direct effect on peripheral nerves.   It is frequently used to treat peripheral neuropathy.   However, this non-pharmacokinetic effect of phenytoin may only be masking symptoms, rather than preventing damage to nerves by misonidazole.

Steroids also may protect peripheral nerves from misonidazole toxicity to some degree.   A lower incidence of peripheral neuro-pathy has been observed in patients with malignant glioma who have been on steroid therapy while receiving misonidazole on a Brain Tumour Study Group (BTSG) protocol (Pistenma, personal communication).

DEVELOPMENT OF NEW COMPOUNDS

Real improvements will likely come only from the synthesis of new radiosensitizers having a number of desirable properties. Lipophilicity, a characteristic allowing peripheral and central nervous system penetration, should be kept low, although some degree of lipophilicity is needed for tumour penetration.   Ideally, electron affinity, primarily responsible for sensitization, should remain as high as possible with minimal toxicity.   Plasma $T_{\frac{1}{2}}$ should be short, but adequate to allow tumour penetration by the drug.   The ideal drug is one that could be infused to maintain a constant level, and then rapidly cleared after irradiation is delivered.   In order to guide the development of hypoxic cell radiosensitizers rationally, the Division of Cancer Treatment (DCT), National Cancer Institute (NCI), initiated a program as part of its comprehensive effort in antineoplastic drug development.   This followed a recommendation by the Committee on Radiation Oncology Studies (C.R.O.S.) in 1976 (10).

Because of basic differences between radiation sensitizers and protectors and cytotoxic drugs, this sensitizer and protector development effort has required extensive modification of the National Cancer Institute Drug Development Program (11).   The radio-sensitizer and protector effort, which spans the entire spectrum from synthesis and screening of potential agents to clinical trials, has been integrated successfully into the Drug Development Program.

EXTRAMURAL ADVISORY COMMITTEE

The inception of this project has been guided by a special ad hoc coordinating committee, the Radiosensitizer/Radioprotector Working Group, serving as an extramural advisory body to the Division of Cancer Treatment (DCT) Radiation Therapy Development Branch.   This committee meets approximately three times per year and serves as the central advisory body during the formative stages of sensitizer development of a sensitizer to facilitate its integration into the ongoing DCT Drug Development Program.

ANALOGUE COMMITTEE

On a day-to-day basis, coordination and monitoring of the radiosensitizer and radioprotector related activities within the Division of Cancer Treatment is vested in a Radiation Sensitizer/ Radiation Protector Analogue Committee.   This committee's primary function is to ensure the smooth flow of compounds (from program or outside sources) through the Drug Development Program and into clinical trials.

TREATMENT LINEAR ARRAY

In order to accomplish this aim, considerable modification of the existing cytotoxic agent development program research logic (Linear Array) has been necessary (12) (Treatment Linear Array for Radiosensitizers, Division of Cancer Treatment, NCI).   The criteria for choosing potential radiation sensitizing agents differ significantly from those which have been established for cytotoxic drugs. This treatment linear array for radiation sensitizers provides for orderly and rapid testing of compounds which promise a better therapeutic ratio.   Initially, interest has focused on electron-affinic hypoxic cell sensitizers, and this is reflected in the selection criteria.   However, the development of agents whose efficacy is dependent upon alternative mechanisms is also being encouraged.

At each stage in the research logic (Linear Array), the decision to continue is made by the Drug Development Decision Network Committee of the DCT based on data presented by NCI and extramural personnel.   Initially, compounds are chosen which:

1.   demonstrate electron affinity;

2.   have measurable lipid/water partition coefficients;

3.   demonstrate in vitro sensitization of hypoxic mammalian cells to radiation;

4.   fail to demonstrate significant sensitization of aerated mammalian cells in vitro to radiation;

5.   have a toxicity (cell kill) that is limited at active levels in vitro for acute times of sensitization;

6.   demonstrate a structure indicative of reasonable stability in solution;

7.   have an LD_{50} determined in the animal to be used for in vivo testing;   and

8. have demonstrated sensitization activity in at least
    one in vivo model tumour at doses below the drug LD_{50}.
    Additional physical and chemical parameters, such as
    solubility, stability, purity and biological activity,
    as well as estimates of quantities needed for further
    testing are determined prior to selection for in vivo
    testing.

Compounds are selected for in vivo testing if the in vitro
screening data show that the agent is superior to the reference
compound (currently misonidazole).   The present DCT radiosensitizer
tumour panel consists of a variety of solid tumours, including C_3H
mammary carcinoma, B16 melanoma, Lewis lung, EMT6, and KHT sarcoma.
It is anticipated that additional tumour models may be necessary in
future testing since the predictive accuracy of the current panel
is not well established.   Preparation by NCI is under way to
establish a facility to complete both in vitro and in vivo testing
of compounds from both NCI and outside sources.

In vivo efficacy must be demonstrated in at least three panel
tumours with different endpoints, i.e. (1) in vivo tumour cell
survival modification, (2) tumour growth delay modification, or (3)
tumour cure dose modification (TCD_{50}).   For each animal strain used,
LD_{50} and other toxicity parameters must be determined.   Controls
without drug and with a current reference radiosensitizer (misonidazole) should be tested under identical experimental conditions
at equimolar (and/or equitoxic) doses.

In cases where a drug demonstrates superior or equivalent
efficacy with acceptable toxicity (potential for increased therapeutic benefits in clinical use), additional evaluation is undertaken for large-scale production feasibility, dosage formulation,
cost factors, and large animal toxicology, including specific studies
directed at detection of neurotoxicity.

INITIAL CLINICAL TRIALS

After the above evaluation has been completed satisfactorily,
promising compounds are entered in Phase I clinical trials to determine the maximum tolerated dose and toxicity for both parenteral and
oral administration initially in single doses and then in multiple
doses.   Subsequently, Phase II studies are initiated in patients
with a variety of solid tumours with a primary objective of determining the feasibility of delivering radiation and sensitizer in the
desired doses and times.   This is extremely important because the
optimal use of hypoxic cell sensitizers and radiation may require
radiation fractionation schemes different from those utilized con-
ventionally.   It is estimated that 20 to 30 patients are necessary
for each Phase II study of each of the several different tumour
types.   Only after these have been completed is it appropriate to

proceed to randomized clinical trials to compare the efficacy of
the combined treatment with radiation sensitizer and radiation
therapy and treatment with conventional radiation therapy.   If
so, it will be necessary to compare the new radiation schedule with
conventional radiation therapy.   Otherwise, what appears to be an
effect of the radiation sensitizer may be due only to the modified
radiation fractionation schedule.

The first compound to be entered into this program, Desmethylmisonidazole, (Ro 07-9963) the major metabolite of misonidazole,
has met all criteria necessary to proceed to Phase I clinical trials
(pharmacology and determination of maximum tolerated doses).   Large
animal studies indicate a twofold lower toxicity than with misonidazole.   Preliminary pharmacologic testing orally indicates
good absorption and a $T_{\frac{1}{2}}$ markedly shorter than misonidazole (Dische,
personal communication).   Full-scale Phase I trials with a form
for parenteral administration in the United States are awaiting the
production of formulated drug, and are expected to begin in late
1980.

SYNTHESIS OF NEW COMPOUNDS

In order to explore fully the potential range of radiation
sensitizing compounds, contracts have been awarded to the Institute
of Cancer Research in Sutton, England, and to the Stanford Research
Institute for synthesis of additional nitroimidazole-type radiosensitizers.   Emphasis has been placed on development of compounds
which would be less lipophilic than misonidazole, and have shorter
plasma half-lives.   Two of these compounds, SR 2508 and SR 2555,
the hydroxyethylamide and dihydroxyethylamide analogues of misonidazole, appear especially promising (13).   Both compounds possess
electron-affinic properties identical to misonidazole, but are highly
hydrophilic.   Both are less toxic and have markedly shorter plasma
$T_{\frac{1}{2}}$ in mice.   After meeting the preceding criteria, both these compounds are undergoing toxicity studies in large animals.   If, as
expected, they prove less toxic than misonidazole, they will likely
enter preliminary clinical trials in late 1982.   As Adams has
reported, several of the compounds synthesised at Sutton also
appear promising in preliminary testing.

OTHER MECHANISMS OF RADIOSENSITIZATION

In addition, other mechanisms of radiosensitization are
currently being investigated.   Evidence from Goffinet and Brown
(14) at Stanford indicate that hepatic dehalogenation of halogenated pyrimidines may not occur as rapidly as previously believed.
Thus, NCI is using a recently developed HPLC assay for BUdR to
evaluate its use by intravenous rather than intraarterial administration of bromodeoxyuridine (BUdR) (Myers, personal communication).

Thus, while current clinical trials are being conducted with misonidazole and metronidazole, a number of less toxic and potentially more efficacious radiosensitizers will likely soon be available.

REFERENCES

1. Report of NCI Radiosensitizer/Radioprotector Working Group. Available from Radiation Development Branch, DCT, NCI (1980).
2. T. H. Wasserman, J. Stetz and T. L. Phillips, Cancer trials of misonidazole in the United States, p.387 in: "Radiation Sensitizers: Their Use in the Clinical Management of Cancer", Cancer Management, Vol.5, ed. L.W. Brady, Masson Publishing USA Inc., New York (1980).
3. S. Dische, M. I. Saunders, I. R. Flockhart, M. E. Lee and P. Anderson, Misonidazole: A drug for trial in radiotherapy and oncology, Int. J. Radiat. Oncol. Biol. Phys. 5:851 (1979).
4. J. G. Schwade, J. M. Strong, D. Gangji and E. Glatstein, Phase I trial of intravenous misonidazole (NSC 261037), Proc. Am. Soc. Clin. Onc. 21:396 (1980).
5. J. G. Schwade, J. M. Strong and D. Gangji, I.V. misonidazole (NSC 261037): report of initial clinical experience, p.414 in: "Radiation Sensitizers: Their Use in the Clinical Management of Cancer", Cancer Management, Vol.5, ed. L.W. Brady, Masson Publishing USA Inc., New York (1980).
6. P. Workman, N. M. Bleehen and C. Wiltshire, Phenytoin shortens the half-life of the hypoxic cell radiosensitizer misonidazole in man: implications for possible reduced toxicity, Br. J. Cancer 41:307 (1980).
7. D. Gangji, D. G. Poplack, J. Schwade, J. H. Wood and J. M. Strong, Misonidazole blood and cerebrospinal fluid kinetics in monkeys following intravenous and intrathecal administration, Eur. J. Cancer 17:29 (1981).
8. J. M. Strong, J. G. Schwade, D. Gangji, D. D. Shoemaker and D. K. Upton, p.73 in: "Radiation Sensitizers: Their Use in the Clinical Management of Cancer", Cancer Management, Vol. 5, ed. L.W. Brady, Masson Publishing USA Inc., New York (1980).
9. T. A. Rich, S. Dische, M. I. Saunders, M. Stratford and A. Michinton, p.411 in: "Radiation Sensitizers: Their Use in the Clinical Management of Cancer", Cancer Management, Vol. 5, ed. L.W. Brady, Masson Publishing USA Inc., New York (1980).
10. Committee for Radiation Oncology Studies Research Plan: Radiation Sensitizers, Cancer 37:2062 (1976).
11. De Vita et al., Cancer Clin. Trials 2:195 (1979).
12. T. L. Phillips, T. H. Wasserman, R. J. Johnson, The hypoxic cell sensitizer program in the US, Br. J. Cancer 37 (Suppl.III): 276 (1978).

13. J. M. Brown and P. Workman, Partition coefficient as a guide
     to the development of radiosensitizers which are less
     toxic than misonidazole, Rad. Res. 82:171 (1980).
14. D. R. Goffinet and J. M. Brown, Comparison of intravenous and
     intra-arterial pyrimidine infusion as a means of radio-
     sensitizing tumours in vivo, Radiology 124:819 (1977).

CLINICAL EXPERIMENTS WITH RADIOSENSITIZING DRUGS IN ITALY

C. Rimondi

Radiotherapy Division
M. Malpighi Hospital, Bologna, Italy

Clinical studies with misonidazole were first started in 1978 when a few researchers obtained the drug from Roche and initiated a double-blind study on a limited number of patients suffering from epithelial malignant tumours sensitive to radiotherapy.

During the Course, Italian researchers have their first opportunity to present their observations and their preliminary results on the association of radiotherapy and misonidazole in glioblastoma of the brain (Ramundo Orlando), head and neck carcinoma (Nervi and coworkers), infiltrating carcinoma of the bladder, inoperable non-oat-cell carcinoma of the lung, and uterus Portio III carcinoma (Busutti and coworkers). The various schemes for association of radiotherapy and misonidazole differ in relation to the particular type of fractionation used, but there is a definite preference for multiple daily fractionation schemes.

Taking into consideration the fact that only a very short time has elapsed since the end of treatment, the results presented here mainly concern tolerance to treatment and intermediate tumour response. Only early data are available on survival rate. Tolerance to radiotherapy plus misonidazole treatment generally appears to be satisfactory; in particular, neurotoxic phenomena of a sensory nature seem to be both rare and of low intensity and are limited to peripheral paresthesia.

Reactive manifestations affecting healthy tissues comprised in the irradiated volume are not different from those observed in the absence of misonidazole. Only in association with multiple daily fractions with doses of 5-6Gy/day does misonidazole seem to increase mucosal reactions. The intermediate responses of tumours, both

247

full and partial, are increased, although not to a great extent.
However, follow-up has not proceeded far enough yet to allow the
evaluation of the effect of such a better response upon the
disease-free interval on the survival rate.

The survey presented shows only a few clinical data, even
though there has been much interest in radiosensitizing drugs.
It is necessary to collect more information so that the potential
of misonidazole in radiotherapy may be more fully explored.   A
few contributions are concerned with the use of metronidazole
which has a few problems of its own with respect to misonidazole.
In particular, its use in the treatment of a few advanced stages
in various sites (Rimondi, Busutti) and in the treatment of soft
tissue sarcomas (Coucourde and coworkers) is discussed.

MULTIPLE DAILY FRACTIONATION (MDF) IN ASSOCIATION WITH MISONIDAZOLE (MIS): A TWO-YEAR EXPERIENCE WITH HEAD AND NECK CANCER

G. Arcangeli[1], F. Mauro[2] and C. Nervi[1] .

(1) Istituto Medico e di Ricerca Scientifica
    00191 Rome, Italy
(2) Comitato Nazionale per l'Energia Nucleare
    00060, Rome, Italy

INTRODUCTION

In our Institution MDF schemes have been introduced several years ago (1,2). One of the main reasons for developing and testing this kind of scheme is the possibility of compressing the radiation dose in time, thus allowing a better exploitation of hypoxic cell radiosensitizers administration within the well-known toxicity limits. Further, other radiobiological criteria may justify the use of non-conventional fractionation per se (and of local hyperthermia) on radioresistant tumours with a presumably high fraction of hypoxic cells.

The addition of MIS to our pilot scheme was therefore a logical consequence to the availability of a routine MDF scheme (three fractions per day, 4 h fractionation interval, 1.6-2 Gy per fraction).

Apart from miscellaneous exploration, our initial approach has been determined by the opportunity for comparing in a quantitatively acceptable way, the schedules and sequences for the various modalities of multi-modalities (radiation, MIS, heat, or the relative combinations) without entering a priori directly into a rigid clinical trial.

TREATMENT OF NECK NODE METASTASES

The basic option has been to treat comparable lesions in the same patient with at least two different modalities. This was obtained by entering into a pilot study 25 patients with multiple (N_2-N_3) neck node metastases.

Materials and Methods

All patients (including those of the historical series with conventional radiotherapy) were irradiated with a 5.7 MeV photon beam from a Neptune Linear Accelerator at a dose of some 3 Gy/min up to a total dose of 40-70 Gy.   Although this is a relatively large dose range, it must be pointed out that only 20% of the lesions received a dose less than 50 or more than 60 Gy.   In the patients treated with MIS, the drug was discontinued at 50 Gy, and the irradiation continued, if necessary.   Patients were generally treated through an anterior field covering the whole neck with protection of the laryngeal region and cervical spine only, or through two cross-firing portals when irradiation of the primary was required.

MIS, obtained by the courtesy of the Prodotti Roche S.p.A. (Milan, Italy), was orally administered in capsules of 100 and 500 mg, according to the dosage reported below.   Ten mg of metoclopramide were given as an anti-nauseant when necessary. Heparinized blood samples were taken every day, 2 h after drug ingestion, in each patient to monitor MIS plasma levels and to avoid undesirably high drug concentration.   In consideration of the neurotoxicity of misonidazole, the patients were examined weekly with special emphasis upon the central and peripheral nervous system, and also for skin and mucous reactions, nausea and vomiting.

The node volume was estimated by accurately measuring the three diameters of the lesion by independent evaluation by two of us (G.A. and C.N.).   Complete regression was defined as macroscopic disappearance of the lesions below the palpable size. Partial regression was defined as that of a lesion shrinking at least 50% within the treatment period.

The lesions were treated according to the following comparative schedules: 1) MDF - 2+1.5+1.5 Gy/day, 4 h interval between fractions, 5 days/week;   2) MDF + hyperthermia (heat at 42-43°C was applied each other day, that is, on day 1, 3 and 5 of each week, for 45 min, immediately after the second daily fraction of MDF, to only one lesion per patient);   3) MDF + MIS (the drug was administered daily, 2 h before the first daily fraction of MDF, at a dose of 1.2 g/m^2, up to a total border dose of 12 g/m^2);   4) MDF + hyperthermia + MIS (as indicated in 2 and 3).   The patients belonging to the historical series of conventional radiotherapy were treated with 2 Gy/day, 5 days/week.

Our TUETT 500 microwave apparatus, described elsewhere (2) was utilized for local hyperthermia and operated at 500 MHz. The measured tumour core temperature was always in the 42-43°C range.   Hyperthermia was administered to only one lesion per patient.

RESULTS

Pharmacology of MIS

The plasma concentration of MIS has been evaluated according to the spectrophotometric method (3), as described elserhere (4).

Before establishing the final dose and dose sequence used in the present work, the relation between the administered dose and the plasma concentration was determined on a preliminary group of patients.   Fig. 1 indicates that this relation is linear and that a dose of at least 1 g/m^2 is necessary to achieve, by 2 h, a plasma level around 50 µg/g which is supposedly the minimum useful concentration (5).

The concentrations as a function of time reported in Fig.2 indicate that the advantage given by a higher dose of day 1 is appreciable but does not justify, from the point of view of the maximum tolerance dose, such an extra use of the drug.

With a daily dose of 1.2 g/m^2, a certain plasma accumulation in the course of the week can be observed and a level of about 50 µg/g can be maintained for the whole week concomitant with the first daily radiation fraction.   Lower dosages are definitely insufficient, therefore the final daily dose was fixed at 1.2 g/m^2.

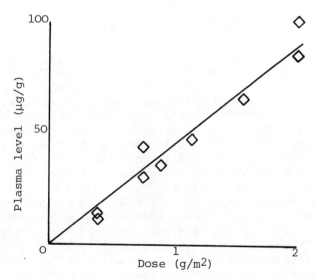

Fig. 1.   Relationship between the misonidazole dose administered to the patient and the plasma level determined 2 h later.

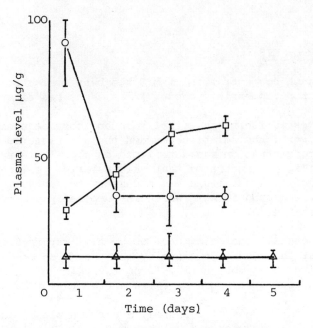

Fig. 2.   Variations of MIS plasma level determined 2 h after
          administration during a weekly course.   Circles:
          2 g/m^2 on day 1 and 0.75 g/m^2 on following days.
          Squares: 1.2 g/m^2 per day.   Triangles: 0.4 g/m^2 per
          day.   Bars indicate range of observed variations
          among patients.

Clinical Results

        Tumour responses, at the end of treatment, 6 and 12 months
are   summarized in Table 1.   The results are compared also with
our historical series of treating the same type of lesions with
conventional fractionation (2 Gy/day).   In these results, the
local control rate, either crude of actuarial, appeared to be much
higher in the cases treated with MDF in respect to those treated
with conventional fractionation.   Multimodality treatments
appeared to be more effective than conventional fractionation or
MDF.   In particular, the best response was obtained when MDF was
combined with both MIS and hyperthermia, with an actuarial control
rate of 80% lesions after 12 months. Because of the low number of
patients available at 12 months, the results in both groups also
treated with hyperthermia, are statistically different only versus
the historical series treated with conventional fractionation alone,
although the results at the end of treatment in the same groups are
significantly higher even versus the control group treated with MDF

Table 1. Results of Multimodality Treatments

TREATMENT	C.R.^{a} at End XRT	C.R. at 6 months	C.R. at 12 months	Crude C.R. at 12 months
1. MDF	15/32 (.47)	14/27 (.52)	7/16 (.43)	7/32 (.22)
2. MDF+HT	21/27 (.78)	17/22 (.77)	11/15 (.73)	11/27 (.41)
3. MDF+MIS	15/22 (.68)	12/18 (.67)	7/12 (.58)	7/22 (.32)
4. MDF+HT+MIS	16/20 (.80)	13/16 (.81)	8/10 (.80)	8/20 (.40)
5. Convent.	14/46 (.30)	11/39 (.28)	6/28 (.21)	6/46 (.13)

$\underline{a}$ C.R. = Complete response

Statistical significance: - end of treatment 1 vs. 2 and 1 vs. 4 p<0.05

2 vs. 5, 3 vs. 5 and 4 vs. 5, 0.05>p>0.01

- 12 months: 2 vs. 5 and 4 vs. 5 p<0.05

alone.   The general pattern of the responses is shown in Fig. 3
where the results are expressed in terms of local control in
surviving patients.

It is interesting to note that the best results were
obtained when hyperthermia was combined with MDF, MDF+MIS, and
that the percentage of control remained at the same level during
the follow-up period, suggesting that recurrence was rarely a
cause of death in these two groups.   Unfortunately, the numerous
deaths of these patients make it difficult to extend the analysis
of the results beyond 12 months.

Toxicity in Patients Exposed to MIS

Contrary to expectations, no neurological symptoms have been
observed.   Only some mild immediate nausea, easily controlled by
metoclopramide, was present at the beginning in 8 of 10 (80%)
patients.   No treatment has yet been discontinued because of
this reason.   However, in 3 of 3 cases treated with MIS and
irradiated with two cross-firing portals, oropharyngeal mucositis

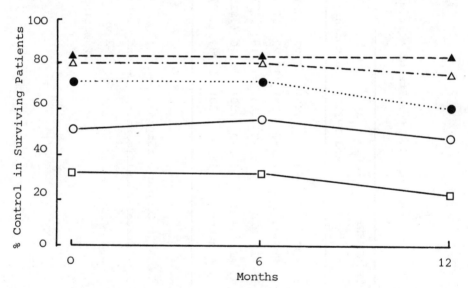

Fig. 3.   Percentage of local control in surviving patients
          following different comparative multimodality treatment
          schedules:

          □ Conventional

          O MDF   △ MDF + HT

          ● MDF + MIS   ▲ MDF + HT + MIS

has been constantly observed earlier, longer and stronger in respect to patients treated with MDF alone or combined with hyperthermia. In these cases, the treatment had to be discontinued at 25-30 Gy, even up to two to three weeks. Our observation on orpharyngeal mucositis seems to suggest several hypotheses: 1) MIS cytotoxicity is not highly selective against hypoxic cells; 2) some hypoxic cells are present in normal tissues; and 3) MIS induces a slowing down of repair processes. Apart from the likelihood of these hypotheses, MIS-induced radiosensitization of at least the normal epithelium should be taken into account.

TREATMENT OF HEAD AND NECK TUMOURS

The previous study showed an appreciable effect in terms of local response by the association of MDF with MIS. Therefore, a second pilot study was initiated on H & N primary tumours. This study soon evolved, together with the studies of other European institutions, into an EORTC feasibility study preliminary to a randomized clinical trial.

From the previous data, it would seem that a multimodality treatment such as MDF + MIS + hyperthermia could be slightly more advantageous. However, we decided to limit the present study to MDF + MIS because of the present difficulties in delivering heat to deep-seated tumours (i.e. oropharynx) and of the necessity of reaching an agreement for an international cooperative protocol.

Materials and Methods

At present, 17 patients have randomly entered the study, 9 for MDF + MIS and 8 for MDF alone. Irradiation characteristics are as described above. The characteristics of the patients are listed in Tables 2, 3 and 4.

Table 2.   MDF/MIS Pilot Study Localization

Supraglottic larynx	1
Paranasal sinus	5
Oropharynx	3
Oral cavity	3
Neck node	1
Nasopharynx	1
Salivary gland	1
Hypopharynx	2

Table 3.   MDF/MIS Pilot Study Histology

Squamous	10
Undiff.	4
Sarcoma	2
Cylindroma	1

Table 4.   MDF/MIS Pilot Study

Nodal Status

NO	9
N1	-
N2	1
N3	6
Unclass.	1

The treatment schedule and doses are indicated in Tables 5 and 6.

Table 5.   MDF/MIS Pilot Study

Misonidazole

1.6 x 3 Gy/day	5 patients
1.8 x 3 Gy/day	4 patients

No misonidazole

1.6 x 3 Gy/day	4 patients
1.8 x 3 Gy/day	4 patients

It should be noted that, in some MIS patients, the treatment schedule had to be modified because of the early mucositis warranting a rest period.   The reasons for these modifications are better explained by the data of Fig. 4 showing the average mucosal reactions.   The observations given in Fig. 4 indicate that, in the case of MDF alone, mucositis occurs earlier but at the same degree as in the case of conventional fractionation.   When MDF is employed with the radiosensitizer, mucositis occurs still earlier and in 4/9 patients with a very evident second mucositis peak. In these patients, it was therefore necessary to give a rest period after 25-36 Gy (instead of 48-54 Gy), and then a second rest period after the occurrence of the second severe mucositis. Accordingly, the overall treatment resulted in a first treatment series, a rest period, a second series, a second rest period and a final "boost".

Clinical Results

The results available at present are reported in Table 7 and in Fig. 5.

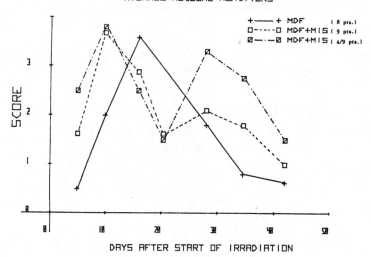

Figure 4.

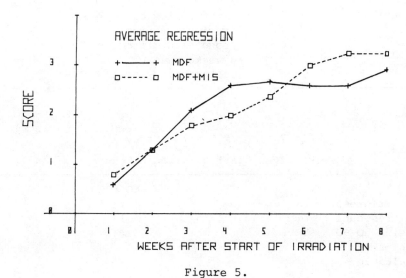

Figure 5.

Table 6.   MDF/MIS Pilot Study

Total Doses

Misonidazole

4 patients: First series of ~ 48 - 54 Gy

   3 patients   2-3 weeks rest
           Boost up to 66-76 Gy

   1 patient   No boost

5 patients: First series of 26-36 Gy
           (series arrested because of
           early confluent mucositis)
           2-3 weeks rest
           Second series up to 48-54 Gy

   4 patients   2-3 weeks rest
           Boost up to 70-74 Gy

   1 patient   No boost

No Misonidazole

7 patients: First series of 48 or 54 Gy

   5 patients   2-3 weeks rest
           Boost up to 70-76 Gy

   2 patients   No boost

1 patient: First series of 28.8 Gy
           (series arrested because of
           pronounced discomfort)
           3 weeks rest
           Second series up to 54 Gy

Table 7.   MDF/MIS Pilot Study

6 weeks after start of irradiation

	NO MISO	MISO
Complete regression	2 (*)	4 (+)
Minimal residual tumour	1	2
Regression 50-90%	4	1
No response	-	1
Not evaluable	1	1

 (*) 4 (8 weeks after start of irradiation)
 (+) 6 (8 weeks after start of irradiation)

There are clearly insufficient data to allow any comparison between protocols, but they are of interest from the point of view of feasibility.   Meanwhile, some patients are being followed up, and new patients are entering the feasibility study.   Of course, statistically valid indications will be available only at the end of the study, but more will be available after the completion of the EORTC randomized trial.

Toxicity in Patients Exposed to MIS

MIS toxicity effects are reported in Table 8.

Table 8. MDF/MIS Pilot Study

Misonidazole Toxicity

$(1.2 \ g/m^2$ per treatment day up to a total of 12 $g/m^2)$	
No reactions	5
Peripheral neuropathy	2
Central and peripheral neuropathy	1
Gastric intolerance	1

They appear similar to those previously reported in the present paper and by other authors, except for the unexpected severe neurotoxicity in one patient.   Such an episode warrants further discussion on the suitable MIS dosage to be used in this kind of protocol (perhaps decreasing the total dose to 10 g/m^2).

CONCLUSION

The results reported above indicate that as MDF is a relatively effective irradiation scheme characterized by the compression of the overall treatment time, the addition of MIS (and, if possible, of local hyperthermia) to the scheme should be taken into consideration.   Our observations on multiple neck node metastases support the possibility of a further enhancement of local control.   Information is being gathered to establish an acceptable protocol, especially as far as mucosal reactions and MIS toxicity are concerned.   The final demonstration of the effectiveness of this kind of scheme can be obtained only by randomized clinical trials, one of which is presently in preparation within the EORTC framework.

REFERENCES

1. G. Arcangeli, F. Mauro, D. Morelli and C. Nervi, Multiple daily
   fractionation in radiotherapy: biological rationale and
   preliminary clinical experiences, Europ. J. Cancer 15:
   1077 (1979).
2. G. Arcangeli, E. Barni, A. Cividalli, F. Mauro, D. Morelli,
   C. Nervi, M. Spano and A. Tabocchini, Effectiveness of
   microwave hyperthermia combined with ionizing radiation:
   Clinical results on neck node metastases, Int. J. Radiat.
   Oncol. Biol. Phys. 6:143 (1980).
3. R. C. Urtasun, J. Sturmwind, H. Rabin, T.R. Band and J.D.
   Chapman, 'High dose' metronidazole: a preliminary pharmacological study prior to its investigational use in
   clinical radiotherapy trials, Br. J. Radiol. 47:297 (1974).
4. G. Arcangeli, A. Barocas, F. Mauro, C. Nervi, M. Spano and
   A. Tabocchini, Multiple daily fractionation (MDF) radiotherapy in association with hyperthermia and/or misonidazole:
   Experimantal and clinical results, Cancer 45:2707 (1980).
5. S. Dische, M.I. Saunders, M.E. Lee, G.E. Adams and I.R.
   Flockhart, Clinical testing of the radiosensitizer Ro 07-
   0582: Experience with multiple doses, Br. J. Cancer 35:567
   (1977).

CLINICAL TRIALS AND PRELIMINARY RESULTS OBTAINED BY ASSOCIATION
OF ELECTROAFFINIC HYPOXIC CELL RADIOSENSITIZING DRUGS
(MISONIDAZOLE AND METRONIDAZOLE) WITH RADIOTHERAPY (TELECOBALT
THERAPY) FOR THE TREATMENT OF SOME TYPES OF NEOPLASTIC DISEASES
AT A LOCALLY ADVANCED STAGE

L. Busutti
Radiotherapy Division
M. Malpighi Hospital, Bologna, Italy

CLINICAL EXPERIMENTS ON THE ASSOCIATION OF RADIOTHERAPY AND
MISONIDAZOLE

a) Bladder Carcinoma - T3 NX MO

The treatment protocol consists of a first part in which
patients undergo Telecobalt therapy with two opposed fields or
with three fields (one anterior and two laterals) around the
pelvic area, including bladder, bulbous urethra and inguinaliliac lymphnodes; daily dose amounts to 1Gy x 3 with four hours
interval between the fractions; weekly dose is 15Gy; total dose
45Gy. Radiation treatment is accompanied by daily administration
of misonidazole in doses of 800mg/m^2 up to a maximum tolerance
dose of 12g/m^2; administration occurs between the third and the
fourth hours before the first exposure to radiation.

The second part of the treatment is chosen on the basis of
the extent of tumour response evaluated radiologically as well as
cystoscopically. In fact, if a 50% reduction of neoplasia is
achieved, radiation therapy is completed by means of a second
treatmend (pendular technique). If on the other hand, the
reductive response of the neoplasia is less than 50% the patient
is proposed for cystectomy.

The purpose of this investigation was to induce a summation
effect of these factors: the predictable and moderate radiosensitizing efficiency of the drug, the physiological multiple

261

fractionation-dependent reoxygenation, the greater repair of
normal tissue damage with respect to neoplastic tissue during the
brief intervals between irradiation sessions.   The study was
initiated in 1979 and was carried out with a double-blind technique
utilizing misonidazole supplied by Hoffmann-La Roche Company.

The preliminary results obtained from a group of 25 patients
(11 of which were treated with misonidazole and 14 with placebo)
show a better response in patients who received MDF and misonidazole.   In this group, we observed 5 complete responses, 4
partial responses, and 2 cases of no response.   In the group
treated with placebo we find two complete responses, 5 partial
responses, 3 cases of no response, while 4 patients are not
evaluable.   As far as toxicity is concerned, misonidazole treatment has been shown to induce 4 cases of mild peripheral neuropathy,
1 case of ototoxicity, 2 cases of cutaneous rash, and 2 cases of
leukopenia.   Only in one case was the treatment discontinued
because of toxicity.

b) Cervix Carcinoma - Stage III

The treatment comprises two parts.   During the first, the
patient undergoes telecobalt therapy by means of two opposed fields
on the pelvic region, intended to cover the internal genitals, the
vagina up to III medium, the inguinaliliac lymphnodes.   Daily
dose is 1Gy x 3 with four hours' interval between single fractions;
weekly dose if 15Gy;   total dose 45Gy.   To the described radiation
treatment a daily administration of misonidazole in single dose is
added.   The dose of 650 mg/m^2 is administered from the first to
the 25th day of the week for three weeks.   The second part of the
treatment, which takes place after an interval of 3 to 4 weeks,
consists of endocavity irradiation carried out by means of a Cs^{137}
source.   Treatments vary according to the general clinical status,
the overall dose being 20Gy at point A.   To this curietherapy,
whenever possible, three administrations of misonidazole in 650mg/
m^2 doses are associated.

The purpose of the investigation, again, is to detect an
increased efficiency of MDF in association with radiosensitizing
drugs.   This study is still in progress and is not randomized.
It was started in 1978 and has involved until now three patients
treated with MDF and metronidazole, 10 treated with MDF and misonidazole.

A comparison with the earlier case studies of our Institute
has shown also in the present case a better short term response
(T reduction) to treatment when MDF is combined with misonidazole.
In fact, we have obtained in 12/13 cases, a reduction of 76% of the
pelvic component of neoplasia and in 8/13 cases a similar reduction
of the vaginal exophytic component.

We have recorded an acceptable tolerance level.   Mild
gastrointestinal conditions were observed in the three cases of
metronidazole treatment;   misonidazole, on the other hand, gave
rise to peripheral neuropathy, which was mild (grades I, II) in
3/10 cases, and more serious (grade III) in 3/10 cases, and to
ototoxicity in 1/10 cases.   In this group no symptoms of
toxicity toward other organs or apparatuses were detected.   In
only one case did toxicity lead to discontinuation of the treatment.

On the basis of the encouraging results obtained, and of the
acceptable tolerance picture, it is suggested to adopt a protocol
of treatment for the carcinoma of portio stage III based on the
parameters given above.

c) Non-Oat-Cell, Non-Resectable Lung Carcinoma

The treatment calls for irradiation (telecobalt therapy) with
two opposed fields of the primary bronchogen infiltrate and of the
mediastinal ipsy and controlateral lymphatic-drainage.   In the
case of localization in upper lobar bronchus, the plan calls for
contemporary bilateral irradiation of the neck lymphnodes。   The
dose is 2Gy per day for 5 days a week for 5 weeks, both on the
mediastinal-hilar region and on the neck nodes.   Successively the
treatment calls for a higher dosage in the region of the primary
bronchogen infiltrate with a dose of 15-20Gy in 1-2 weeks.   The
radiation treatment is accompanied by the administration of misonidazole at a daily dose of 480 mg/m^2 from the first to the fifth
days of the week for five weeks.

The purpose of the investigation is to verify whether the
association of radiotherapy and misonidazole can improve the local
control of pulmonary neoplasia with respect to the radiotherapy
treatment alone。   The study was carried out with a double-blind
technique and was initiated in 1979 utilizing misonidazole supplied
by Hoffmann-La Roche Company。

The preliminary results obtained from a group of 17 patients
(10 of which were treated with misonidazole and 7 with placebo)
show a detectable increase in percentage of objective response, as
evaluated radiologically 30 days after the end of treatment.

In the group treated with misonidazole we had partial response
in 8/10 patients and no response in 2/10, in the control group there
were 2/7 with partial response and 5/7 with no response.   As far
as toxicity is concerned, misonidazole induced mild peripheral
neuropathy in four cases, cutaneous rash in two cases。   Only in
one case was treatment discontinued because of toxicity.

d) Concluding Remarks on the Cases Presented

31 patients underwent radiotherapy in association with misonidazole administration.   26 of these showed an objective favourable response (5 had a complete remission as proven histologically)
and 5 showed no response.

As far as toxicity goes, we point out that as indicated in
Table 1, in 5/31 cases no major symptom was observed, while in
1/31, hyporexia and nausea developed, that in 14/31 cases, signs
of peripheral toxicity were present, in 2/31, ototoxicity occurred
and finally in 4/31 cases, abnormal cutaneous and/or mucous rash
appeared.

Table 1.   General Toxicity of Misonidazole

	Bladder 10 pt.	Bronchus 10 pt.	Portio 10 pt.
Hyporexia and nausea	-	1	-
Peripheral neuropathy	4	4(1s)	6
Ototoxicity	1	-	1
Rash	2(1s)	2	-
Sphincterial bladder abnormality	2	-	-
Leukopenia	2	-	1

Table 2.   Neurotoxicity of Misonidazole
Total number of patients = 31

Grade	0	-	no symptoms	15
Grade	I	-	paresthesia limited to fingers and fingertips	5
Grade	II	-	paresthesia of the palm of the hand and of the sole of the foot	6
Grade	III	-	paresthesia extended to forearms and calves	3
Grade	IV	-	ototoxicity	2
			Total	31

A more detailed analysis presented in Table 2 shows that the neurotoxicity problems, which are by far the most common ones, can be subdivided: grade I = 5, grade II = 6, grade III = 3, grade IV (ototoxicity) = 2.

The duration of the symptoms is very variable, from 3 to 13 weeks and is not affected to a significant extent by medical therapy. The appearance is early for patients treated with MDF, due probably to the short time span of drug administration, it is late in those patients that take smaller doses of the drug in more than three weeks, but this factor does not modify the intensity (grade) of symptoms, as is borne out by the data in Figure 1.

More difficult to interpret is the appearance of leukopenia (3/31) and sphincterial bladder abnormality (2/31) which is probably related to the pathological case examined (carcinoma of the bladder).

In two cases (2/31) the treatment (radiation + misonidazole) could not be completed according to the schedule because of toxic signs (1 cutaneous rash, 1 neurotoxicity grade III).

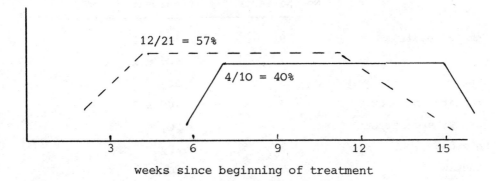

weeks since beginning of treatment

Fig. 1. Duration of neurotoxicity symptoms from misonidazole

CLINICAL EXPERIMENTS ON THE ASSOCIATION OF RADIOTHERAPY AND METRONIDAZOLE

The fairly inhomogeneous group comprised 37 patients having locally advanced neoplasia and in some cases with metastasis and subdivided as follows.

Patients treated with metronidazole in single doses of $4g/m^2$ orally, 4 hours before radiation treatment, every other day up to an overall dose of 48-68g. in association with MDF telecobalt therapy: neoplasia of female pelvis - 8 patients; ORL - 7 patients;

prostate and bladder - 7 patients.

Patients treated with metronidazole according to the scheme reported above, but in association with conventional fractionation telecobalt therapy.   Neoplasia of the lung - 5 patients;   soft tissue sarcomas - 4 patients;   melanoblastoma - 3 patients;   other sites - 3 patients.   See Table 3 for a summary.

The treatments which were completed according to the proposed schedule were 28/37, while 9/37 were discontinued.   Of the latter, 4/9 were interrupted due to the patients' refusal to go on beyond the first administration, as seen in Table 4.

Response to treatment was favourable in 18/28, i.e. 64% of the cases, that is the modification of objective neoplastic response greater than or equal to 50%, while no response was observed in 10/28, i.e. 35.7% of the cases.

Table 3.   Patients Treated with Radiotherapy and Metronidazole

	No. patients	Fractionation RxT
Female pelvis	8	1Gy x 3
ORL	7	1Gy x 2
Lung	5	2Gy
Prostate, bladder	7	1Gy x 3
Soft tissue sarcoma	4	2Gy
Melanoma	3	2Gy
Others	3	2Gy
Total	37	

Table 4.   Radiotherapy and Metronidazole

Completed treatment   = 28

Non-completed treatment =   9 (24.3%) out of which discontinued
                            due to patients' refusal after
                            first administration

It is true that the data are difficult to evaluate due to the small number of patients treated, but a prevalence of responders is apparent especially in gynaecological neoplasia, ORL and prostate-bladder neoplasia (on the whole, 12 favourable responses against 5 cases of no response). This is shown in Table 5.

The fact that this group of patients were subject to MDF scheme seems to indicate that beside the better tissue reoxygenation connected with hyperfractionation what might be operating here is the advantageous exploitation of the persistence of the drug in the blood allowed by the repeated daily radiotherapy application.

Metronidazole administration took place every other day and was preceded and followed by antiemetic medication, since gastro-enteral tolerance is the most serious limitation to the use of the drug.

An examination of the 37 patients in relation to toxicity symptoms showed:

- nausea in 29/37 cases (12 = grade I; 8 = grade II)
- vomiting in 12/37 (8 = grade I; 4 = grade II)
- headache in 4/37 .

Table 5. Metronidazole Toxicity

	Grade I	Grade II	Total
Nausea	12/37	8/37	20/37
Vomiting	8/37	4/37	12/37
Headache	4/37	–	4/37
Neuropathy	1/37	–	1/37
Abnormal skin reaction	4/37	–	4/37
Leukopenia	–	–	–

Nausea, headache, vomiting:	grade I - duration up to 8 hours. grade II - duration up to 24 hours.
Neuropathy:	grade I - paresthesia of fingertips (hand and foot).
Abnormal skin reaction:	erythema.

Table 6. Response Evaluation after Radiotherapy and Metronidazole

	PR	NR	NV
Pelvis	5	2	1
ORL	3	1	2
Lung	3	2	1
Prostate and bladder	4	2	1
Soft tissue sarcomas	2	2	–
Melanoblastoma	1	1	1
Others	–	–	3
Total	18/28 34%	10/28 35.7%	

Cutaneous and mucosal reactions were also present in 4/37 patients and appeared more intense than expected.   Gastroenteral toxicity symptoms generally attained their maximum level at 7 hours after administration, which seems to indicate, at least in some instances, an interference with radiation treatment.

In summary, the clinical studies presented here seem to suggest an effectiveness of metronidazole in association with radiotherapy, which might receive confirmation from a more selected case group and in a randomized study.

The clinical knowledge of the drug, its easy availability in form of tablets, powder, granules, its toxicity, which is a predictable, reversible and short-term effect, its long persistency in the blood and the ease of diffusion in hypoxic cells in tissues, constitute from our point of view a very good motivation for more detailed studies.

CONTROL OF THE IMMUNOLOGICAL STATUS OF NEOPLASTIC PATIENTS UNDER-GOING TELECOBALT THERAPY IN ASSOCIATION WITH RADIOSENSITIZERS

A. Petralia

Radiotherapy Division
M. Malpighi Hospital, Bologna, Italy

For about three years, immunological checks on neoplastic patients undergoing radiation treatments have been performed. Checks are carried out before, during and at the end of the irradiation cycle, and afterwards at different times, over a period of one year. One of the checks routinely carried out on blood samples is the study of rosettes and the lymphocyte mitogen stimulation (LMS). More recently, such immunological controls were extended to neoplasia patients to which radiosensitizers were administered during radiotherapeutic treatment. From a preliminary analysis of the data hitherto collected, no significant variation of immunological status seems to single out the patients subjected to radiation treatment in association with nitroimidazoles with respect to those undergoing radiotherapy alone. In this way it is hoped to detect any change in immunological status that might be induced by the imidazoles.

The number of persons examined is small and the study is still underway, so that only preliminary indications can be assessed.

ACKNOWLEDGEMENTS

This work was supported by Grant N.8001 63496 of the finalized project "Control of the Tumour Growth".

THE ASSOCIATION OF RADIOTHERAPY WITH RADIOSENSITIZING DRUGS IN THE TREATMENT OF SOFT TISSUE SARCOMAS (PRELIMINARY STUDIES)

F. Coucourde, G. F. Frezza, P. Frezza, F. Fortunato,
D. Zarrilli, G. Cornella, M. Pergola and P. Silvestro

Istituto per lo Studio dei Tumori "Sen Pascale"
Naples, Italy

We have started clinical studies involving the use of radio-sensitizing drugs for patients suffering from soft tissue sarcomas. The patients belonged to three categories, i.e. they had active neoplasia either because they were considered inoperable, or because they had refused radical surgial intervention, or finally because they had received surgery but not radically.

Diagnoses were always ascertained by histology.   The age of eligible patients varied from 12 to 68.   Patients presenting with pathology of the gastroenteral apparatus and those with life expectancy of less than 6 months were excluded.   Patients who had already undergone radical surgery, radiation treatment and anti-blastic chemotherapy, were also excluded.   Because of the gastric toxicity and neurotoxicity already reported in the literature for radiosensitizers, we have worked out a treatment scheme character-ized by high radiation doses and by long time-interval fractiona-tion.   This method permits variation of the treatment and to space out administration.   It is our opinion it also has a better chance of controlling neoplasias, in particular, those commonly called "radioresistant", since it allows for a better cell survival ratio, i.e. the ratio between initial and final cells, within the neoplasia, of the order of 10^{-10}, 10^{-11} (as was recently evidenced in work by Ellis).

Our Health Physics agency has worked out a mathematical model for the optimization of radiotherapy fractionation for certain types of tumours such as carcinomas, sarcomas, and melanomas. The model which can be considered a first order approximation to a multidimensional relation of much greater complexity, but has definite value as groundwork for future refinements of the method,

Table 1. Description of cases

Patient (initials)	Sex	Age	Site	Histology	Flagyl dose	RT	Response
L.A.	F	62	Knee (relapse)	Fibrous	4g x 6	700 rad x 6	Considerable reduction
A.C.	F	53	Right supraclavear cavity	Malignant mesenchimal	"	"	Necrosis, drastic reduction, radiodermite
A.A.	F	17	Left lung metastasis	Malignant synovialoma	"	"	X-ray detected drastic reduction
M.M.	M	14	Hilum-pulmonar mass	Soft tissue sarcoma metastasis	"	"	X-ray detected disappearance
S.L.	F	69	Perineal relapse	Leiomyosarcoma	"	"	Full regression
B.F.	M	19	Extended axillary relapse	Leiomyo	"	"	1/3 reduction of initial volume
G.A.	F	50	Pubic region sarcoma with osteolysis	Soft tissue sarcoma	"	"	Stationary status

is based on the assumption of exponential growth for tumours and
on the knowledge of the relevant survival curves.   The model can
supply, not only an optimized method which minimizes cell survival
for tumours with respect to maximum tolerance of adjacent healthy
tissues, but also a continuous guarantee for treatment for which
various choices can be compared and the one best suited for a
particular clinical case selected.

Coming to the case of soft tissue sarcomas we recall that our
protocol before the introduction of radiosensitizing drugs, called
for an association of radiotherapy and chemotherapy with the following schedule 6-7000 rad with 200 rad fractions per day, five days a
week; chemotherapy, initiated at the same time as radiotherapy and
continuing after its termination, with actinomycin (cosmegen),
adriblastina, vincristina and endoxan.   Such a chemotherapeutic
scheme has not been modified after the introduction of radiosensitizers into the protocol.

Our studies have been limited, but we have not detected neurotoxicity among our patients.   All patients presented on the day
of drug administration with dyspeptic symptoms, especially of the
gastric type, which were well controlled within 24-48 hours with
suitable gastro-protective antiemetic and hydrating therapeutic
agents.

As far as therapeutic response is concerned, we noted that
the greatest reduction of neoplastic mass is achieved after the
first or second radiotherapy session.   The patients who were
treated according to the previous scheme are presently undergoing
chemotherapy and they all present a stabilization of neoplastic
masses.

Taking into consideration the results obtained and, in
particular, the reduction of neoplastic mass achieved after the
first radiotherapy sessions, and keeping in mind that the patients
are also undergoing chemotherapy, we are now studying the possibility of spacing further apart the fractions of radiation dose
and varying the dose of each fraction.   This development is based
on the hypothesis that after the first session a selection of
radioresistant cellular clones may be formed, whereby they enter
G_1 phase from G^0 and are prompted into multiplication by a
"recruiting" phenomenon due to the necrosis of radiosensitive
cells.

In the Table we have summarized the treated cancers and the
more significant results.

ACKNOWLEDGEMENTS

    This work was carried out under the sponsorship of Progetto
Finalizato "Neoplastic growth control" Contract No. 8001 82796 of
the CNR.

PARTICIPANTS

(C - conference only)

D. AMADORI
Ospedali Civile-Oncologia
Forli, Italy.

L. BABINI
Istituto di Radiologica
e de Radio "L. Galvani"
Universita di Bologna
Policlinico "S. Orsola"
Bologna, Italy.

R. BADIELLO
Laboratorio FRAE
CNR
Via Castaguoli 3
Bologna, Italy.

R. BALDUCCI
Cattedra di Chimica Generale
ed Inorganica
Facoltà Farmacia
Università di Bologna
Bologna, Italy.

S. BAR-POLLAK
National Institute of Oncology
H-1118 Budapest
Otthon u. 27
Hungary

A. C. BENINI
Istituto di scienze Chimiche
Facoltà di Farmacia
Università di Bologna
Via S. Donato 15
Bologna, Italy.

T. BERGAMI
Divisione di Radioterapia
Ospedale "M. Malpighi"
V. le Albertoni 15
Bologna, Italy.

G. BERTOCCHI (C)
Istituto Chimico "G. Ciamician"
Universita di Bologna
Via Selmi 2
Bologna 40126
Italy.

M. BIGNARDI
Ospedale del Circolo Varese
Via Borri 57
Varese 21100, Italy.

R. H. BISBY
Cockroft Building
University of Salford
Salford M5 4WT, UK.

A. BLOTTA
Divisione di Radioterapia
Ospedale "M. Malpighi"
V. le Albertoni 15
Bologna, Italy.

M. BOTTCHER
Universität Hamburg
D-2059 Büchen
Weisenweg, Germany.

A. BOZZI
Istituto di Chimica Biologica
Università degli Studi
P. le Aldo Moro
Rome, Italy.

L. CIONINI
Istituto di Radiologia
Policlinico
Università di Firenze
Firenze 50134, Italy.

C. CLARKE
Institute of Cancer Research
Clifton Avenue
Sutton, Surrey, UK.

L.A. COHEN (C)
Department of Health
National Institutes of Health
Building 4, Room 330
Bethesda
Maryland 20014, USA.

F. COUCOURDE
Istituto Tumori
Fondazione Pascale
Napoli 80100, Italy.

D. COVIC
Central Institute for Tumours
and Allied Diseases Zagreb
Ilica 197
Zagreb 41000, Yugoslavia.

S. DAL FIOR
Reparto di Radioterapia
Ospedale Civile
Vicenza 36100, Italy.

M. D'ANGELANTONIO
Cattedra di Chimica Generale
Istituto di Scienze Chimiche
Facoltà di Farmacia
Via S. Donato 15
Bologna, Italy.

S. DE GARIS
F. Hoffmann-La Roche
CH-4002
Basel, Switzerland.

G. DE GIULI
Presidente, SARO-SISM
Istituto di Radiologica Medica
Università degli Studi
V. le Morgagni-Careggi
Firenze 50134, Italy.

D. DE MARIA
Istituto di Radiologia
Università degli Studi
Modena 41100, Italy.

E. EMILIANI
Istituto di Radioterapia
"L. Galvani"
Policlinico "S. Orsola"
Via Massarenti 9
Bologna 40126, Italy.

P. ENGSTROM (C)
AB Leo Rhodia
Fack, S-251 00
Helsingborg, Sweden.

M.G. FABRINI
Istituto di Radiologia
Università di Pisa
P.za Gorgona 21
Marina di Pisa
Pisa 56100, Italy.

F. FASANO
Divisione di Radioterapia
Ospedale "M. Malpighi"
Bologna, Italy.

F. FORTUNATO
Fisica Sanitaria
Fondazione Sen. Pascale
Via M. Semmola 1
Napoli 80100, Italy.

F.C. GARDINI
Casa di Cura
Villa Torri
V. le Filopanti 12
Bologna 40126, Italy.

P. GOLDMAN
Beth Israel Hospital
330 Brookline Avenue
Boston
Massachusetts 02215
USA.

G. GRASHEV
Tumor Radiobiology Laboratory
The National Center of Oncology
Plovdivsko Pole 6
Sofia 11-56, Bulgaria.

M.G. GRILLI
Istituto di Scienze Chimiche
Facoltà di Farmacia
Università di Bologna
Via S. Donato 15
Bologna 40127, Italy.

H. HAKKOUSH
Radiotherapy Department
National Cancer Institute
Kars El Aini Street
Fom El Khaling
Cairo, Egypt.

C. HOUEE-LEVIN
Laboratoire de Chimie-Physique
Université Paris V
45 rue des Saints-Peres
75270 Paris Cedex 06
France.

W.R. INCH
The Ontario Cancer Foundation
London Clinic
Victoria Hospital
South Street
London, Ontario N6A 4G5
Canada.

A.M.M. JOKIPII (C)
Department of Serology
and Bacteriology
University of Helsinki
Helsinki, Finland.

L. JOKIPII (C)
Department of Serology
and Bacteriology
University of Helsinki
Helsinki, Finland.

J.S. KEINTHLY (C)
Cornell University Medical School
Department of Medicine
Division of International Medicine
1300 York Avenue
New York 10021, USA.

R.C. KNIGHT
Department of Applied Biology
North East London Polytechnic
Romford Road
London E15 4LZ, UK.

R.J. KNOX
Chemotherapy Research Unit
North East London Polytechnic
Romford Road
London E15 4LZ, UK.

F. LANCEWICZ
Istituto di Oncologia
"Felice Addarii" di Bologna
Via E. Duse 7
Bologna 40100, Italy.

G.C. LANCINI
Lepetit
Via Durando 38
Milano 20158, Italy.

M.A. LELLI
Viale dei Mille 72
Cesenatico
Forli 47100, Italy.

I. LENOX-SMITH
Roche Products Ltd.
P.O.Box 8
Welwyn Garden City
Herts AL7 3AY, UK.

L. LEONARDI
Divisione di Radioterapia
Ospedale "M. Malpighi"
V. le Albertoni 15
Bologna 40100, Italy.

H. MA'
Institute of Cancer Research
Clifton Avenue
Sutton, Surrey SM2 5PX, UK.

G. MAGNONI
Arcispedale S. Anna
Istituto di Radiologia
Via G. da Carpi 6
Ferrara 44100, Italy.

L. MAHOOD
Department of Biochemistry
Brunel University
Uxbridge, Middlesex, UK.

M. MAKROPOULOU
Institute of Medicine and
Pharmacology
Department of Biophysics
Bd. Petru Groza 8
Bucharest, Romania.

C. MALTONI
Istituto di Oncologia
"F. Addarii"
Policlinico S. Orsola
Bologna, Italy.

T.R. MARTEN
Roche Products Ltd.
Welwyn Garden City
Herts AL7 3AY, UK.

F. MONDINI
Istituto di Scienze Chimiche
Facoltà di Farmacia
Università di Bologna
Via S. Donato 15
Bologna 40127, Italy.

C. NERVI
Department of Radiation Oncology
Clinica Villa Flaminia
Via L. Bodio 58
Roma 00100, Italy.

I. NILSSON-EHLE (C)
Hospital of Lund
Lund, Sweden.

C.E. NORD (C)
National Bacteriological Lab.
Stockholm
S-105 21 Stockholm, Sweden.

L. OLIVETTI
Spedali Civili di Brescia
Istituto del Radio
"O. Alberti"
Brescia 25100, Italy.

P. PACINI
Servizio di Radioterapia
Arcispedale S. Maria Nuova
V. le Morgagni-careggi
Firenze 50134, Italy.

M. PASINI
Istituto di Scienze Chimiche
Facoltà di Farmacia
Università di Bologna
Bologna 40127, Italy.

V.T. PASQUINELLI
Istituto di Radioterapia
Ospedale S. Orsola
Università
Via Massarenti 9
Bologna 40126, Italy.

C. PISONI
Farmitalia - Carlo Erba
Via Imbonati 24
Milano 20159, Italy.

G. PIZZI
Divisione di Radioterapia
Ospedale Civile
Padova 35100, Italy.

M. QUINTILLIANI
Laboratorio di Biologia
CNEN
Casaccia
Roma, Italy.

A.V. REYNOLDS (C)
The School of Pharmacy
University of London
Department of Pharmaceutics
29/39 Brunswick Square
London WC1N 1AX, England.

T. RIPA (C)
Department of Clinical
Bacteriology
Lanssjukhuset
S-301 85 Halmstad, Sweden.

P.T. RISSANEN (C)
Radiotherapy Clinic
University Central Hospital
Haartmaninkatu 4
00290 Helsinki 29
Finland.

L. ROCCHI
Ospedale Civile Cesena
Centro Tumori
Cesena
Forli, Italy.

D. ROWLEY
Department of Applied Biology
North East London Polytechnic
Romford Road
London E15 ALZ, UK.

D. RUBIN
National Heart, Lung and Blood
Institute
Building 31, Room 5A03
9000 Rockville Pike
Bethesda
Maryland 20205, USA.

G. SEMERANO
Via Stellini 8
Padova 35100, Italy.

R.A. SMITH
Department of Biology
Medical and Biological Sciences
Building
Bassett Crescent East
Southampton SO9 3TU, UK.

T. SOYLEMEZ
Institut fur Biophysics
und Elektronenmikroskopie
der Universität Düsseldorf
D-4000 Düsseldorf
Mooren Strasse 5, Germany.

M. SPANO
Dosimetria Biofisica
CNEN
Casaccia
Via Anguillarese Km. 1300
Roma 00100, Italy.

D. SPINELLI
Cattedra di Chimica Organica
Facoltà di Farmacia
Università di Bologna
Via Zanolini 4
Bologna 40216, Italy.

R. SRIDHAR
Biomembrane Research Lab.
825 Northeast 13th Street
Oklahoma City
Oklahoma 73104, USA.

R. STAGNI
Istituto di Scienze Chimiche
Facolta di Farmacia
Universita di Bologna
Via S. Donato 15
Bologna 40127, Italy.

M.R.L. STRATFORD
CRC Gray Laboratory
Mount Vernon Hospital
Northwood
Middlesex HA6 2RN, UK.

J. SUWINSKI (C)
Institute of Organic Chemistry
and Technology
Silesian Polytechnical Univ.
Gliwice 44-100, Poland.

M. TAMBA
Laboratorio FRAE
CNR
Via Castaguoli 3
Bologna 40126, Italy.

P. TAMULEVICIUS
Istitut fur Strahlen Biol
Universität-Klinikum Essen
45 Essen
Hufelanstrasse 55
W. Germany.

E. TEKAVCIC
Institute of Oncology
61000 Ljubljana
Vrazov TRG 4, Yugoslavia.

R. TEMPLETON
May & Baker Ltd
Pharmacology
Dagenham
Essex RM1 OXS, UK.

B. URSING (C)
Department of Infectious
Diseases
University Hospital
S-221 85 Lund, Sweden.

A.Y. WIJNMAALEN
Rotterdamsch Radio-Therap.
Institute
Groene Hilledijk
3075 EA Rotterdam, Holland.

R.L. WILLSON
Department of Biochemistry
Brunel University
Uxbridge
Middlesex UB8 2QH, UK.

E. WINKELMANN (C)
Hoechst AG
Pharma Synthese G 838
Postfach 80 03 20
6130 Frankfurt/Main 80
W. Germany.

S. YASHVIR
Jawaharlal Nehru University
School of Life Sciences
New Mehrauli Road
New Delhi - 110067, India.

A. YERUSHALMI
Weizmann Institute of Sciences
P.O.Box 26
Rehovot, Israel.

K.L. YEUNG
Texas Medical Centre
Houston
Texas 77030, USA.